Symptom Management in Advanced Cancer

Third edition

Robert Twycross DM, FRCP, FRCR

Macmillan Clinical Reader in Palliative Medicine,
University of Oxford
Consultant Physician, Sir Michael Sobell House,
Churchill Hospital, Oxford
Director, WHO Collaborating Centre for
Palliative Cancer Care, Oxford

Andrew Wilcock DM, FRCP

Macmillan Senior Lecturer in Palliative Medicine and
Medical Oncology, University of Nottingham
Consultant Physician,
Hayward House Macmillan Specialist Palliative Care Unit,
Nottingham City Hospital NHS Trust,
Nottingham

RADCLIFFE MEDICAL PRESS

© 2001 Robert Twycross and Andrew Wilcock

Radcliffe Medical Press Ltd
18 Marcham Road, Abingdon, Oxon, OX14 1AA

First edition 1995
Second edition 1997

British Library Cataloguing in Publication Data

A catalogue record for this book is available from the British Library.

ISBN 1 85775 510 3

Typeset by Advance Typesetting Ltd, Oxon
Printed and bound by TJ International Ltd, Padstow, Cornwall

Contents

Preface

Symptom Management in Advanced Cancer is written primarily for doctors. It provides a framework of knowledge which will enable the clinician to develop a scientific approach to the management of symptoms in advanced cancer. The book will also be of value to nurses working with cancer patients, particularly in palliative care.

In this third edition, the authorship has been extended in order to cope with the rapidly expanding body of published information and to ensure continuity for the future. In addition, we have introduced the convention of substituting 'they' and 'theirs' for 'he/she' and 'his/hers', even though the associated verb is singular. International non-proprietary names (INNs) are used throughout the book; few proprietary names are included. Readers are directed to their own national and local formularies to confirm which drugs are locally available.

There are major changes to eight chapters; two others have been removed – *Oral morphine in advanced cancer* (published separately by Beaconsfield Publishers, ISBN 0 906584 45 0) and *Drug profiles* (subsumed into the *Palliative Care Formulary* by Twycross R, Wilcock A and Thorp S (1998) Radcliffe Medical Press, ISBN 1 85775 264 3). By way of compensation, a new final chapter of guidelines has been added. These are fluid rather than solid and mainly reflect clinical practice at Sobell House at the time of writing. If desired, they can be modified by other palliative care services to reflect their own practice and distributed locally.

The support provided by Meg Roberts, librarian at Sir Michael Sobell House, has been invaluable. We thank Karen Allen for preparing the typescript for publication and Susan Brown, copy-editor, for her painstaking attention to detail.

Robert Twycross
Andrew Wilcock
March 2001

Acknowledgements

The contents of a textbook can never be wholly original. Much information and help has been received from our colleagues, Ray Corcoran, Vincent Crosby, Mary Miller and Michael Minton, and from many others. We are particularly grateful to the following for their help with individual chapters:

Alimentary symptoms, Claud Regnard, Oxford University Press (for permission to reproduce Table 3.6);

Respiratory symptoms, Anne Tattersfield;

Psychological symptoms, Aslög Malmberg;

Haematological symptoms, Miriam Johnson, David Keeling (for providing the content of Figures 7.2 and 7.4), Tim Littlewood, David Morgan;

Neurological symptoms, John Newsom-Davis;

Skin care, George Cherry (for permission to reproduce Plate 3), ConvaTec (for permission to reproduce Plates 2 and 4), Tim Dale, Jenny Millward (for permission to reproduce Plate 1), Wendy Osborne, Angie Perrin, Mary Walding, Fran Woodhouse;

Lymphoedema, Gail Close, Karen Jenns, Vaughan Keeley;

Clinical guidelines, Bruce Foggo.

Getting the most out of *Symptom Management in Advanced Cancer*

The literature on symptom management in advanced cancer is now immense, and it is impossible for any one person (or indeed two) to be familiar with all of it. *Symptom Management in Advanced Cancer* is an account mainly of the measures used clinically by two palliative care physicians.

The reader is warned that many drugs used regularly in palliative care are used 'beyond the licence'/'off label'. For example, few drugs are licensed for use by continuous subcutaneous infusion (CSCI) but many are given this way. Because of the costs involved, it is unlikely that this situation will ever be rectified. Unlicensed use is highlighted occasionally in *Symptom Management in Advanced Cancer*; for more information, see the *Palliative Care Formulary* and, of course, the manufacturers' Product Information Leaflet/Datasheet.

Physicians have a duty in common law to act with reasonable care and skill in a manner consistent with the practice of professional colleagues of similar standing. Thus, when prescribing outside the terms of a licence, doctors must be fully informed about the actions and uses of the drug and be assured of the quality of the particular product.

Symptom Management in Advanced Cancer and the *Palliative Care Formulary* are companion volumes. When more detailed information is required about a drug, it will often be found in the *Palliative Care Formulary*. Use should also be made of www.palliativedrugs.com which contains the master version for the *Palliative Care Formulary*. This is updated regularly and is free to use. The site includes a bulletin board for the exchange of information and advice, and a regular e-mail newsletter.

Drug names

For about 150 drugs marketed in the UK, the recommended International Non-proprietary Name (rINN) differs from the British Approved Name (BAN). Following a European Union Directive, the use of BANs will be discontinued and all drugs marketed in the UK will be known by their rINNs. For drugs where there is a high risk to health from possible confusion, there will be a 5-year transition period during which both the rINN and the BAN must be used (Table 1). In the case of adrenaline (BAN), an exception has been made; it will continue to have priority over epinephrine (rINN), i.e. it will be prescribed as *adrenaline (epinephrine)*.

Table I   Main drugs for which both BAN and rINN must be used

BAN	rINN
Adrenaline	Epinephrine
Amethocaine	Tetracaine
Bendrofluazide	Bendroflumethiazide
Benzhexol	Trihexyphenidyl
Chlorpheniramine	Chlorphenamine
Dicyclomine	Dicycloverine
Dothiepin	Dosulepin
Frusemide	Furosemide
Lignocaine	Lidocaine
Methotrimeprazine	Levomepromazine
Mitozantrone	Mitoxantrone
Noradrenaline	Norepinephrine
Procaine penicillin	Procaine benzylpenicillin
Salcatonin	Calcitonin (salmon)
Trimeprazine	Alimemazine

For many drugs, the change is slight (e.g. danthron → dantron) but for others the rINN is very different (e.g. methotrimeprazine → levomepromazine). Certain general rules apply:

- 'ph' becomes 'f' (e.g. cephradine → cefradine)
- 'th' becomes 't' (e.g. indomethacin → indometacin)
- 'y' becomes 'i' (e.g. napsylate → napsilate).

Inevitably perhaps there are exceptions, e.g. amitriptyline which is unchanged. The main drugs affected are listed in Table 2.

Table 2 Main drugs affected by European Union Directive on rINN

BAN	rINN
Bendrofluazide	Bendroflumethiazide
Amylobarbitone	Amobarbital
Amoxycillin	Amoxicillin
Beclomethasone	Beclometasone
Benorylate	Benorilate
Benzathine penicillin	Benzathine benzylpenicillin
Benztropine	Benzatropine
Cephalexin (etc.)	Cefalexin (etc.)
Chlormethiazole	Clomethiazole
Cholestyramine	Colestyramine
Cyclosporin	Ciclosporin
Danthron	Dantron
Dexamphetamine	Dexamfetamine
Dienoestrol	Dienestrol
Dimethicone	Dimeticone
Glycopyrronium	Glycopyrrolate
Guaiphenesin	Guaifenesin
Hexamine hippurate	Methenamine hippurate

continued opposite

BAN	rINN
Indomethacin	Indometacin
Oestradiol	Estradiol
Oxethazaine	Oxetacaine
Phenobarbitone	Phenobarbital
Sodium cromoglycate	Sodium cromoglicate
Stilboestrol	Diethylstilbestrol
Sulphasalazine	Sulfasalazine
Sulphathiazole	Sulfathiazole
Thyroxine	Levothyroxine
Vitamin A	Retinol

Outside Europe, it is important to note several differences between rINNs and USANs, i.e. the 'adopted' names used in the USA (Table 3). Note also that:

- diamorphine (available only in the UK) = di-acetylmorphine = heroin
- hyoscine = scopolamine
- liquid paraffin = mineral oil.

Table 3   Important differences between rINNs and USANs

rINN	USAN
Dimeticone[a]	Simethicone
Dextropropoxyphene	Propoxyphene
Paracetamol	Acetaminophen
Pethidine	Meperidine

a   in some countries, dimeticone is called (di)methylpolysiloxane.

A complete list of drugs affected by the new regulations is contained in the preliminary section of the *British National Formulary*.

Common abbreviations

General

BNF	British National Formulary
BP	British Pharmacopoeia
IASP	International Association for the Study of Pain
UK	United Kingdom
USA	United States of America
USP	United States Pharmacopoeia
WHO	World Health Organization

Medical

CNS	central nervous system
COPD	chronic obstructive pulmonary disease
COX	cyclo-oxygenase
CSF	cerebrospinal fluid
CT	computed tomography
DVT	deep vein thrombosis
5HT	5-hydroxytryptamine (serotonin)
H_1, H_2	histamine type 1, type 2 receptors
IVC	inferior vena cava
LFT	liver function tests
MAOI(s)	mono-amine oxidase inhibitor(s)
MRI	magnetic resonance imaging
NMDA	N-methyl D-aspartate
NSAID(s)	non-steroidal anti-inflammatory drug(s)

PCA   patient-controlled analgesia

PG(s)   prostaglandin(s)

PPI   proton-pump inhibitor

RIMA(s)   reversible inhibitor(s) of mono-amine oxidase type A

SSRI(s)   selective serotonin re-uptake inhibitor(s)

SVC   superior vena cava

TENS   transcutaneous electrical nerve stimulation

Drug administration

a.c.   ante cibum (before food)

b.d.   bis die (twice daily); alternative, b.i.d.

CSCI   continuous subcutaneous infusion

ED   epidural

IM   intramuscular

IT   intrathecal

IV   intravenous

m/r   modified-release; alternative, slow-release

o.d.   omni die (daily, once a day)

o.m.   omni mane (in the morning)

o.n.   omni nocte (at bedtime)

p.c.   post cibum (after food)

PO   per os, by mouth

PR   per rectum

p.r.n.   pro re nata (as needed, when required)

q.d.s.   quater die sumendus (four times a day); alternative, q.i.d.

q4h   quarta quaque hora (every 4 hours)

SC   subcutaneous

SL   sublingual

stat	immediately
TD	transdermal
t.d.s.	ter die sumendus (three times a day); alternative, t.i.d.

Units

cm	centimetre(s)
cps	cycles per sec
g	gram(s)
Gy	Gray(s), a measure of radiation
h	hour(s)
Hg	mercury
IU	international unit(s)
kg	kilogram(s)
L	litre(s)
mg	milligram(s)
ml	millilitre(s)
mm	millimetre(s)
mmol	millimole(s)
min	minute(s)
µg	microgram, alternative, mcg

1 General principles

Biopsychosocial care · Ethical considerations
Symptom management · As death approaches

Biopsychosocial care

Care of the dying extends far beyond pain and symptom management. It includes supporting:

- the patient as he adjusts to his decreasing physical ability and as he mourns in anticipation the loss of family, friends and all that is familiar

- the family as they adjust to the fact that one of them is dying.

Although psychologically demanding for doctors, nurses and other carers, it is potentially one of the most rewarding of their responsibilities. One of the keys to success is an attitude of partnership between the caring team and the patient and family (Box 1.A).

Box 1.A Partnership with the patient	
Be courteous	Explain
Be polite	Agree priorities and goals
Be honest	Discuss treatment options
Do not be condescending	Accept treatment refusal
Listen	

To be maximally supportive, it is also necessary to show that you care about the patient as a person, and that you are not only concerned about physical symptoms. Beginning consultations with an open question is one way of doing this. For example:

'Where would you like to begin?'

'How are you feeling today?'

'How have you been coping since we last met?'

An enquiry from time to time about how the family is coping is also interpreted by the patient as an indication of your general interest and concern. Finally, at the end of the consultation, ask the patient if there are any questions he would like to ask you.

Ethical considerations

Cardinal principles

The cardinal principles which underpin all clinical practice, including palliative care, are:

- respect for patient autonomy (patient choice)

- beneficence (do good)

- non-maleficence (minimize harm)

- justice (fair use of available resources).[1]

These four principles need to be applied against the background of respect for life and an acceptance of the ultimate inevitability of death.[2] Thus in practice, there are three dichotomies which need to be held in balance:

- the potential benefits of treatment versus the potential risks and burdens

- striving to preserve life but, when the burdens of life-sustaining treatments outweigh the potential benefits, withdrawing or withholding such treatments and providing comfort in dying

- individual needs versus the needs of society.

Patient autonomy

Doctors often act as if patients have an obligation to accept treatment which is recommended. However, legally a person is not obliged to accept medical treatment, even if refusal may result in an earlier death. Doctors have an obligation, therefore, to discuss treatment options and their implications with patients.

Without consent, a doctor risks being found liable in battery. If a patient lacks capacity to give or withhold consent, a doctor's legal obligation is to treat in what he perceives as the patient's best interests. Severe depression, delirium (acute confusional state) or dementia are common causes of lack of capacity to give consent. A doctor, in common with any citizen, can restrain even a competent person in an emergency to prevent, for example, a crime or damage to other people.

Principle of double effect

The principle of double effect has been described in various ways.[1,3–5] In essence the principle states that:

> A single act having two possible foreseen effects, one good and one harmful, is not always morally prohibited if the harmful effect is not intended.

This is a universal principle without which the practice of medicine would be impossible. It follows inevitably from the fact that all treatment has an inherent risk. However, most discussions of the principle of double effect focus on the use of morphine or similar drugs to relieve pain in terminally ill patients. This gives the false impression that the use of morphine in this circumstance is a high risk strategy. When correctly used, morphine (and other strong opioids) are very safe drugs, safer than non-steroidal anti-inflammatory drugs, which are widely prescribed with impunity.[6,7] The use of both classes of analgesic is justified on the basis that the benefits of pain relief far outweigh the risk of serious adverse effects. Indeed, clinical experience suggests that those whose pain is relieved live longer than would have been the case if they had continued to be exhausted and demoralized by severe unremitting pain.

The situation in the UK is encapsulated in a classic legal judgment:

> 'A doctor who is aiding the sick and the dying does not have to calculate in minutes or even in hours, and perhaps not in days or weeks, the effect upon a patient's life of the medicines which he administers or else be in peril of a charge of murder. If the first purpose of medicine, the restoration of health, can no longer be achieved, there is still much for a doctor to do, and he is entitled to do all that is proper and necessary to relieve pain and suffering, even if the measures he takes may incidentally shorten life.'[8]

Similar sentiments have been expressed in other countries, and reflect a broad international consensus.

However, the intended aim of treatment must be the relief of suffering and not the patient's death. Although a greater risk is acceptable in more extreme circumstances, it remains axiomatic that effective measures which carry less risk to life will generally be used. Thus, in an extreme situation, although it

may occasionally be necessary and acceptable to render a patient unconscious, it remains unacceptable and unnecessary to cause death deliberately
(euthanasia). Indeed, palliative care and euthanasia are essentially mutually
exclusive philosophies.

Appropriate treatment

'Treatment that does not provide net benefit to the patient may, ethically
and legally, be withheld or withdrawn and the goal of medicine should
shift to the palliation of symptoms.'[9]

Doctors must keep in mind the fundamental fact that all patients must die
eventually. Part of the skill of medicine, therefore, is to decide when to allow
death to occur without further impediment. A doctor is not obliged legally or
ethically to preserve life 'at all costs'. Priorities change when a patient is
clearly dying. There is no obligation to employ treatments if their use can best
be described as prolonging the process of dying.[10,11] A doctor has neither a
duty nor the right to prescribe a lingering death. In palliative care, the primary
aim of treatment is not to prolong life but to make the life which remains as
comfortable and as meaningful as possible.

However, it is not a question of to treat or not to treat but what is the most
appropriate treatment given the patient's biological prospects and his
personal and social circumstances? Appropriate treatment for an acutely ill
patient may be inappropriate in the dying (Figures 1.1 and 1.2). Nasogastric
tubes, IV infusions, antibiotics, cardiac resuscitation, and artificial respiration
are all primarily support measures for use in acute or acute-on-chronic
illnesses to assist a patient through the initial crisis towards recovery of
health. The use of these measures in patients who are irreversibly close to
death is generally inappropriate (and therefore bad practice) because the
burdens of such treatments exceed their potential benefits.

Medical care is a continuum, ranging from complete cure at one end
to symptom relief at the other. Many types of treatment span the entire
spectrum, notably radiotherapy and, to a lesser extent, chemotherapy and
surgery. It is important to keep the therapeutic aim clearly in mind when
employing any from of treatment. In deciding what is appropriate, the key
points to bear in mind are:

- the patient's biological prospects
- the therapeutic aim and benefits of each treatment
- the adverse effects of treatment
- the need not to prescribe a lingering death.

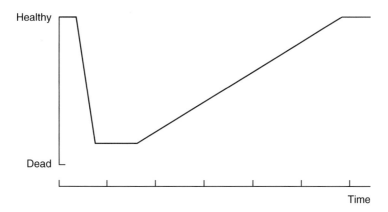

Figure 1.1   A graphical representation of acute illness. Biological prospects are generally good. Acute resuscitative measures are important and enable the patient to survive the initial crisis. Recovery is aided by the natural forces of healing: rehabilitation is completed by the patient on his own, without continued medical support.

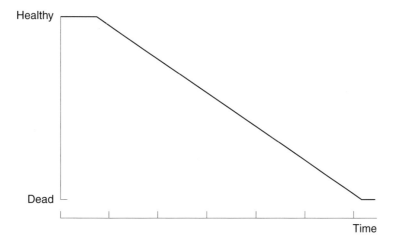

Figure 1.2   A graphical representation of terminal illness. Biological prospects progressively worsen. Acute and terminal illnesses are therefore distinct pathophysiological entities. Therapeutic interventions which can best be described as prolonging the distress of dying are futile and inappropriate.

Although the possibility of unexpected improvement or recovery should not be totally ignored, there are many occasions when it is appropriate to 'give death a chance'.

As death draws near, interest in hydration and nutrition often becomes minimal, and it is inappropriate to force someone to accept food and fluid.

The patient's disinterest or positive disinclination is part of the process of letting go.

Symptom management

The scientific approach to symptom management can be encapsulated in the acronym 'EEMMA'.

- Evaluation: *diagnosis of each symptom before treatment*
- Explanation: *explanation to the patient before treatment*
- Management: *individualized treatment*
- Monitoring: *continuing review of the impact of treatment*
- Attention to detail: *no unwarranted assumptions.*

Evaluation

A wide range of symptoms is experienced by patients with advanced cancer, but no symptom occurs invariably.[12] Evaluation, which must always precede treatment, is based on *probability and pattern recognition*. For example, hiccup in advanced cancer is mostly associated with gastric stasis or distension, and the most common cause of pruritus is dry skin.

What is the cause of the symptom?

The cancer itself is not always the cause of a symptom. Causal factors include:

- the *cancer* itself
- anticancer or other *treatment*
- cancer-related *debility*
- a *concurrent disorder.*

Some symptoms are caused by several factors. All symptoms are made worse by insomnia, exhaustion, anxiety and depression.

What is the underlying pathological mechanism?

Even when the cancer is responsible, a symptom may be caused by different mechanisms, e.g. vomiting from hypercalcaemia and from raised intracranial pressure. Treatment varies accordingly.

What has been tried and failed?

This helps in planning the most appropriate management strategy by excluding certain treatment options, provided they were used optimally. If not, a further trial of therapy may be indicated.

What is the impact of the symptom on the patient's life?

The following questions will help determine how big an impact a symptom is having on the patient's life:

'How much does [the symptom] affect your life?'

'What makes it worse and what makes it better?'

'Is it worse at any particular time of the day or night?'

'Does it disturb your sleep at all?'

Explanation

Explain the underlying mechanism(s) in simple terms

Treatment begins with an explanation by the doctor of the reason(s) for the symptom. This knowledge does much to reduce the psychological impact of the symptom on the sufferer, for example 'The shortness of breath is caused partly by cancer itself and partly by the fluid at the base of the right lung. In addition, you are anaemic.'

If explanation is omitted, the patient may continue to think that his condition is shrouded in mystery. This is frightening because 'even the doctors don't know what's going on'.

Discuss treatment options with the patient

Whenever possible, the doctor and the patient should decide together on the immediate course of action. Few things are more damaging to a person's self-esteem than to be excluded from discussions about one's self.

Explain the treatment to the family

Discussion with close relatives generally enlists their cooperation and helps to re-inforce symptom management strategies. This is particularly important when the patient is at home. If actively involved in supporting the patient the family have a right to be informed, subject to the patient's approval. However, it is important not to let the family take over. Whenever possible, the patient's wishes should prevail.

Management

Management falls into three categories:

- correct the correctable
- non-drug treatment
- drug treatment.

By adopting an appropriate multimodality approach, although the underlying disease cannot be cured, it is generally possible to obtain significant, even complete, relief. Achievable goals should be identified and agreed with the patient. For example, with inoperable intestinal obstruction, because it is not always possible to relieve vomiting completely, it is better initially to aim to reduce it to, say, 1–2 times a day. It may also be necessary to compromise so as to avoid unacceptable adverse effects. For example, drug-induced dry mouth or visual disturbance may limit the dose escalation of an anti-muscarinic drug (e.g. amitriptyline, hyoscine).

Although many symptoms respond to a combination of non-drug and drug measures, often the main part of the management of anorexia, weakness and fatigue, for example, is helping the patient (and family) accept the irreversible physical limitations of terminal disease.

Correct the correctable

Palliative care often includes disorder-specific treatment – when it is practical and not disproportionately burdensome. For example, patients with breathlessness and bronchospasm benefit from bronchodilator therapy. Likewise, aqueous cream applied topically will relieve pruritus associated with dry skin.

Non-drug treatment

Examples of non-drug treatment are contained in the sections dealing with individual symptoms. Relaxation therapy is an example of a non-drug treatment with wide applicability.

Drug treatment

Prescribe drugs prophylactically for persistent symptoms

When treating a persistent symptom with a drug, it should be administered regularly on a prophylactic basis. The use of drugs as needed (p.r.n.) instead of regularly is the cause of much unrelieved distress.

Keep drug treatment as straightforward as possible

When an additional drug is considered, ask the following questions:

'What is the treatment goal?'

'How can it be monitored?'

'What is the risk of adverse effects?'

'What is the risk of drug interactions?'

'Is it possible to stop any of the current medications?'

Written advice is essential

Precise guidelines are necessary to achieve maximum patient cooperation. 'Take as much as you like, as often as you like' is a recipe for anxiety, poor symptom relief and maximum adverse effects. The drug regimen should be written out in full for the patient and his family to work from (Figures 1.3 and 1.4). Times to be taken, names of drugs, reason for use (for pain, for bowels etc.) and dose (*x* ml, *y* tablets) should all be stated. Also the patient should be advised how to obtain further supplies, for example from his general practitioner.

Seek a colleague's advice in seemingly intractable situations

No one can be an expert in all aspects of patient care. For example, the management of an unusual genito-urinary problem is likely to be enhanced by advice from a urologist or gynaecologist.

Never say 'I have tried everything' or 'there's nothing more I can do'

It is generally possible to develop a repertoire of alternative measures. Although it is important not to promise too much, it is important to assure the patient that you are going to stand by him and do all you can to help, for example 'No promises but we'll do our best'.

Instead of expecting immediate complete relief, be prepared to chip away at symptoms a little at a time. When tackled in this way it is often surprising how much can be achieved with determination and persistence.

SIR MICHAEL SOBELL HOUSE

Name *Mary Smith*   Date *August 15, 1997*

TABLETS/MEDICINES	2 am	On waking	10 am	12 pm	6 pm	Bedtime	PURPOSE
ORAMORPH (2mg in 1ml)		10ml	10ml	10ml	10ml	20ml	pain relief
METOCLOPRAMIDE (10mg tablet)		1	1	1	1	1	anti-sickness
FLURBIPROFEN (100mg capsule)			1			1	pain relief
AMITRIPTYLINE (50mg tablet)						1	for sleep and to help mood
CO-DANTHRUSATE (capsules)			2			2	for bowels

If troublesome pain   take extra 10ml of ORAMORPH between regular doses.

If bowels constipated   increase CO-DANTHRUSATE to *3 capsules* twice a day.

Figure 1.3   Take-home medication chart (q4h).

SIR MICHAEL SOBELL HOUSE

Name *John Bull*   Date *August 15, 1997*

TABLETS/MEDICINES	Breakfast	Midday meal	Evening meal	Bedtime	PURPOSE
ASILONE (suspension)	10ml	10ml	10ml	10ml	for hiccup
MORPHINE slow release (100mg tablet)	1			1	pain relief
FLURBIPROFEN slow release (200mg capsule)	1				pain relief
HALOPERIDOL (1.5mg tablet)				1	anti-sickness
CO-DANTHRUSATE (capsules)	2			2	for bowels
TEMAZEPAM (20mg tablet)				1	for sleeping

If troublesome pain   take liquid morphine (ORAMORPH 2mg in 1ml) 15ml up to every 3 hours.

If troublesome hiccup   take extra 10ml of ASILONE up to every 2 hours.

Figure 1.4 Take-home medication chart (q.d.s).

Monitoring

Review! review! review!

Patients vary and it is not always possible to predict the optimum dose of opioids, laxatives and psychotropic drugs. Adverse effects put drug compliance in jeopardy. Adjustments will be necessary, particularly initially. This should be anticipated and arrangements made for ongoing supervision. Further, cancer is a progressive disease, and new symptoms occur. These must be dealt with urgently.

Attention to detail

Attention to detail makes all the difference to palliative care; without it success may be forfeited and patients suffer needlessly. Attention to detail requires an inquisitive mind, one which repeatedly asks 'Why?'

'Why is this patient with breast cancer vomiting? She's not taking morphine; she's not hypercalcaemic. Why is she vomiting?'

'This patient with cancer of the pancreas has pain in the neck. It does not fit with the typical pattern of metastatic spread. Why does he have pain there?'

It is important not to make unwarranted assumptions. Remember: to *ass-u-me* means to make an *ass* of *u* and *me*.[13]

Attention to detail is important at every stage; in evaluation, explanation (e.g. avoid jargon, use simple language), when deciding management (e.g. drug regimens which are easy to follow, providing written advice) and when monitoring the impact of the treatment. Attention to detail is equally important in relation to the non-physical aspects of care; all symptoms are exacerbated by anxiety and fear.

As death approaches

With increasing weakness, the patient is faced with the fact that death is inevitable and imminent. Support and companionship are of paramount importance at this time. Explanation is essential:

'This often happens   [The doctor understands]
in an illness like yours.'

'When the body is short of energy   [The patient understands]
it takes a lot more effort to do even
simple jobs. This means you'll need
to rest more in order to restock your
limited energy supply.'

For the patient who has not yet come to terms with the situation:

'I think a few quiet days in bed are called for. If tomorrow or the next day you are feeling more energetic, of course you can get up but, for the moment, bed is probably the best place for you.'	[Not destroying hope, breaking bad news gently, giving the patient permission to let go]

For the spouse and close family:

'This weakness is normal. The cancer is like a parasite and is sapping all his energy.'	[The patient is not to blame. Also he is not odd or bad]
'I think the illness is beginning to win.'	[Time is short]

However, it is often difficult for a doctor to be sure that a patient has reached their last few days.[14,15] Weight loss of >8kg over the previous 6 months, a plasma albumin concentration of <35g/L and a plasma lactate dehydrogenase concentration of >600IU/L are helpful objective prognostic factors but only in terms of weeks or months, not days.[16]

Unless there is a reversible cause, in a progressive disease like cancer, patients probably have a prognosis of only a few days when they become:

- profoundly weak
- bedbound
- semicomatose
- unable to take tablets or have great difficulty swallowing them
- unable to take more than sips of water.[17,18]

Although you may feel powerless in the face of rapidly approaching death, patients are generally more realistic. They know you cannot perform a miracle and time is limited. Despite possibly having nothing new to offer, it is important to:

- continue to visit
- quietly indicate that 'At this stage the important thing is to keep you as comfortable as possible'
- simplify medication: 'Now that your husband is not so well, he can probably manage without the heart tablets'
- arrange for medication to be given SL, PR or SC, preferably by CSCI, when the patient cannot swallow

- continue to inform the family of the changing situation
  'He's very weak now, but may still live for several days'
  'Although he seems better today, he's still very weak. He could quickly deteriorate and die within a few days'
- control agitation even if it results in sedation
- listen to the nurses.

'Slowly, I learn about the importance of powerlessness.

I experience it in my own life and I live with it in my work.

The secret is not to be afraid of it – not to run away.

The dying know we are not God.

All they ask is that we do not desert them.'[19]

References

1   Beauchamp T and Childress J (1994) *Principles of Biomedical Ethics.* Oxford University Press, New York, pp 206–11.
2   Gillon R (1994) Medical ethics: four principles plus attention to scope. *British Medical Journal.* **309**:184–8.
3   Dunphy K (1998) Sedation and the smoking gun: double effect on trial. *Progress in Palliative Care.* **6**:209–12.
4   Thorns A (1998) A review of the doctrine of double effect. *European Journal of Palliative Care.* **5**:117–20.
5   Randall F and Downie R (1999) *Palliative Care Ethics. A companion for all specialties.* Oxford University Press, Oxford, pp 119–21.
6   Armstrong C and Blower A (1987) Nonsteroidal anti-inflammatory drugs and life threatening complications of peptic ulceration. *Gut.* **28**:527–32.
7   Hawkey C (1999) COX-2-inhibitors. *Lancet.* **353**:307–14.
8   Devlin P (1985) *Easing the Passing. The trial of Dr John Bodkin Adams.* The Bodley Head, London, pp 171–82.
9   BMA (1999) *Withholding or Withdrawing Life-prolonging Medical Treatment. Guidance for decision making.* BMA, London.
10 Gillon R (1999) End-of-life decisions. *Journal of Medical Ethics.* **25**:435–6.
11 London D (2000) Withdrawing and withholding life-prolonging medical treatment from adult patients. *Journal of the Royal College of Physicians of London.* **34**:122–4.
12 Walsh D *et al.* (2000) The symptoms of advanced cancer: relationship to age, gender, and performance status in 1000 patients. *Supportive Care in Cancer.* **8**:175–9.

13   Gordon L (1997) *If You Really Loved Me*. Science & Behaviour Books, Palo Alto.

14   Christakis N and Lamont E (2000) Extent and determinants of error in doctors' prognoses in terminally ill patients: prospective cohort study. *British Medical Journal*. **320**:469–73.

15   Vigano A *et al.* (2000) Survival prediction in terminal cancer patients: a systematic review of the medical literature. *Palliative Medicine*. **14**:363–74.

16   Vigano A *et al.* (2000) Clinical survival predictors in patients with advanced cancer. *Archives of Internal Medicine*. **160**:861–8.

17   Ellershaw JE *et al.* (1995) Dehydration and the dying patient. *Journal of Pain and Symptom Management*. **10**:192–7.

18   Higgs R (1999) The diagnosis of dying. *Journal of the Royal College of Physicians of London*. **33**:110–12.

19   Cassidy S (1988) *Sharing the Darkness*. Darton, Longman and Todd, London.

2 Pain relief

Pain

> 'Pain is what the patient says hurts.'

Pain is an unpleasant *sensory* and *emotional* experience associated with actual or potential tissue damage or described in terms of such damage.[1] In other words, pain is a *somatopsychic* phenomenon which is modulated by:

- the patient's *mood*
- the patient's *morale*
- the *meaning* of the pain for the patient.

The meaning of persistent pain in advanced cancer is 'I am incurable; I am going to die'. Common factors affecting pain threshold are shown in Table 2.1. Because pain is multidimensional, it is helpful to think in terms of *total pain*, encompassing physical, psychological, social and spiritual aspects of suffering (Figure 2.1).

People with chronic pain generally do not look in pain because of the absence of autonomic concomitants (Table 2.2). In cancer, acute pain concomitants may be evident particularly if the pain is severe and of recent onset, or is paroxysmal.

Evaluation

Pain and advanced cancer are not synonymous:

- 3/4 of patients experience pain
- 1/4 of patients do not experience pain.[2,3]

Table 2.1   Factors affecting pain sensation

Pain increased	Pain decreased
Discomfort	Relief of other symptoms
Insomnia	Sleep
Fatigue	Understanding
Anxiety	Companionship
Fear	Creative activity
Anger	Relaxation
Sadness	Reduction in anxiety
Depression	Elevation of mood
Boredom	
Mental isolation	
Social abandonment	

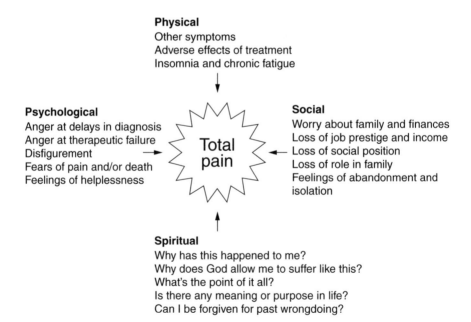

Physical
Other symptoms
Adverse effects of treatment
Insomnia and chronic fatigue

Psychological
Anger at delays in diagnosis
Anger at therapeutic failure
Disfigurement
Fears of pain and/or death
Feelings of helplessness

Total pain

Social
Worry about family and finances
Loss of job prestige and income
Loss of social position
Loss of role in family
Feelings of abandonment and isolation

Spiritual
Why has this happened to me?
Why does God allow me to suffer like this?
What's the point of it all?
Is there any meaning or purpose in life?
Can I be forgiven for past wrongdoing?

Figure 2.1   The four dimensions of pain.

Table 2.2 Temporal classification of pain

	Acute	Chronic	
Time course	Transient	Persistent	
Meaning to patient	Positive draws attention to injury or illness	Negative serves no useful purpose	Positive patient obtains secondary gain
Concomitants	Fight or flight pupillary dilation increased sweating tachypnoea tachycardia shunting of blood from viscera to muscles	Vegetative sleep disturbance anorexia decreased libido no pleasure in life constipation somatic pre-occupation personality change lethargy	

Multiple concurrent pains are common in those who have pain. Approximately:

- 1/3 has a single pain
- 1/3 has two pains
- 1/3 has three or more pains.[4]

Evaluation is a multidimensional process (Figure 2.2). It is partly sequential and partly synchronous. It begins by asking the patient to identify the *location* of the pain ('Where exactly is your pain?') and its *duration* ('When did it start?'). Then while the patient describes the pain (Box 2.A), the physician reflects on:

- the cause of the pain (cancer *v* non-cancer)
- the underlying mechanism (pathological *v* functional; nociceptive *v* neuropathic)
- the contribution of non-physical factors.

For patients who describe episodic (intermittent) pain, it is important to differentiate between:

- *predictable (incident) pain*, an exacerbation of pain caused by weight-bearing and activity which may or may not be associated with a background of constant (through controlled) pain at the same location[5]

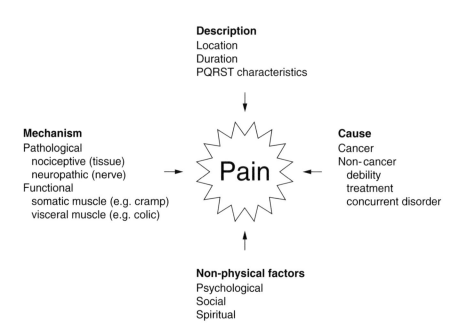

Description
Location
Duration
PQRST characteristics

Mechanism
Pathological
  nociceptive (tissue)
  neuropathic (nerve)
Functional
  somatic muscle (e.g. cramp)
  visceral muscle (e.g. colic)

Cause
Cancer
Non-cancer
  debility
  treatment
  concurrent disorder

Non-physical factors
Psychological
Social
Spiritual

Figure 2.2   The four dimensions of pain evaluation.

Box 2.A   The PQRST characteristics of pain

Palliative factors	'What makes it better?'
Provocative factors	'What makes it worse?'
Quality	'What exactly is it like?'
Radiation	'Does it spread anywhere?'
Severity	'How severe is it?'
	'How much does it affect your life?'
Temporal factors	'Is it there all the time or does it come and go?'
	'Is it worse at any particular time of the day or night?'

In practice it may be better to begin with T and end with P, i.e. TSRQP!

- *unexpected (unpredictable) pain,* spontaneous pain unrelated to weight-bearing or activity, e.g. colic, stabbing pain associated with nerve injury

- *end-of-dose failure,* occurs shortly before the next dose of regular analgesics is due; it generally responds to an increase in the analgesic dose

Some patients will have more than one type of pain (*mixed episodic pains*). If these pains occur despite regular strong opioid therapy, they are often called *break-through pain.*

Causes of pain

Pain in advanced cancer can be grouped into four causal categories:

- the *cancer* itself, e.g. soft tissue, visceral, bone, neuropathic

- anticancer or other *treatment,* e.g. chemotherapy-related mucositis

- cancer-related *debility,* e.g. constipation, muscle tension/spasm

- a *concurrent disorder,* e.g. spondylosis, osteo-arthritis.

In 15% of patients with advanced cancer and pain, none of their pain is caused by the cancer itself.[4]

Mechanisms of pain

It is important to distinguish between *functional* and *pathological* pains (Figure 2.3). Functional muscle pains are part of everybody's general life experience and are common in patients with advanced cancer. For example:

- somatic muscle–tension pains, e.g. tension headache, cramp, myofascial

- visceral muscle–tension pains, e.g. distension and colic.

Myofascial pain is a specific form of cramp related to myofascial trigger points.[6] These occur most commonly in the muscles of the pectoral girdle and neck, and are likely to be more troublesome in physically debilitated and anxious people (Figure 2.4).[7]

Pathological pains can be divided into:

- nociceptive, associated with tissue distortion or injury

- neuropathic, associated with nerve compression or injury (Figure 2.3).

Pain in an area of abnormal or absent sensation is always neuropathic.

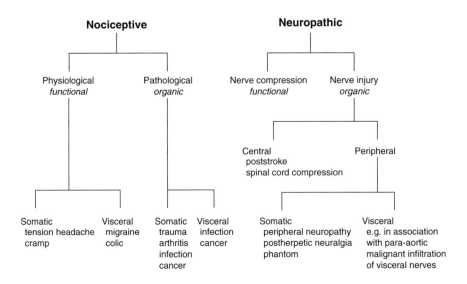

Figure 2.3 Classification of pain.

There are many potential causes of neuropathic pain in cancer (Box 2.B). When caused by cancer, nerve compression generally precedes nerve injury. Nerve compression manifests as a deep ache of variable intensity in a neurodermatomal distribution. In contrast, peripheral nerve injury pain tends to be superficial and burning ± a spontaneous stabbing (lancinating) component (Box 2.C). These characteristic features stem from several pathological changes in the nervous system:

- neuronal hyperexcitability and spontaneous activity at the site of injury

- a cascade of neurochemical and physiological changes in the CNS, particularly in the dorsal horn of the spinal cord ('central sensitization').[8]

The relative importance of the various mechanisms differs between patients, and probably accounts for different responses to drug treatment.[9] Nerve injury does not always result in pain; with identical lesions, only a minority develops pain, suggesting a genetic factor.

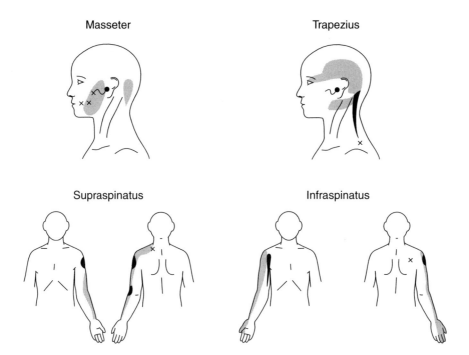

Figure 2.4   Selected trigger points and associated patterns of myofascial pain.[7]
Site of pain ■□ ;   trigger area X.

Box 2.B   Causes of neuropathic pain in advanced cancer

Cancer
Nerve compression/infiltration
Plexopathy
Spinal cord compression
Thalamic tumour

Anticancer or other treatment
Chronic surgical incisional pain
Phantom limb pain
Chemotherapy → peripheral neuropathy
Radiation fibrosis → plexopathy

Debility
Postherpetic neuralgia

Concurrent disorders
Diabetic neuropathy
Poststroke pain

Box 2.C   Clinical features of nerve injury pain

Distribution
If a peripheral nerve lesion, neurodermatomal.

If central, an area of pain within a larger area of abnormal sensation or dysfunction.

Quality
One or all of the following:

• superficial burning/stinging pain, particularly if a peripheral lesion

• spontaneous stabbing/lancinating pain

• a deep ache.

Concomitants
Often there is:

• allodynia (light touch exacerbates pain), e.g. unable to bear clothing on the affected area

• a sensory deficit, generally numbness.

Occasionally there is a sympathetic component manifesting as:

• cutaneous vasodilation → increased skin temperature

• sweating.

Patients also become exhausted and demoralized, particularly if there is insomnia.

Relief from analgesics
About $\frac{1}{2}$ of nerve injury pains caused by cancer respond to the combined use of a NSAID and a strong opioid; the rest need adjuvant analgesics.[10]

If there is a sympathetic component, a regional sympathetic block may help.

Non-physical factors

Non-physical factors always influence pain intensity. Psychosocial evaluation is therefore important. The ability to facilitate the expression of patient's fears and anxieties is crucial to success in cancer pain management. In some patients, the help of a clinical psychologist or psycho-oncologist may be necessary if the patient seems to be using pain to express otherwise inexpressible negative emotions ('somatization').

Explanation

Given that many patients have pain which is not caused by the cancer, the positive value of an explanation of the causes and mechanisms of their pains is self-evident. In relation to neuropathic pain which is not responding to standard analgesics, it is important to tell the patient that:

- nerve compression pain 'often needs cortisone as well as painkillers'

- nerve injury pain 'sometimes does not respond to painkillers like aspirin and morphine ... Because of this we need to start a different type of painkiller ... The first step is to get you a good night's sleep'.

Management

Different types of pain may well need different types of treatment (Table 2.3). A broad-spectrum multimodal approach is often necessary (Box 2.D). For pain caused by the cancer itself, drugs generally give adequate relief provided the right drugs are administered in the right doses at the right time intervals. It is often best to aim at progressive pain relief:

- relief at night
- relief at rest during the day
- relief on movement (not always completely possible).

If anticancer treatment is recommended, analgesics should be given until the treatment ameliorates the pain; this may take several weeks. It is important to avoid various forms of bad practice (Box 2.E).

Correct the correctable

Radiotherapy

This should be considered whenever pain is caused by a bone metastasis or nerve compression.[11] A single dose treatment with 6–10Gy is often possible,

Table 2.3 Mechanisms of pain and implications for treatment

Type of pain	Mechanism	Examples	Response to opioids	Typical Treatment
Nociceptive	Stimulation of nerve endings			
muscle spasm		Cramp	−	Muscle relaxant
somatic		Soft tissue, bone pain	±	NSAID ± opioid
visceral		Liver capsule pain	+	Opioid ± NSAID
Neuropathic				
nerve compression	Stimulation of nervi nervorum		±	Opioid + corticosteroid (if cancer)
nerve injury de-afferentation pain	Peripheral nerve injury	Neuroma or nerve infiltration, e.g. brachial or lumbosacral plexus		Opioid; NSAID (if cancer); tricyclic antidepressant; anti-epileptic; local anaesthetic congener; NMDA-receptor-channel blocker; spinal analgesia; TENS
central pain	CNS injury	Spinal cord compression or poststroke pain	±	

a TENS = transcutaneous electrical nerve stimulation.

Box 2.D Pain management in cancer

Explanation to reduce the psychological impact of pain

Modification of the pathological process
Radiation therapy
Hormone therapy
Chemotherapy
Surgery

Analgesics
Non-opioid (antipyretic)
Opioid
Adjuvant
  corticosteroids
  antidepressants
  anti-epileptics
  muscle relaxants
  antispasmodics

Non-drug methods
Physical
  heat pads
  TENS

Psychological
Relaxation
Cognitive–behavioural therapy
Psychodynamic therapy

Interruption of pain pathways
Local anaesthesia
  lidocaine
  bupivacaine
Neurolysis
  chemical, e.g. alcohol, phenol
  cryotherapy
  thermocoagulation
Neurosurgery
  cervical cordotomy

Modification of way of life and environment
Avoid pain-precipitating activities
Immobilization of the painful part
  cervical collar
  surgical corset
  slings
  orthopaedic surgery
Walking aid
Wheelchair
Hoist

---

particularly in peripheral sites.[12] Radiation reduces pain in 90% of patients with bone pain and in half of these there is complete relief.[13] Recalcification occurs in most of these. Radiation is also beneficial in several other situations (Box 2.F). It is generally inappropriate in patients with a very short prognosis, i.e. <2 weeks.

Bisphosphonates

Bisphosphonates are osteoclast inhibitors and are used to relieve metastatic bone pain which persists despite analgesics and radiotherapy ± orthopaedic surgery. Published data relate mainly to breast cancer and myeloma, for

---

Box 2.E   Bad practice in cancer pain management

Failure to distinguish between pains caused by cancer and pain related to other causes.

Failure to evaluate each pain individually and to plan treatment accordingly.

Failure to use non-drug treatments, particularly for muscle spasm pain.

Failure to use a NSAID and an opioid in combination.

Ignorance about adjuvant analgesics, notably antidepressants and anti-epileptics.

A *laissez-faire* attitude to drug times and to education of the patient and family.

Changing to an alternative analgesic before optimizing the dose and timing of the previous analgesic.

Combining analgesics inappropriately, e.g. two weak opioids or a strong opioid and a weak opioid.

Failure to appreciate that a mixed agonist-antagonist such as pentazocine should not be used in conjunction with codeine and morphine.

Reluctance to prescribe morphine.

Changing from another strong opioid, e.g. buprenorphine or oxycodone, to an inadequate dose of morphine.

Reducing the interval between administrations instead of increasing the dose.

Using injections when oral medication is possible.

Failure to monitor and control adverse effects, particularly constipation.

Lack of attention to psychosocial issues.

Failure to listen to the patient.

---

which both pamidronate and clodronate are licensed for use; benefit is also seen with other cancers.[15–19] Recommended regimens include:

- pamidronate 90–120mg in 500ml 0.9% saline IV over 1–2h[20]
- clodronate 600–1500mg in 500ml 0.9% saline IV over 4h.[21]

Clodronate can also be given SC in 1L 0.9% saline over 6–12h ± hyaluronidase 150–300IU.[22] Swelling, erythema or bruising occurs in about 25%.

Benefit is seen in about 50% of patients, typically in 7–14 days, and may last for 2–3 months. Benefit may be seen only after a second treatment but, if there is no response after two treatments, nothing is gained by further use. In those who respond, continue to treat p.r.n. for as long as there is benefit.

Box 2.F   Indications for radiation therapy in symptom management ('BUMP')[14]

Bleeding	**Mass effect/compression**
Haemoptysis	SVC obstruction
Haematuria	Oesophagus (dysphagia)
Vaginal	Brachial plexus
	Lumbosacral plexus
Ulceration	Cauda equina
Superficial	Spinal cord
Mucosal	Brain
oronasopharyngeal	
rectal	**Pain**
	Bone metastases
	Plexopathy

When bisphosphonates are being used prophylactically to reduce the long-term complications of metastatic bone disease, an appropriate regimen is pamidronate 60–90mg IV every 3–4 weeks or clodronate 1600mg PO o.d.[16,23–25]

Non-drug treatment

The perception of pain requires both consciousness and attention. Pain is worse when it occupies a person's whole attention. Activity, particularly when creative, does much more than pass the time; it diminishes pain. Further, professional time spent exploring a patient's worries and fears is time well spent, and relates directly to pain management.

Since the advent of spinal analgesia (see p.55) and the increased use of local anaesthetic and corticosteroid injections, procedures which destroy nerves have become almost obsolete in the UK. At many centres, a coeliac plexus block with alcohol for epigastric visceral pain is the only neurolytic block still used and only infrequently.

Internal fixation or the insertion of a prosthesis should be considered if a pathological fracture of a long bone threatens or occurs. This obviates the need for prolonged bed rest and pain is much reduced. Fracture is unlikely when >25% of the cortex of a long bone has been eroded, but when >75% is eroded, the bone is so weak that it often fractures spontaneously.[26] Thus, provided the patient's general condition warrants it, prophylactic internal fixation of a long bone should be considered when there is:

- increasing pain
- destruction of >50% of the cortex radiologically.

Some patients continue to experience pain on movement despite analgesics, other drugs, radiotherapy and nerve blocks. Here, the situation is often improved by suggesting modifications to the patient's way of life and environment. This is where the help of a physiotherapist and an occupational therapist is invaluable.

Relief should be evaluated in relation to each pain. If there is severe anxiety and/or depression, it may take 3–4 weeks to achieve maximum benefit. Re-evaluation is a continuing necessity; old pains may get worse and new ones develop.

Drug treatment

For convenience, analgesics are divided into three classes:

- non-opioid (antipyretic)
- opioid
- adjuvant.

Paracetamol, NSAIDs and opioids all have peripheral and central effects, although to a different extent.[27,28] Adjuvant analgesics act in various ways. Antidepressants and anti-epileptics act mainly by activating the inhibitory (GABA) system in the dorsal horn of the spinal cord and inhibiting the excitatory (glutamate) system.

Other adjuvants include:

- drugs to control the adverse effects of analgesics, e.g. laxatives, anti-emetics
- psychotropic medication, e.g. night sedatives, anxiolytics, antidepressants.

The principles governing analgesic use have been encapsulated in a series of slogans by the World Health Organization:[29,30]

- *by the mouth,* the oral route is the standard route for analgesics, including morphine and other strong opioids

- *by the clock,* persistent pain requires preventive therapy. Analgesics should be given regularly and prophylactically; as needed medication is irrational and inhumane (Figure 2.5)

- *by the ladder,* use the 3-step analgesic ladder (Figure 2.6). If after optimizing the dose a drug fails to give adequate relief, move up the ladder; do not move sideways in the same efficacy group

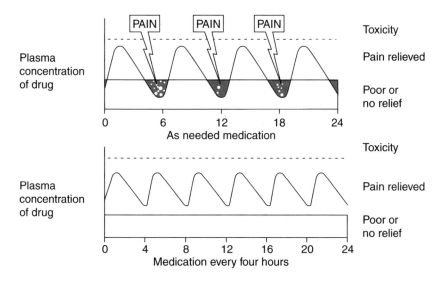

Figure 2.5   A comparison of as needed (p.r.n.) dosing and regular q4h morphine.

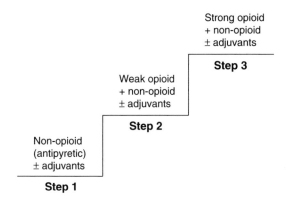

Figure 2.6   The World Health Organization 3-step analgesic ladder for cancer pain.

- *individualized treatment*, the right dose is the one which relieves the pain; if necessary doses should be titrated upwards until the pain is relieved or adverse effects prevent further escalation.

A key concept underlying the analgesic ladder is 'broad-spectrum analgesia', i.e. drugs from each of the three classes of analgesic are used appropriately, either singly or in combination, to maximize their impact (Figure 2.7). Relief with morphine and other opioids is often limited in the presence of central sensitization. This occurs when there is peripheral hyperexcitability as a result of inflammation or nerve injury (Figure 2.8). This is why it is important to use a NSAID and an opioid in combination for most cancer pains, particularly bone and soft tissue pain but also for cancer nerve injury pain.

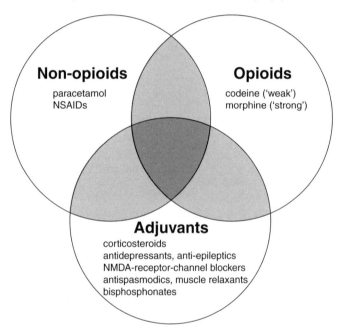

Figure 2.7   Broad-spectrum analgesia; drugs from different categories are used singly or in combination according to the type of pain and response to treatment.

Non-opioid analgesics

The non-opioid (antipyretic) analgesics comprise:

- paracetamol/acetaminophen

- non-steroidal anti-inflammatory drugs (NSAIDs).

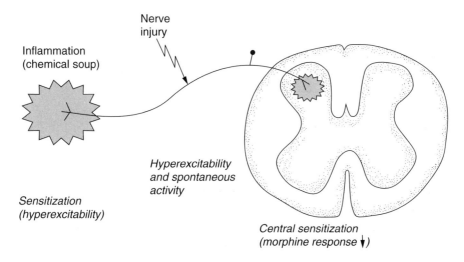

Figure 2.8 Peripheral sensitization leads to central sensitization and a reduced response to opioids.

Paracetamol

The mechanism of action of paracetamol is still not fully understood.[31] It inhibits cyclo-oxygenase (COX) in the brain.[32,33] Although it has a peripheral analgesic effect,[34] it does not have an anti-inflammatory effect in inflamed joints. Paracetamol also interacts with the central L-arginine-nitric oxide, serotonergic and opioidergic systems.[35,36]

The following features distinguish paracetamol from NSAIDs:

- adverse effects are uncommon

- does not injure the gastric mucosa, although it may cause non-specific dyspepsia

- is well-tolerated by patients with peptic ulcers

- does not affect plasma uric acid concentration.

Paracetamol also has no effect on platelet function. It can be taken by 2/3 of patients who are hypersensitive to aspirin.[37] NSAIDs and paracetamol can be used together with an additive effect. The main drawback with paracetamol is the frequency of administration, generally q6h, and its potential for hepatotoxicity.[31]

NSAIDs

NSAIDs are of particular benefit for pains associated with inflammation, e.g. soft tissue infiltration and bone metastases. Because inflammation leads to central sensitization and increased pain, NSAIDs sometimes play a crucial role in relieving cancer-related neuropathic pain.[38]

Ibuprofen, diclofenac and naproxen are the most widely used NSAIDs in palliative care in the UK. Flurbiprofen is the preferred NSAID at Sobell House; diclofenac at Hayward House. This could change now that less gastrotoxic selective COX-2 inhibitors are available (*see below*). The central analgesic effects of NSAIDs have not been fully elucidated and clinically important differences could still emerge.[27]

NSAIDs inhibit COX, an important enzyme in the arachidonic acid cascade which results in the production of tissue and inflammatory PGs.[32] Inhibition of PG synthesis does not account for the total analgesic effect of NSAIDs, although it appears to explain most of their adverse effects. Thus, in post-dental extraction pain, most weak COX inhibitors are significantly superior to aspirin and most strong COX inhibitors are inferior.[39]

COX exists in two forms. COX-1 is present in all normal tissues (and is described as *constitutive*), whereas COX-2 is normally undetectable in most tissues but massively induced by inflammation (Figure 2.9). By using selective COX-2 inhibitors, gastric toxicity is reduced.[40,41] However, COX-1 inhibition alone does not explain the differential impact of NSAIDs on the gastro-intestinal tract; uncoupling of oxidative phosphorylation is possibly more important.[42] Further, COX-2 is normally present in the kidney and the possibility that selective COX-2 inhibitors (like the non-selective NSAIDs) may cause renal dysfunction must not be ignored.

NSAIDs differ in their effect on platelet function. In patients undergoing chemotherapy or with thrombocytopenia from other cause, it is best to use a NSAID which has no effect on platelet function (Table 2.4). Most NSAIDs, and sometimes paracetamol, induce bronchospasm in certain patients. *Choline salicylate, choline magnesium trisalicylate, azapropazone, nimesulide* and *benzydamine (oral rinse)* do not. Meloxicam (preferential COX-2 inhibitor) and celecoxib and rofecoxib (selective COX-2 inhibitors) are also generally safe in this respect.[43]

Note:

- aspirin may cause tinnitus and deafness, particularly in patients with a low plasma albumin
- aspirin and salicylates have a hypoglycaemic effect, e.g. aspirin $\geqslant$1200mg/24h; occasionally it may be necessary to reduce the dose of insulin or oral hypoglycaemic agent[44]

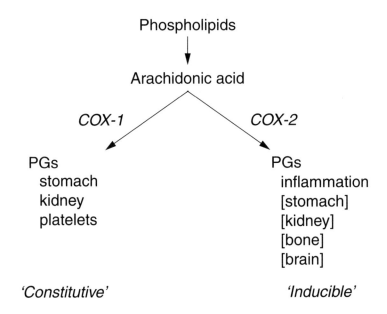

Figure 2.9   Cyclo-oxygenase (COX) and the production of prostaglandins (PGs).

Table 2.4   NSAIDs and platelet function

Drug	Effect on platelets	Comment
Aspirin	+	*Irreversible* platelet dysfunction (acetylation of platelet COX-1)
Non-acetylated salicylates	–	No effect at recommended doses (choline magnesium trisalicylate, diflunisal, salsalate)
Non-selective COX inhibitors	+	Reversible platelet dysfunction (includes most NSAIDs)
Preferential COX-2 inhibitors	–	Diclofenac,[a] meloxicam, nimesulide (when used in typical doses)
Selective COX-2 inhibitors	–	Celecoxib,[b] rofecoxib

a   diclofenac is traditionally classed as a non-selective NSAID but is a preferential COX-2 inhibitor in some assays.[45] Although it is a potent reversible inhibitor of platelet aggregation *in vitro*, typical oral doses do not effect platelet function *in vivo*[46]

b   more preferential than selective *in vivo*.[47]

- aspirin *antagonizes* uricosuric agents
- all NSAIDs cause salt and water retention which may result in ankle oedema; they therefore *antagonize* the action of diuretics
- NSAIDs may cause renal failure (acute or acute-on-chronic), particularly in patients with hypovolaemia from any cause, e.g. diuretics, fever, dehydration, vomiting, diarrhoea, haemorrhage, surgery
- NSAIDs may also cause interstitial nephritis (± nephrotic syndrome or papillary necrosis); this is sporadic and unpredictable.

Choice of NSAID

This depends on several factors, e.g. availability, fashion, local guidelines, cost, frequency of administration, individual toxicity and response (Box 2.G and Table 2.5).

Box 2.G Typical NSAID regimens			
Ibuprofen	400–800mg t.d.s.	Naproxen	250–500mg b.d.
Diclofenac sodium	50mg t.d.s.	Diflunisal	250–500mg b.d.
Diclofenac sodium m/r	150–200mg o.d.[a]	Meloxicam	15mg o.d.
	75–100mg b.d.[a]	Celecoxib	200mg o.d.–b.d.
Flurbiprofen	50–100mg b.d.	Nimesulide	100mg b.d.
Flurbiprofen m/r	200mg o.d.	Rofecoxib	25mg o.d.

a   the UK licence is for ≤150mg/day.

Table 2.5 Risk of NSAID-related gastroduodenal toxicity

Minimal	*Low*	*Intermediate*	*Highest*
Rofecoxib	Meloxicam	Diflunisal	Azapropazone
Celecoxib	Nimesulide	Flurbiprofen	Ketorolac
	Diclofenac	Indometacin	
	Ibuprofen	Ketoprofen	
		Naproxen	
		Piroxicam	

Diclofenac 150mg or ketorolac 30–90mg/24h by CSCI is used at some centres when parenteral administration is necessary.[48,49] Tenoxicam 20mg SC/IM o.d. is a useful alternative and may obviate the need for a second syringe driver in a patient requiring multiple drugs (see p.384).

Piroxicam 20mg, given as a Feldene Melt tablet, is another option; this dissolves rapidly and completely if placed on the tongue or in the mouth. However, absorption is gastro-intestinal which means that Feldene Melt tablets can be used only in patients who can swallow their saliva.

Weak opioids

The division of opioids into 'weak' and 'strong' is to a certain extent arbitrary (Table 2.6). By IM injection, most weak opioids can provide analgesia approximately equivalent to morphine 10mg. However, codeine, dextro-propoxyphene and dihydrocodeine are not used parenterally. Pentazocine is *not* recommended; it is short-acting and often causes psychotomimetic effects, e.g. hallucinations, feelings of unreality, dysphoria.

Table 2.6   Weak opioids

Drug	Bio-availability	Time to maximum concentration	Plasma halflife	Duration of analgesia	Potency ratio with codeine
	(%)	(h)	(h)	(h)[a]	
Codeine	40 (12–84)	1–2	2.5–3.5	4–5	1
Dextropro-poxyphene	40	2–2.5	6–12[b]	6–8	7/8[c]
Dihydrocodeine	20	1.6–1.8	3.5–4.5	3–4	4/3
Pentazocine	20	1	3	2–3	(1)[d]
Tramadol	70	2	6	4–6	(2)[d]

a   when used in general doses for mild–moderate pain
b   increases >50% in the elderly
c   multiple doses; single dose = $^1/_2$–$^2/_3$
d   estimated on the basis of potency ratio with morphine.

Weak opioids are said to have a ceiling effect for analgesia. This is an oversimplification; mixed agonist–antagonists such as pentazocine have a true ceiling effect but the maximum dose of a weak opioid agonist is determined by a disproportionate increase in adverse effects, particularly nausea and vomiting, if the dose is increased beyond a certain level. The following general rules should be observed:

- a weak opioid should be *added* to a non-opioid, not substituted for one

- if a weak opioid is inadequate when given regularly in an optimal dose, change to morphine (or an alternative strong opioid)

- do not 'kangaroo' from weak opioid to weak opioid.

Codeine is about 1/10 as potent as morphine and is partly a prodrug of morphine. *About 10% of the population cannot convert codeine to morphine.*[50] However, those who obtain little analgesic benefit from codeine experience the same incidence of adverse effects.[51]

In the UK, there are various compound preparations (Table 2.7). Dihydrocodeine is widely used either alone or as a compound preparation. It is analgesic in its own right and, like codeine, has an active metabolite, dihydromorphine.[52] Co-proxamol is the weak opioid preparation of choice at many palliative care centres; it is less constipating than codeine and dihydrocodeine. Dextropropoxyphene is also available alone in capsules containing the equivalent of 65mg of the hydrochloride salt.[53] There is no difference between these drugs in terms of efficacy.

Table 2.7   Commonly used weak opioid compound preparations (UK)

Generic name	Drug content	
	Weak opioid	*Non-opioid*
Co-codaprin 8/400	Codeine 8mg	Aspirin 400mg
Co-codamol 8/500	Codeine 8mg	Paracetamol 500mg
Co-codamol 30/500	Codeine 30mg	Paracetamol 500mg
Co-dydramol 10/500	Dihydrocodeine 10mg	Paracetamol 500mg
Co-proxamol 32.5/325	Dextropropoxyphene hydrochloride 32.5mg	Paracetamol 325mg

Tramadol

Tramadol forms a bridge between the classic weak and the classic strong opioids and is used at some centres. By injection, it is 1/10 as potent as morphine.[54] By mouth, it is more potent because of its high oral bio-availability and is about 1/5 as potent as morphine.[55]

Tramadol has a dual mechanism of action, partly via opioid receptors and partly (like a tricyclic antidepressant) by blocking the presynaptic re-uptake of 5HT (serotonin) and noradrenaline (norepinephrine). However, unlike the tricyclic antidepressants, tramadol does not have antimuscarinic or anti-depressant properties. The dual analgesic action is synergistic. Adverse opioid effects are significantly less than with codeine and morphine.[54] It is less constipating.[56]

It is uncertain whether tramadol is more effective in neuropathic pain than other opioids.[9] One trial reports a significant reduction in allodynia.[57] There is circumstantial evidence that tramadol lowers seizure threshold. It should therefore be used with caution in patients with a history of epilepsy and in those taking other medication which lowers seizure threshold, e.g. tricyclic antidepressants and SSRIs.

Strong opioids

Strong opioids exist to be given, not merely to be withheld; their use is dictated by therapeutic need and response, not by brevity of prognosis.

Pain is a physiological antagonist to the central depressant effects of opioids.

Strong opioids do *not* cause clinically important respiratory depression in patients in pain.[58] Naloxone, a specific opioid antagonist, is rarely needed in palliative care. In contrast to postoperative patients, cancer patients with pain:

- have generally been receiving a weak opioid for sometime, i.e. are not opioid naive
- take medication by mouth (slower absorption, lower peak concentration)
- titrate the dose upwards step by step (less likelihood of an excessive dose being given).

The relationship of the therapeutic dose to the lethal dose of a strong opioid (the therapeutic ratio) is greater than commonly supposed. For example, patients who take a double dose of morphine at bedtime are no more likely to die during the night than those who do not.[59]

Tolerance to strong opioids is not a practical problem.[60] Psychological dependence (addiction) to morphine is rare in patients.[61,62] Physical dependence does not prevent a reduction in the dose of morphine if the patient's pain ameliorates, e.g. as a result of radiotherapy or a nerve block.[63]

Strong opioids are not the panacea for cancer pain; generally they are best administered with a non-opioid. Further, even combined use does not guarantee success, particularly with neuropathic pain and if the psycho-social dimension of suffering is ignored. Other reasons for poor relief include:

- underdosing (failure to titrate the dose upwards)
- poor patient compliance (patient not taking medication)
- poor alimentary absorption because of vomiting.

Oral morphine

Guidelines 2.1: Starting patients on oral morphine (p.376).

Morphine by mouth is the global strong opioid of choice for cancer pain.[30,64] It is administered as tablets, e.g. 10mg, 20mg, or in aqueous solutions, e.g. 2mg in 1ml. An increasing range of m/r preparations is available, i.e. tablets, capsules, suspensions. Most are administered b.d., some o.d. There are no generic m/r morphine tablets, but the pharmacokinetic profiles of different proprietary brands are broadly similar.[65] If changing from PO to SC/IV, give 1/3–1/2 of the PO dose.[66]

The main metabolites of morphine are morphine-3-glucuronide (M3G) and morphine-6-glucuronide (M6G). M3G is not analgesic but M6G is *more potent* than morphine. Both glucuronides cumulate in renal failure. This results in a prolonged duration of action, with a danger of severe sedation and respiratory depression if the dose or frequency of administration is not reduced.

Initial dose titration with IV morphine

Initial dose titration with small boluses of IV morphine provides a method of rapidly determining morphine-responsiveness, e.g. in 30–40min (Box 2.H). This approach is ideal in countries where patients travel long distances and cannot readily return for monitoring. IV *patient-controlled analgesia* (PCA) can be used but is more costly, requires inpatient admission and takes ≤10h to achieve relief.[67]

Box 2.H   Dose titration with IV morphine (Calicut, India)[68]

Prerequisites

Pain, i.e. ≥5/10 on a numerical scale.

Likelihood of a partial or complete response to morphine.[a]

Method

Obtain venous access with a butterfly cannula.

Give metoclopramide 10mg IV routinely.

Dilute the contents of 15mg morphine ampoule in a 10ml syringe.[b]

Inject 1.5mg every 10min until the patient is pain-free or complains of sedation.

If patients experience nausea, give additional metoclopramide 5mg IV.

Results

Dose required (with approximate percentages):

   1.5–4.5mg (40%)   10.5–15mg (15%)

   6–9mg (40%)   >15mg (5%).

Complete relief in 80%; none in 1%.

Drop outs 2%

Adverse effects: sedation 32%; other 3%.

Ongoing treatment

Prescribe a dose of PO morphine q4h which is similar to the IV requirement, rounded to the nearest 5mg, i.e. relief with morphine 3–6mg IV → 5mg PO etc; the minimum dose is 5mg q4h.

Instruct patients to take p.r.n. doses and to adjust the dose the next day if necessary.

---

a   most patients will already be taking a NSAID

b   ampoule strength is determined by local availability.

Diamorphine

Diamorphine hydrochloride (di-acetylmorphine, heroin) is available for medicinal use only in the UK. It is much more soluble than morphine sulphate/hydrochloride and large amounts can be given in a very small volume. It is used instead of morphine when injections are necessary.

IV diamorphine is twice as potent as IV morphine.[69,70] By this route, its initial effects are mediated by the primary metabolite, mono-acetylmorphine.[71] However, by mouth diamorphine is virtually a prodrug for morphine because of its rapid de-acetylation.[72] When changing to SC diamorphine, give 1/3 of the PO dose of morphine, and adjust as necessary.[66]

Alternative strong opioids

Guidelines 2.2: Switching opioids (p.378).

There are multiple opioid receptor subtypes in the CNS and elsewhere, including the dorsal horn of the spinal cord; μ, κ and δ opioid receptors are all involved in analgesia. Opioids differ from each other in terms of intrinsic activity, receptor site affinity, and concomitant non-opioid effects. These properties can be utilized in patients who are intolerant of morphine by switching to an alternative opioid (Table 2.8).[73] The initial dose of the second opioid depends on the relative potency of the two drugs (Table 2.9).

Some patients who are taking high-dose morphine manifest evidence of hyperexcitability, i.e. myoclonus, allodynia, hyperalgesia. The main causal factor seems to be a cumulation of morphine-3-glucuronide which indirectly antagonizes the analgesic effect of morphine, i.e. not via opioid receptors.[78] Thus when switching from morphine because of hyperexcitability, a lower than expected dose of the alternative opioid is needed.[76,79]

For example, single doses of IM morphine and methadone given post-operatively are approximately equipotent.[80] However, when changing to methadone from high-dose morphine, the dose of methadone is likely to be 5–10 times less (Box 2.I).[81] Indeed, cases have been reported on the internet of patients still in pain on, e.g. morphine 10g/24h PO who have experienced complete relief after a single dose of methadone 10mg PO. It is necessary to have locally agreed guidelines for switching from morphine to methadone which take account of such experiences (*see* p.378).

Table 2.8   Potential intolerable effects of morphine

Type	Effects	Initial action	Comment
Gastric stasis	Epigastric fullness, flatulence, anorexia, hiccup, persistent nausea	Metoclopramide 10–20mg q4h	If the problem persists, switch to an alternative opioid
Sedation	Intolerable persistent sedation	Reduce dose of morphine; consider methylphenidate 10mg o.d.–b.d.	Sedation may be caused by other factors; stimulant rarely appropriate
Cognitive failure	Agitated delirium with hallucinations	Reduce dose of morphine and/or prescribe haloperidol 3–5mg stat and o.n.; if necessary switch to an alternative opioid	Some patients develop intractable delirium with one opioid but not with an alternative opioid
Myoclonus	Multifocal twitching ± jerking of limbs	Reduce dose of morphine but revert to former dose if pain recurs; consider a benzodiazepine	Unusual with typical oral doses; more common with high dose IV and spinal morphine
Hyperexcitability	Abdominal muscle spasms, symmetrical jerking of legs, whole-body allodynia, hyperalgesia (manifests as excruciating pain)	Prescribe a benzodiazepine stat; reduce morphine dose; consider switching to an alternative opioid	Seen in patients receiving IT or high-dose IV morphine; occasionally with typical PO and SC doses[74,75]
Vestibular stimulation	Incapacitating movement-induced nausea and vomiting	Cyclizine or dimenhydrinate or promethazine 25–50mg t.d.s.–q6h	Rare; try an alternative opioid or levomepromazine
Histamine release cutaneous	Pruritus	Oral antihistamine, e.g. chlorphenamine 4mg b.d.–t.d.s.	If the pruritus does not settle in a few days, switch to an alternative opioid
bronchial	Bronchoconstriction → dyspnoea	IV/IM antihistamine, e.g. chlorphenamine 5–10mg, and a bronchodilator	Rare. Switch to a chemically distinct opioid immediately, e.g. methadone

Table 2.9 Approximate oral analgesic equivalence to morphine[a]

Analgesic	Potency ratio with morphine	Duration of action (h)[b]
Codeine		
Dihydrocodeine	1/10	3–6
Dextropropoxyphene		
Pethidine	1/8	2–4
Tramadol	1/5[c]	4–6
Dipipanone (in Diconal UK)	1/2	4–6
Papaveretum	2/3[d]	3–5
Oxycodone	1.5–2[c]	4–5
Dextromoramide (UK)	[2][e]	2–3
Levorphanol (USA)	5	4–6
Methadone	5–10[f]	8–12
Hydromorphone	7.5	4–5
Buprenorphine (sublingual)	60	6–8
Fentanyl (transdermal)	100–150[g]	72

a multiply dose of opioid by its potency ratio to determine the equivalent dose of morphine sulphate

b dependent in part on the severity of pain and on the dose; often longer-lasting in the very elderly and those with renal dysfunction

c tramadol and oxycodone are both relatively more potent by mouth because of high bio-availability; parenteral potency ratios with morphine are 1/10 and 3/4 respectively.

d papaveretum (strong opium) is standardized to contain 50% morphine base; potency expressed in relation to morphine sulphate

e dextromoramide: a single 5mg dose is equivalent to morphine 15mg in terms of peak effect but is shorter-acting; overall potency ratio adjusted accordingly

f methadone: a single 5mg dose is equivalent to morphine 7.5mg. However, its long plasma halflife and its broad-spectrum receptor affinity result in a much higher than expected potency ratio when given repeatedly[76]

g the manufacturers in UK state 150; in Germany they state 100.[77]

A similar disparity has been reported with TD fentanyl and PO morphine, e.g. still in pain on TD fentanyl 1mg/h (100μg/h ×10) but out of pain when given morphine 10mg SC. The explanation may lie in differences in lipophilicity (Box 2.1). Because morphine is poorly lipophilic and fentanyl highly lipophilic, their distribution in the body is different.[82]

Box 2.1   Possible reasons for 'opioid inequivalence'

Morphine (μ-receptor agonist)
Oral bio-availability 30%
Halflife 1.5–4.5h
Antagonized by M3G
Low lipophilicity
Greater penetration into spinal cord after spinal application[82]

Methadone (μ- and δ-receptor agonist)[a]
Oral bio-availability 80%
Halflife ranges from about 8–80h
Glutamate (NMDA) receptor-channel blockade
Serotonin re-uptake blockade
Lipophilic

Fentanyl (μ-receptor agonist)
Transdermal bio-availability 100%
Halflife 3–4h after IV injection
Highly lipophilic
Greater non-specific binding to CNS lipids[82]

---

a   gene knockout animal studies cast doubt on methadone's δ-receptor status.[83]

Pethidine and dextromoramide have little place in cancer pain management because of short durations of action. Because it has a rapid onset of action, some centres use dextromoramide SL/PO for episodic pain in patients taking regular morphine or prophylactically before a painful procedure. However, at other centres patients are given either an additional dose of morphine or the procedure is timed for 1h after a regular q4h dose of morphine or 2–3h after m/r morphine.

Buprenorphine

Buprenorphine is a potent partial μ-receptor agonist, δ-receptor agonist and κ-receptor antagonist. It is an alternative to oral morphine in the low-to-middle part of morphine's dose range. In low doses, buprenorphine and morphine are additive in their effects; at very high doses, antagonism by buprenorphine may occur. However, there is no need to prescribe both; use one or the other.

Buprenorphine is available as a *sublingual* tablet; swallowing the tablet reduces bio-availability. It needs to be given only t.d.s. With daily doses of over 3mg, patients may prefer to take fewer tablets more often, i.e. q6h.

It is generally considered that there is an analgesic ceiling at a daily dose of 3–5mg, equivalent to 180–300mg of oral morphine/24h. In some countries, 1.6mg is regarded as the ceiling daily dose. Whether this represents genetic differences or local custom is not clear.

Buprenorphine is a strong opioid, not an alternative to codeine or other weak opioid. Like morphine, therefore, it should generally be used only when a weak opioid has failed. Assuming the previous regular use of a weak opioid, patients should commence on 200μg t.d.s. with the advice that: 'If it is not more effective than your previous tablets take a further 200μg after 1h, and 400μg t.d.s. after that'.

When changing to morphine, multiply the total daily dose of buprenorphine by 60. If the pain was previously poorly controlled, multiply by 100. Adverse effects, e.g. nausea, vomiting, constipation, drowsiness, need to be monitored as with morphine. It is not widely used in palliative care.

Fentanyl

Guidelines 2.3: Transdermal fentanyl (p.380).

Fentanyl is a potent μ-receptor agonist. It is widely used by injection as a peri-operative analgesic. Transdermal (TD) patches are available for cancer pain.[84,85] These deliver 25, 50, 75 or 100μg/h over 3 days. Patients who have not previously taken morphine or other strong opioids should always be started on the lowest dose, i.e. 25μg/h.[86]

In some patients the potency ratio for PO morphine and TD fentanyl may be only half that recommended by the manufacturer, i.e. 70 rather than 150.[77] Accordingly, some centres use a conversion factor of 100 to determine the initial patch strength.[77] After removal of a patch, the elimination plasma halflife is almost 24h,[87] compared with 3–4h after a single IV injection.[88]

If effective analgesia does not last for 3 days, the correct response is to increase the patch strength. Even so, a few patients do best if the patch is changed every 2 days. High fever and exposure of TD patches to external heat sources, e.g. heat pads and electric blankets, may increase the rate of delivery of fentanyl.

TD fentanyl is less constipating than morphine.[85,89] Thus, when converting from morphine to fentanyl, the dose of laxative should be halved and subsequently adjusted according to need (Figure 2.10).[90] Some patients experience withdrawal symptoms when changed from PO morphine to TD fentanyl despite satisfactory pain relief, i.e. colic, diarrhoea and nausea together with sweating and restlessness. These symptoms are easily treatable by using rescue doses of morphine until they resolve after a few days.

TD fentanyl can be continued until the death of the patient, and the dose varied as necessary. Rescue medication will continue to be ordinary morphine tablets or solution (or an alternative strong opioid preparation). When a patient is no longer able to swallow oral medication, most essential drugs are given PR or parenterally, e.g. by CSCI. Although there is no need to change TD fentanyl, it is important to give adequate rescue doses of diamorphine (in the UK) or an alternative strong opioid (Box 2.J).

Oral transmucosal fentanyl citrate (OTFC) is available in some countries for break-through pain; it is expensive.[91]

Hydromorphone

Hydromorphone is an analogue of morphine with similar pharmacokinetic and pharmacodynamic properties. By mouth and by injection it is about 7.5 times more potent than morphine.[92] As with morphine, there is wide inter-patient variation in bio-availability. The main metabolite is hydromorphone-3-glucuronide; hydromorphone-6-glucuronide is not formed.[93] Hydromorphone provides useful analgesia for about 4h.

Hydromorphone is available in many countries in a range of preparations for oral and parenteral administration. In the UK, hydromorphone is available as:

- ordinary capsules, 1.3 and 2.6mg (= morphine 10 and 20mg)
- m/r capsules, 2, 4, 8, 16 and 24mg (= m/r morphine 15, 30, 60, 120 and 180mg).

In some countries hydromorphone is available in high potency ampoules containing 10mg/ml and 20mg/ml to facilitate use by CSCI.

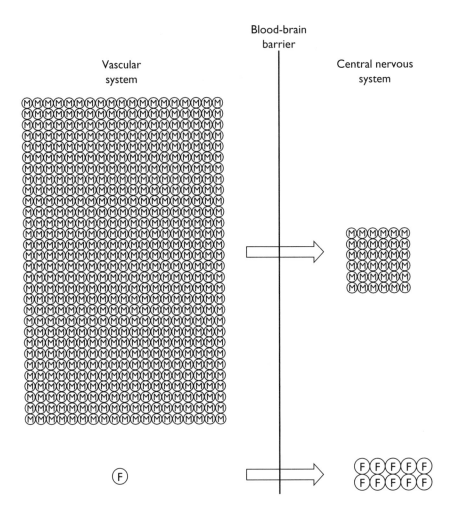

Figure 2.10   Distribution of equipotent doses of morphine and fentanyl in the vascular and central nervous systems based on animal data.[90] Converting from oral or parenteral morphine to transdermal or parenteral fentanyl will result in a massive decrease in opioid molecules outside the CNS. This will result in less constipation and could, in physically-dependent subjects, precipitate peripherally-mediated withdrawal symptoms.

Box 2.J   Parenteral rescue medication for patients receiving TD fentanyl

---

Divide the delivery rate ('patch size') of TD fentanyl (μg/h):

  by 3 and give as SC morphine (mg)

  by 5 and give as SC diamorphine (mg)

  by 15 and give as SC hydromorphone (mg).

Methadone

Guidelines 2.4: Use of methadone (p.382).

Methadone is a μ-receptor, and possibly a δ-receptor agonist,[94] a NMDA-receptor-channel blocker[95] and a presynaptic blocker of serotonin reuptake.[96] Some patients with pain who obtain poor relief and severe adverse effects (drowsiness, delirium, nausea and vomiting) with a non-opioid and morphine, obtain good relief with relatively low doses of methadone and few adverse effects.[97,98] Methadone is less constipating than morphine.[99]

Methadone is also useful in patients with renal failure who develop excessive drowsiness and/or delirium with morphine because of cumulation of M6G. Methadone does not have a comparable active metabolite and it is not greatly affected by renal failure.

The plasma halflife of methadone ranges from about 8–80h.[100] It is reduced by urinary acidification and prolonged by urinary alkalination.[101] Cumulation is a potential problem for most patients and therefore dose titration is different with morphine.[98,102–105]

Methadone is sometimes given by CSCI; it causes significant local inflammation in many patients necessitating site rotation and possibly other measures (*see* p.384).[106] Methadone can also be given IV.[107] Most centres in the UK use the guidelines proposed by Morley and Makin (*see* p.382).[98]

Oxycodone

Oxycodone is a κ- and μ-agonist with similar properties to morphine.[108,109] It appears to cause less sedation, delirium, vomiting and pruritus than morphine but more constipation.[73,110,111]

Although oxycodone has no clinically important active metabolites, the maximum plasma concentration increases by 50% in renal failure causing more sedation.[112] It has a plasma halflife of about 3.5h, which is prolonged by about 1h in renal failure. Parenterally it is about 3/4 as potent as morphine.[112] However, oral bio-availability is 2/3 or more, compared with about 1/3 for morphine. This means that oxycodone by mouth is about 1.5–2 times more potent than oral morphine.[113,114] Like morphine, in most patients oxycodone is best given q4h.

Oxycodone is partly metabolized to oxymorphone, a strong opioid analgesic which by injection is 10 times more potent than morphine. The bio-transformation is mediated by cytochrome CYP2D6. After blocking this by quinidine, the effects of oxycodone in volunteers are unchanged, indicating that oxycodone is an analgesic in its own right, and that the contribution by oxymorphone is small.[115]

Oxycodone is available in the UK in various preparations:

- ordinary capsules, 5, 10 and 20mg (= morphine 7.5–10, 15–20 and 30–40mg)
- solution, 1mg/ml (= morphine 1.5–2mg/ml)
- concentrated solution, 10mg/ml (= morphine 15–20mg/ml)
- m/r tablets, 10, 20 and 40mg (= m/r morphine 15–20, 30–40 and 60–80mg).

Oxycodone pectinate 30mg suppositories are available in the UK and Canada. These are given q8h. Oxycodone pectinate 30mg *q8h* is equivalent to morphine 15mg *q4h*. Oxycodone hydrochloride 5mg suppositories are available in the USA; these are equivalent to morphine 10mg and are given q4h.

Spinal morphine

If given epidurally (ED) or intrathecally (IT), a much lower dose of morphine has a much greater analgesic effect because of the proximity to the opioid receptors in the dorsal horn of the spinal cord. The ED dose is about 1/10 and the IT dose 1/100 of the dose of PO morphine. Adverse effects are correspondingly reduced. In the UK, <5% of cancer patients needing morphine receive it spinally.

The main indications for spinal morphine are:

- intractable pain despite the appropriate combined use of standard and adjuvant analgesics
- intolerable adverse effects with systemic opioids.

To increase the effect of spinal analgesia in neuropathic pain, morphine is often combined with bupivacaine, and sometimes clonidine.

Naloxone

Naloxone is a potent opioid antagonist. The *British National Formulary* contains two entries for it. One relates to overdosage by addicts and recommends *0.8–2mg* IV every 2–3min up to a total of 10mg if necessary, with the possibility of an ongoing IV infusion. The other relates to reversal of iatrogenic respiratory depression. In this circumstance, *100–200µg* IV should be given, with increments of *100µg* every 2min until respiratory function is satisfactory. Further doses should be given after 1–2h by IM injection if there is concern that further absorption of the opioid will result in delayed respiratory depression. Even lower doses are sometimes recommended (Box 2.K).

Box 2.K Naloxone for iatrogenic opioid overdose (based on the recommendations of the American Pain Society)[116]

If respiratory rate ≥8/min and the patient easily rousable and not cyanosed, adopt a policy of 'wait and see'; consider reducing or omitting the next regular dose of morphine.

If respiratory rate ≤8/min, patient unrousable and/or cyanosed:

  dilute a standard ampoule containing naloxone 400µg to 10ml with saline for injection

  administer 0.5ml (20µg) IV every 2min until the patient's respiratory status is satisfactory

  further boluses may be necessary because naloxone is shorter-acting than morphine (and other opioids).

It is important *not* to measure response by level of consciousness because total antagonism will cause a return of severe pain with hyperalgesia and, if physically-dependent, severe physical withdrawal symptoms and marked agitation. However, for respiratory depression with epidural morphine, it is safe to give 400µg. In this circumstance, naloxone reverses respiratory depression without reversing analgesia.[117]

Adjuvant analgesics

Adjuvant analgesics are a miscellaneous group of drugs which relieve pain in specific circumstances. They include:

• corticosteroids

- antidepressants
- anti-epileptics
- NMDA-receptor-channel blockers
- antispasmodics
- muscle relaxants.

Corticosteroids

Corticosteroids (and radiotherapy) are helpful for pain *and* weakness associated with:

- nerve root/nerve trunk compression, e.g. dexamethasone 4–8mg o.d.
- spinal cord compression, e.g. dexamethasone 12–20mg o.d. and sometimes more[118] (Figure 2.11).

Corticosteroids are not helpful in pure non-cancer nerve injury pain, e.g. chronic postoperative scar pain, postherpetic neuralgia. However, with

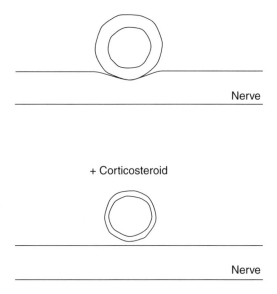

Figure 2.11   Possible mechanism of action of corticosteroids in relief of nerve compression pain. Total tumour mass = neoplasm + surrounding inflammation. General anti-inflammatory effect of corticosteroid reduces total tumour mass resulting in reduction of pain.

cancer-related nerve injury pain, if there is associated limb weakness a 5–7 day trial of dexamethasone may well show benefit.

Antidepressants and anti-epileptics

Nerve injury pains do not always respond to the combined use of a NSAID and a strong opioid.[10] Antidepressants and anti-epileptics are often of benefit (Figure 2.12). These:

- enhance descending inhibitory pathways *or*

- dampen down the hyperexcitability of damaged peripheral nerves *or*

- inhibit the glutamate-excitatory system in the dorsal horn *or*

- enhance the GABA-inhibitory system in the dorsal horn.

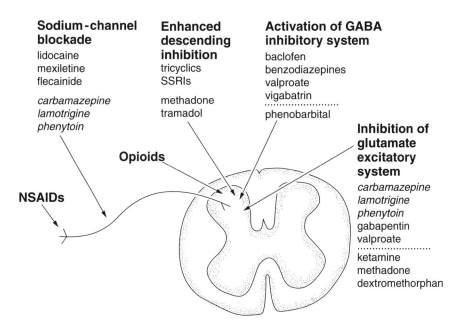

Figure 2.12 Primary site of action of analgesics and adjuvant analgesics on peripheral nerves and the dorsal horn of the spinal cord. Drugs in italics act both peripherally and centrally. Drugs below the dotted lines are channel blockers at their respective receptor-channel complex.

The analgesic action of the antidepressants relates to the blocking of the presynaptic re-uptake of noradrenaline (norepinephrine) and serotonin (5HT) (Figure 2.13). Generally, antidepressants with an impact on both mono-amine systems have a greater analgesic effect than SSRIs.[9,119,120] Amitriptyline 25–75mg o.n. (an antidepressant) and sodium valproate 400–1000mg o.n. (an anti-epileptic) are often used either singly or together.[121,122] Generally these should be given in combination with morphine and a NSAID if the nerve injury pain is associated with an infiltrating cancer.[38,123,124] but may well be effective alone in 'pure' nerve injury pain, e.g. chronic surgical incision pain, postherpetic neuralgia.

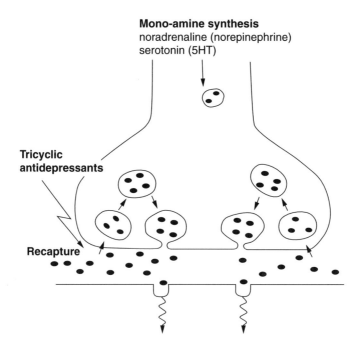

Figure 2.13 Tricyclic antidepressants potentiate two descending spinal inhibitory pathways (one noradrenergic, the other serotonergic) by blocking presynaptic re-uptake. They also potentiate opioid analgesia by a serotonergic mechanism in the brain stem.

Gabapentin, marketed principally as an add-on anti-epileptic, is also licensed for treating neuropathic pain. It binds to a specific site in the CNS, gabapentin-binding protein (GBP) and probably acts as a calcium-channel blocker.[125] However, it is distinct from the traditional calcium-channel blockers used in cardiology in that it is relatively free from adverse effects and therefore much better tolerated. In addition to the central action, gabapentin suppresses the ectopic nerve activity which is a feature of nerve injury pain. The effective dose varies between 100–1200mg t.d.s.[126,127] Like many drugs acting on the CNS, gabapentin can cause drowsiness and dose increases are best made slowly in debilitated patients, e.g. every 3–4 days.[128]

It is important to establish a straightforward practical scheme for neuropathic pain management, selecting only one or two drugs from each category of agents (Figure 2.14).[129,130] About 90% of patients with nerve injury pain respond well to the systematic use of non-opioids, opioids and adjuvant analgesics.[10] The remainder require spinal analgesia (e.g. morphine + bupivacaine ± clonidine) or a neurolytic procedure to obtain adequate relief. Some patients derive benefit from other non-drug measures, e.g. TENS.

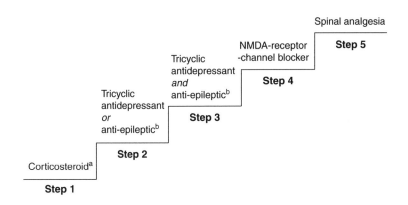

Figure 2.14 Adjuvant analgesics for neuropathic pain. If caused by cancer, use only if the pain does not respond to the combined use of a NSAID and a strong opioid.
a   a trial of a corticosteroid is important when neuropathic pain is associated with limb weakness
b   some centres use mexiletine, a local anaesthetic congener and cardiac anti-arrhythmic drug which blocks sodium channels, as an alternative to an anti-epileptic.[129,130]

Relief is not an 'all or none' phenomenon. The crucial first step in many cases is to help the patient obtain a good night's sleep. The second is to reduce pain intensity and allodynia to a bearable level during the day. Initially there may be marked diurnal variation in the relief achieved, with more prolonged periods with less or no pain rather than a decrease in worst pain intensity round-the-clock.

The patient should be warned that major benefit often takes a week or more to manifest, although improvement in sleep should occur immediately. Adverse drug effects tend to be the limiting therapeutic factor.

NMDA-receptor-channel blockers

NMDA-receptor-channel blockers are used most commonly when neuropathic pain does not respond well to standard analgesics together with an antidepressant and an anti-epileptic. They include:

- methadone (see p.382)[98,131]

- ketamine[132–134]

- amantadine, e.g. 100mg PO b.d.[135,136]

Ketamine

Ketamine is an anaesthetic induction agent. Its plasma halflife is about 3h, and it has an active metabolite, norketamine, with a halflife of 12h.[137] PO doses of ketamine yield lower plasma ketamine concentrations but higher norketamine ones; in chronic use norketamine may be the main analgesic agent. Its use IV, SC or PO as an analgesic is beyond the manufacturer's licence.[138]

Dose recommendations vary considerably but ketamine is often started in a low dose PO (Box 2.L), or even SL.[139] Ketamine is unusual in that the PO doses are often much lower than those given SC. Psychotomimetic effects are common and are treated with haloperidol, diazepam or midazolam.[140] Ketamine has been used IV with fentanyl and midazolam to control intractable pain and agitation.[141,142]

Patients should be supplied with 1ml graduated syringes and advised to leave two needles (one as an air vent) inserted in the bung of a ketamine vial; sterility is not necessary for PO administration. Use 10mg/ml or 20mg/ml; 50mg/ml is too bitter. Long-term success, i.e. both pain relief and tolerable adverse effects, varies from <20% to about 50%.[132,139,143]

Box 2.L   Dose recommendations for ketamine

PO[144–146]

Use direct from vial or dilute for convenience to 50mg/5ml.

Patient adds flavouring of choice to mask the bitter taste:

starting dose 2–25mg t.d.s.–q.d.s. and p.r.n. (equivalent to 0.4–5mg SC)

increase the dose in steps of 6–25mg; maximum reported PO dose is 200mg q.d.s.[146,147]

give a smaller dose more frequently if psychotomimetic phenomena or drowsiness occur which does not respond to a reduction in opioid.

CSCI[144,148,149]

Because ketamine is irritant, dilute with sodium chloride 0.9% to the largest volume possible (i.e. for a Graseby syringe driver, 18ml in a 30ml luerlock syringe given over 12–24h). Ketamine is compatible with dexamethasone (low-dose), diamorphine, haloperidol, levomepromazine, metoclopramide, midazolam:

starting dose 0.1–0.5mg/kg/h, typically 150–200mg/24h

increase by 50–100mg/24h; maximum reported dose is 2.4g/24h[150]

Inflammation at infusion site may be helped by hydrocortisone 1% cream or by adding dexamethasone 0.5–1mg to the infusion (dilute in 5–10ml sodium chloride 0.9% and then add ketamine).

Antispasmodics

Antispasmodics is the term given to antimuscarinic drugs used to relieve visceral distension pain and colic. In advanced cancer, there is little place for 'weak' antispasmodics such as dicycloverine (dicyclomine) and mebeverine. In the UK, hyoscine *butylbromide* is widely regarded as the antispasmodic of choice. This is given by SC injection, i.e. 20mg stat and p.r.n., and 40–160mg by CSCI. In the USA, where hyoscine *butylbromide* is not available, SC glycopyrrolate can be substituted, e.g. 200–400µg stat and p.r.n., and 600–1200µg/24h by CSCI.

Muscle relaxants

For painful muscle spasm (cramp) and myofascial pain, the correct approach is:

- explanation
- physical therapy (local heat and massage)
- diazepam and relaxation therapy
- injection of the trigger points with local anaesthetic and a corticosteroid (e.g. bupivacaine 0.5% and depot methylprednisolone 80mg).

However severe, morphine is not indicated for the relief of cramp and trigger point pains because it is ineffective.

Alternative routes of administration

Guidelines 2.5: Use of syringe drivers at Sobell House (p.384).

Not all patients are able to swallow tablets or capsules and those experiencing nausea and vomiting may not be able to retain them. A range of alternative routes is available. In practice, choice is largely determined by commercial availability (Figure 2.15).

'Sprinkling' refers to the practice of emptying the contents of a m/r morphine *capsule* onto a teaspoon of semisolid food immediately before swallowing, e.g. apple sauce, puree, jam, yoghurt, ice-cream. Although sachets of

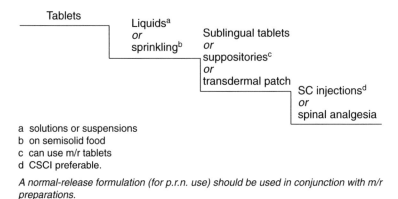

a solutions or suspensions
b on semisolid food
c can use m/r tablets
d CSCI preferable.

A normal-release formulation (for p.r.n. use) should be used in conjunction with m/r preparations.

Figure 2.15 Alternative routes of administration.

m/r morphine granules are available for use as a suspension, they are much more expensive.

Various buccal and sublingual tablets are available, e.g. piroxicam and buprenorphine. Lingual piroxicam (Feldene Melt) is in fact a soluble oral preparation, i.e. the dissolved tablet still has to be swallowed. On the other hand, SL buprenorphine is absorbed locally, and swallowing it results in a major loss of efficacy because of first-pass hepatic metabolism. Oral transmucosal fentanyl citrate (OTFC) is used at some centres for break-through pain.[151]

Morphine is slowly absorbed through the buccal mucosa.[151] However, it was successfully used in the past by this route in moribund patients being cared for at home. M/r morphine suppositories for o.d. or b.d. use makes PR administration more feasible.[152] Although not licensed for this route, m/r morphine tablets have been used PR to provide emergency analgesia in moribund patients.

Battery-driven portable syringe drivers are a convenient method for administering many drugs by CSCI to patients with severe nausea and vomiting, or who cannot swallow medication for various reasons.[138] The advantages of CSCI infusion include:

- better control of nausea and vomiting (guarantees drug absorption)
- constant analgesia (no peaks or troughs)
- generally reloaded once in 24h (saves nurses' time)
- comfort and confidence (minimal number of injections)
- does not limit mobility (lightweight and compact).

The most common choices for infusion are:

- upper chest (intercostal plane)
- upper arm (outer aspect)
- abdomen
- thighs.

If the infusion causes painful local inflammation, consider the following options:

- change the needle site prophylactically, e.g. daily
- reduce the quantity of the irritant drug or increase the volume infused

- change to an alternative drug, e.g. cyclizine to hyoscine *butylbromide*
- give the irritant drug IM or PR
- use a plastic cannula instead of a metal needle
- give a stat injection of hydrocortisone sodium succinate 25–50mg through the butterfly needle and add the same amount to the syringe (not used by the authors)
- give a stat injection of hyaluronidase 1500IU through the butterfly needle and add the same amount to the syringe (not used by the authors).

More information about CSCI, can be found in the *Palliative Care Formulary*[138] or at www.palliativedrugs.com. In patients with venous access, e.g. a Hickman line, the IV route is an obvious alternative but CSCI is generally preferable.

Topical morphine

Nociceptive afferent nerve fibres contain peripheral opioid receptors which are silent except in the presence of local inflammation.[153,154] This property is exploited in joint surgery where morphine is given intra-articularly at the end of the operation.[155] Topical morphine has also been used successfully to relieve otherwise intractable pain associated with cutaneous ulceration, often sacral decubitus.[156–158] Generally it is given as a 0.1% (1mg/ml) gel (in Intrasite). A higher dose may be necessary, e.g. 0.3–0.5%, in other situations:

- oral mucositis
- vaginal inflammation associated with a fistula
- rectal ulceration.[157]

The amount of gel applied varies according to the size and the site of the ulcer but is typically 5–10ml applied b.d.–t.d.s. The topical morphine is kept in place with:

- a non-absorbable pad or dressing, e.g. Opsite
- gauze coated with petroleum jelly.

References

1   IASP Task Force on Taxonomy (1994) *Classification of chronic pain*. IASP Press, Seattle.

2   Kane R *et al.* (1984) A randomized controlled trial of hospice care. *Lancet* **1**:890–4.
3   Bonica J (1990) Cancer pain: current status and future needs. In: J Bonica (ed) *The Management of Pain.* Lea & Febiger, Philadelphia, pp 400–55.
4   Grond S *et al.* (1996) Assessment of cancer pain: a prospective evaluation in 2266 cancer patients referred to a pain service. *Pain.* **64**:107–14.
5   Douglas I *et al.* (2000) Central issues in the management of temporal variation in cancer pain. In: R Hillier, I Finlay, J Welsh *et al.* (eds) *The Effective Management of Cancer Pain.* Aesculapius Medical Press, London, pp 93–106.
6   IASP (1986) Subcommittee on Taxonomy. Classification of chronic pain. *Pain.* 1–225.
7   Travell J and Rinzler S (1952) The myofascial genesis of pain. *Postgraduate Medicine (Minneapolis).* **11**:425–34.
8   Baron R (2000) Peripheral neuropathic pain: from mechanisms to symptoms. *Clinical Journal of Pain.* **16**:S12–20.
9   Sindrup S and Jensen T (1999) Efficacy of pharmacological treatments of neuropathic pain: an update and effect related to mechanism of drug action. *Pain.* **83**:389–400.
10 Grond S *et al.* (1999) Assessment and treatment of neuropathic cancer pain following WHO guidelines. *Pain.* **79**:15–20.
11 Hoskin PJ (1995) Radiotherapy in the management of bone pain. *Clinical Orthopaedics.* **312**:105–19.
12 Bone Pain Trial Working Party (1999) 8 Gy single fraction radiotherapy for the treatment of metastatic skeletal pain: randomized comparison with a multi-fraction schedule over 12 months of patient follow-up. *Radiotherapy and Oncology.* **52**:111–21.
13 Hoegler D (1997) Radiotherapy for palliation of symptoms in incurable cancer. *Current Problems in Cancer.* **21**:129–83.
14 George R (1999) Personal communication.
15 Ernst OS *et al.* (1992) A double-blind, crossover trial of intravenous clodronate in metastatic bone pain. *Journal of Pain and Symptom Management.* **7**:4–11.
16 Robertson AG *et al.* (1995) Effect of oral clodronate on metastatic bone pain: a double-blind, placebo-controlled study. *Journal of Clinical Oncology.* **13**:2427–30.
17 Ernst D *et al.* (1997) A randomized, controlled trial of intravenous clodronate in patients with metastatic bone disease and pain. *Journal of Pain and Symptom Management.* **13**:319–26.
18 Lipton A *et al.* (2000) Pamidronate prevents skeletal complications and is effective palliative treatment in women with breast carcinoma and osteolytic bone metastases. *Cancer.* **88**:1082–90.
19 Mannix K *et al.* (2000) Using bisphosphonates to control the pain of bone metastases: evidence-based guidelines for palliative care. *Palliative Medicine.* **14**:455–61.
20 Hillner B *et al.* (2000) American Society of Clinical Oncology guideline on the role of bisphosphonates in breast cancer. American Society of Clinical Oncology Bisphosphonates Expert Panel. *Journal of Clinical Oncology.* **18**:1378–91.
21 Vorreuther R (1993) Biphosphonates as an adjunct to palliative therapy of bone metastases from prostatic carcinoma. A pilot study on clodronate. *British Journal of Urology.* **72**:792–5.

22 Walker P *et al.* (1997) Subcutaneous clodronate: a study evaluating efficacy in hypercalcaemia of malignancy and local toxicity. *Annals of Oncology.* **8**: 915–6.

23 Vinholes J *et al.* (1996) Metabolic effects of pamidronate in patients with metastatic bone disease. *European Journal of Cancer.* **5**:159–75.

24 Cascinu S *et al.* (1998) Different doses of pamidronate in patients with painful osteolytic bone metastases. *Supportive Care in Cancer.* **6**:139–43.

25 McCloskey E *et al.* (1998) A randomized trial of the effect of clodronate on skeletal morbidity in multiple myeloma. *British Journal of Haematology.* **100**:317–25.

26 Fidler M (1973) Prophylactic internal fixation of secondary neoplastic deposits in long bones. *British Medical Journal.* **1**:341–3.

27 Yaksh T *et al.* (1998) Mechanism of action of nonsteroidal anti-inflammatory drugs. *Cancer Investigation.* **16**:509–27.

28 Stein C (1993) Peripheral mechanisms of opioid analgesia. *Anesthesia and Analgesia.* **76**:182–91.

29 World Health Organization (1986) *Cancer Pain Relief.* WHO, Geneva.

30 World Health Organization (1996) *Cancer Pain Relief: with a guide to opioid availability.* WHO, Geneva.

31 Twycross R *et al.* (2000) Paracetamol. *Progress in Palliative Care.* **8**:198–202.

32 Flower RJ and Vane JR (1972) Inhibition of prostaglandin synthetase in brain explains the anti-pyretic activity of paracetamol. *Nature.* **240**:410–11.

33 Simmons D *et al.* (1999) Induction of an acetaminophen-sensitive cyclooxygenase with reduced sensitivity to nonsteroidal antiinflammatory drugs. *Proceedings of the National Academy of Science USA.* **96**:3275–80.

34 Moore U *et al.* (1992) The efficacy of locally applied aspirin and acetaminophen in postoperative pain after third molar surgery. *Clinical Pharmacology and Therapeutics.* **52**:292–6.

35 Bjorkman R *et al.* (1994) Acetaminophen (paracetamol) blocks spinal hyperalgesia induced by NMDA and substance P. *Pain.* **57**:259–64.

36 Pini L *et al.* (1997) Naloxone-reversible antinociception by paracetamol in the rat. *Journal of Pharmacology and Experimental Therapeutics.* **280**:934–40.

37 Settipane R *et al.* (1995) Prevalence of cross-sensitivity with acetaminophen in aspirin-sensitive asthmatic subjects. *Journal of Allergy and Clinical Immunology.* **96**:480–5.

38 Dellemijn P *et al.* (1994) Medical therapy of malignant nerve pain. A randomised double-blind explanatory trial with naproxen versus slow-release morphine. *European Journal of Cancer.* **30A**:1244–50.

39 McCormack K and Brune K (1991) Dissociation between the antinociceptive and anti-inflammatory effects of the nonsteroidal anti-inflammatory drugs. A survey of their analgesic efficacy. *Drugs.* **41**:533–47.

40 Simon L *et al.* (2000) Anti-inflammatory and upper gastrointestinal effects of celecoxib in rheumatoid arthritis. *Journal of the American Medical Association.* **282**:1921–8.

41 Langman M *et al.* (2000) Adverse upper gastrointestinal effects of rofecoxib compared with NSAIDs. *Journal of the American Medical Association.* **282**:1929–33.

42 Somasundaran S *et al.* (1995) The biochemical basis of nonsteroidal anti-inflammatory drug-induced damage to the gastrointestinal tract: a review and a hypothesis. *Scandinavian Journal of Gastroenterology.* **30**:289–99.

43 Bennett A (2000) The importance of COX-2 inhibition for aspirin induced asthma. *Thorax.* **55**:S54–S56.

44 Stockley I (1999) Hypoglycaemic agents and salicylates. In: I Stockley (ed) *Textbook of Drug Interactions, 5th edition.* Pharmaceutical Press, London, pp 528–9.

45 Patrignani P *et al.* (1997) Differential inhibition of human prostaglandin endoperoxide synthase-1 and -2 by nonsteroidal anti-inflammatory drugs. *Journal of Physiology and Pharmacology.* **48**:623–31.

46 Todd P and Sorkin E (1988) Diclofenac sodium: a reappraisal of its pharmacodynamic and pharmacokinetic properties, and therapeutic efficacy. *Drugs.* **35**:244–85.

47 Warner T *et al.* (1999) Nonsteroidal drug selectivities for cyclo-oxygenase-1 rather than cyclo-oxygenase-2 are associated with human gastrointestinal toxicity: a full in vitro analysis. *Proceedings of the National Academy of Science USA.* **96**:7563–8.

48 Middleton RK *et al.* (1996) Ketorolac continuous infusion: a case report and review of the literature. *Journal of Pain and Symptom Management.* **12**:190–4.

49 Hughes A *et al.* (1997) Ketorolac: continuous subcutaneous infusion for cancer pain. *Journal of Pain and Symptom Management.* **13**:315–7.

50 Hanks G and Cherry N (1997) Opioid analgesic therapy. In: D Doyle, G Hanks and N MacDonald (eds) *Oxford Textbook of Palliative Medicine.* Oxford University Press, Oxford, pp 331–5.

51 Eckhardt K *et al.* (1998) Same incidence of adverse drug events after codeine administration irrespective of the genetically determined differences in morphine formation. *Pain.* **76**:27–33.

52 Ammon S *et al.* (1999) Pharmacokinetics of dihydrocodeine and its active metabolite after single and multiple oral dosing. *British Journal of Clinical Pharmacology.* **48**:317–22.

53 Mercadante S *et al.* (1998) Dextropropoxyphene versus morphine in opioid-naive cancer patients with pain. *Journal of Pain and Symptom Management.* **15**:76–81.

54 Vickers M *et al.* (1992) Tramadol: pain relief by an opioid without depression of respiration. *Anaesthesia.* **47**:291–6.

55 Wilder-Smith C *et al.* (1994) Oral tramadol and morphine for strong cancer-related pain. *Annals of Oncology.* **5**:141–6.

56 Wilder-Smith C and Bettiga A (1997) The analgesic tramadol has minimal effect on gastrointestinal motor function. *British Journal of Clinical Pharmacology.* **43**:71–5.

57 Sindrup S *et al.* (1999) Tramadol relieves pain and allodynia in polyneuropathy: a randomised, double-blind, controlled trial. *Pain.* **83**:85–90.

58 Borgbjerg FM *et al.* (1996) Experimental pain stimulates respiration and attenuates morphine-induced respiratory depression: a controlled study in human volunteers. *Pain.* **64**:123–8.

59 Regnard CFB and Badger C (1987) Opioids, sleep and the time of death. *Palliative Medicine.* **1**:107–10.

60 Collin E *et al.* (1993) Is disease progression the major factor in morphine 'tolerance' in cancer pain treatment? *Pain.* **55**:319–26.

61 Passik S and Portenoy R (1998) Substance abuse issues in palliative care. In: A Berger (ed) *Principles and Practice of Supportive Oncology*. Lippincott-Raven, Philadelphia, pp 513–29.

62 Joranson D *et al.* (2000) Trends in medical use and abuse of opioid analgesics. *Journal of the American Medical Association*. **283**:1710–14.

63 Twycross RG and Wald SJ (1976) Longterm use of diamorphine in advanced cancer. In: DA-F J J Bonica (ed) *Advances in Pain Research and Therapy. Vol 1*. Raven Press, New York, pp 653–61.

64 Twycross R (1997) *Oral Morphine in Advanced Cancer*. Beaconsfield Publishers, Beaconsfield.

65 Collins S *et al.* (1998) Peak plasma concentrations after oral morphine: a systematic review. *Journal of Pain and Symptom Management*. **16**:388–402.

66 Hanks GW *et al.* (1996) Morphine in cancer pain: modes of administration. *British Medical Journal*. **312**:823–6.

67 Radbruch L *et al.* (1999) Intravenous titration with morphine for severe cancer pain: report of 28 cases. *Clinical Journal of Pain*. **15**:173–8.

68 Kumar K *et al.* (2000) Intravenous morphine for emergency treatment of cancer pain. *Palliative Medicine*. **14**:183–8.

69 Smith GM *et al.* (1962) Subjective effects of heroin and morphine in normal subjects. *Journal of Pharmacology and Experimental Therapeutics*. **136**: 47–52.

70 Loan WB *et al.* (1969) Studies of drugs given before anaesthesia. XVII. The natural and semi-synthetic opiates. *British Journal of Anaesthesia*. **41**:57–63.

71 Wright CI and Barbour FA (1935) The respiratory effects of morphine, codeine and related substances. *Journal of Pharmacology and Experimental Therapeutics*. **54**:25–33.

72 Twycross RG (1977) Choice of strong analgesic in terminal cancer: diamorphine or morphine? *Pain*. **3**:93–104.

73 Ashby M *et al.* (1999) Opioid substitution to reduce adverse effects in cancer pain management. *Medical Journal of Australia*. **170**:68–71.

74 Sjogren P *et al.* (1993) Hyperalgesia and myoclonus in terminal cancer patients treated with continuous intravenous morphine. *Pain*. **55**:93–7.

75 Sjogren P *et al.* (1994) Disappearance of morphine-induced hyperalgesia after discontinuing or substituting morphine with other opioid antagonists. *Pain*. **59**:313–6.

76 Bruera E *et al.* (1996) Opioid rotation in patients with cancer pain. *Cancer*. **78**:852–7.

77 Donner B *et al.* (1996) Direct conversion from oral morphine to transdermal fentanyl: a multicenter study in patients with cancer pain. *Pain*. **64**:527–34.

78 Bartlett S *et al.* (1994) Pharmacology of morphine and morphine-3-glucuronide at opioid, excitatory amino acid, GABA and glycine binding sites. *Pharmacology and Toxicology*. **75**:73–81.

79 Lawlor P *et al.* (1998) Dose ratio between morphine and methadone in patients with cancer pain. *Cancer*. **82**:1167–73.

80 Beaver WT *et al.* (1967) A clinical comparison of the analgesic effects of methadone and morphine administered intramuscularly, and of orally and parenterally administered methadone. *Clinical Pharmacology and Therapeutics*. **8**:415–26.

81   Gagnon B and Bruera E (1999) Differences in the ratios of morphine to methadone in patients with neuropathic pain versus non-neuropathic pain. *Journal of Pain and Symptom Management.* **18**:120–5.

82   Bernards CM (1999) Clinical implications of physicochemical properties of opioids. In: C Stein (ed) *Opioids in Pain Control.* Cambridge University Press, Cambridge, pp 166–87.

83   Morley (2000) Personal communication.

84   Gourlay GK *et al.* (1989) The transdermal administration of fentanyl in the treatment of post-operative pain: pharmacokinetics and pharmacodynamic effects. *Pain.* **37**:193–202.

85   Ahmedzai S and Brooks D (1997) Transdermal fentanyl versus sustained-release oral morphine in cancer pain: preference, efficacy and quality of life. *Journal of Pain and Symptom Management.* **13**:254–61.

86   Vielvoye-Kerkmeer A *et al.* (2000) Transdermal fentanyl in opioid-naive cancer pain patients: an open trial using transdermal fentanyl for the treatment of chronic cancer pain in opioid-naive patients and a group using codeine. *Journal of Pain and Symptom Management.* **19**:185–92.

87   Portenoy RK *et al.* (1993) Transdermal fentanyl for cancer pain. *Anesthesiology.* **78**:36–43.

88   Hammack JE and Loprinzi CL (1994) Use of orally administered opioids for cancer-related pain. *Mayo Clinic Proceedings.* **69**:384–90.

89   Radbruch L *et al.* (2000) Constipation and the use of laxatives: a comparison between transdermal fentanyl and oral morphine. *Palliative Medicine.* **14**:111–19.

90   Herz A and Teschemacher H-J (1971) Activities and sites of antinociceptive action of morphine-like analgesics and kinetics of distribution following intravenous, intracerebral and intraventricular application. *Advances in Drug Research.* **6**:79–119.

91   Lichtor J *et al.* (1999) The relative potency of oral transmucosal fentanyl citrate compared with intravenous morphine in the treatment of moderate to severe postoperative pain. *Anesthesia and Analgesia.* **89**:732–8.

92   Moriarty M *et al.* (1999) A randomised crossover comparison of controlled release hydromorphone tablets with controlled release morphine tablets in patients with cancer pain. *Journal of Clinical Research.* **2**:1–8.

93   Babul N and Darke AC (1992) Putative role of hydromorphone metabolites in myoclonus. *Pain.* **51**:260–1.

94   Raynor K *et al.* (1994) Pharmacological characterization of the cloned kappa-, delta-, and mu-opioid receptors. *Molecular Pharmacology.* **45**:330–4.

95   Gorman A *et al.* (1997) The d- and l-isomers of methadone bind to the non-competitive site on the N-methyl-D-aspartate (NMDA) receptor in rat forebrain and spinal cord. *Neuroscience Letters.* **223**:5–8.

96   Codd E *et al.* (1995) Serotonin and norepinephrine uptake inhibiting activity of centrally acting analgesics: structural determinants and role in antinociception. *Journal of Pharmacology and Experimental Therapeutics.* **274**:1263–70.

97   Manfredi P *et al.* (1997) Intravenous methadone for cancer pain unrelieved by morphine and hydromorphone: clinical observations. *Pain.* **70**:99–101.

98   Morley J and Makin M (1998) The use of methadone in cancer pain poorly responsive to other opioids. *Pain Reviews.* **5**:51–8.

99 Daeninck P and Bruera E (1999) Reduction in constipation and laxative requirements following opioid rotation to methadone: a report of four cases. *Journal of Pain and Symptom Management.* **18**:303–9.

100 Sawe J (1986) High dose morphine and methadone in cancer patients: clinical pharmacokinetic consideration of oral treatment. *Clinical Pharmacology.* **11**:87–106.

101 Nilsson MI *et al.* (1982) Pharmacokinetics of methadone during maintenance treatment: adaptive changes during the induction phase. *European Journal of Clinical Pharmarcology.* **22**:343–9.

102 Ripamonti C *et al.* (1997) An update on the clinical use of methadone in cancer pain. *Pain.* **70**:109–15.

103 Hagen N and Wasylenko E (1999) Methadone: outpatient titration and monitoring strategies in cancer patients. *Journal of Pain and Symptom Management.* **18**:369–75.

104 Mercadante S *et al.* (1999) Rapid switching from morphine to methadone in cancer patients with poor response to morphine. *Journal of Clinical Oncology.* **17**:3307–12.

105 Scholes C *et al.* (1999) Methadone titration in opioid-resistant cancer pain. *European Journal of Cancer Care.* **8**:26–9.

106 Mathew P and Storey P (1999) Subcutaneous methadone in terminally ill patients: manageable local toxicity. *Journal of Pain and Symptom Management.* **18**:49–52.

107 Fitzgibbon D and Ready L (1997) Intravenous high-dose methadone administered by patient controlled analgesia and continuous infusion for the treatment of cancer pain refractory to high-dose morphine. *Pain.* **73**:259–61.

108 Glare PA and Walsh TD (1993) Dose-ranging study of oxycodone for chronic pain in advanced cancer. *Journal of Clinical Oncology.* **11**:973–8.

109 Poyhia R *et al.* (1993) Oxycodone: an alternative to morphine for cancer pain. A review. *Journal of Pain and Symptom Management.* **8**:63–7.

110 Heiskanen T and Kalso E (1997) Controlled-release oxycodone and morphine in cancer related pain. *Pain.* **73**:37–45.

111 Mucci-LoRusso P *et al.* (1998) Controlled-release oxycodone compared with controlled-release morphine in the treatment of cancer pain: a randomized, double-blind, parallel-group study. *European Journal of Pain.* **2**:239–49.

112 Kaiko R *et al.* (1996) Clinical pharmacokinetics of controlled-release oxycodone in renal impairment. *Clinical Pharmacology and Therapeutics.* **59**:130.

113 Heiskanen T *et al.* (1996) Double-blind, randomised, repeated dose, crossover comparison of controlled-release oxycodone and controlled-release morphine in cancer pain. 1: pharmacodynamic profile. In: *Abstracts of 8th World Congress on Pain.* IASP Press, Seattle, pp 17–18.

114 Kaiko R *et al.* (1996) Analgesic onset and potency of oral controlled-release (CR) oxycodone and controlled-release morphine. *Clinical Pharmacology and Therapeutics.* **59**:130.

115 Heiskanen T *et al.* (1998) Effects of blocking CYP2D6 on oxycodone. *Clinical Pharmacology and Therapeutics.* **64**:603–11.

116 Max MB *et al.* (1992) *Principles of analgesic use in the treatment of acute pain and cancer pain.* American Pain Society, Skokie, Illinois, p.12.

117 Korbon G *et al.* (1985) Intramuscular naloxone reverses the side effects of epidural morphine while preserving analgesia. *Regional Anaesthesia.* **10**:16–20.

118 Loblaw D and Laperriere N (1998) Emergency treatment of malignant extradural spinal cord compression: an evidence-based guideline. *Journal of Clinical Oncology.* **16**:1613–24.

119 Onghena P and Houdenhove BV (1992) Antidepressant-induced analgesia in chronic non malignant pain: a meta-analysis of 39 placebo-controlled trials. *Pain.* **49**:205–19.

120 Ansari A (2000) The efficacy of newer antidepressants in the treatment of chronic pain: a review of current literature. *Harvard Review Psychiatry.* **7**:257–77.

121 McQuay H *et al.* (1995) Anticonvulsant drugs for management of pain: a systematic review. *British Medical Journal.* **311**:1047–52.

122 McQuay H *et al.* (1996) A systematic review of antidepressants in neuropathic pain. *Pain.* **68**:217–27.

123 Ripamonti C *et al.* (1996) Continuous subcutaneous infusion of ketorolac in cancer neuropathic pain unresponsive to opioid and adjuvant drugs. A case report. *Tumori.* **82**:413–15.

124 Dellemijn P (1999) Are opioids effective in relieving neuropathic pain? *Pain.* **80**:453–62.

125 Chizh B *et al.* (1999) The race to control pain: more participants, more targets. *Trends in Pharmacological Sciences.* **20**:354–7.

126 Rowbotham M *et al.* (1998) Gabapentin for the treatment of postherpetic neuralgia. *Journal of the American Medical Association.* **280**:1837–42.

127 Caraceni A *et al.* (1999) Gabapentin as an adjuvant to opioid analgesia for neuropathic cancer pain. *Journal of Pain and Symptom Management.* **17**:441–5.

128 Rosner H *et al.* (1996) Gabapentin adjunctive therapy in neuropathic pain states. *Clinical Journal of Pain.* **12**:56–68.

129 Chabal C *et al.* (1992) The use of oral mexiletine for the treatment of pain after peripheral nerve injury. *Anaesthesiology.* **76**:513–17.

130 Chong S *et al.* (1997) Pilot study evaluating local anesthetics administered systemically for treatment of pain in patients with advanced cancer. *Journal of Pain and Symptom Management.* **13**:112–17.

131 Gannon C (1997) The use of methadone in the care of the dying. *European Journal of Palliative Care.* **4**:152–8.

132 Enarson M *et al.* (1999) Clinical experience with oral ketamine. *Journal of Pain and Symptom Management.* **17**:384–6.

133 Fine P (1999) Low-dose ketamine in the management of opioid nonresponsive terminal cancer. *Journal of Pain and Symptom Management.* **17**:296–300.

134 Finlay I (1999) Ketamine and its role in cancer pain. *Pain Reviews.* **6**:303–13.

135 Kornhuber J *et al.* (1995) Therapeutic brain concentration of the NMDA receptor antagonist amantadine. *Neuropharmacology.* **34**:713–21.

136 Pud D *et al.* (1998) The NMDA receptor antagonist amantadine reduces surgical neuropathic pain in cancer patients: a double blind, randomized, placebo controlled trial. *Pain.* **75**:349–54.

137 Domino E *et al.* (1984) Ketamine kinetics in unmedicated and diazepam premedicated subjects. *Clinical Pharmacology and Therapeutics.* **36**:645–53.

138 Twycross R *et al.* (1998) *Palliative Care Formulary.* Radcliffe Medical Press, Oxford.

139 Batchelor G (1999) Ketamine in neuropathic pain. *The Pain Society Newsletter.* **1**:19.

140 Fisher K and Hagen N (1999) Analgesic effect of oral ketamine in chronic neuropathic pain of spinal origin: a case report. *Journal of Pain and Symptom Management.* **18**:61–6.

141 Berger J *et al.* (2000) Ketamine-fentanyl-midazolam infusion for the control of symptoms in terminal life care. *American Journal of Hospice and Palliative Care.* **17**:127–32.

142 Enck R (2000) A ketamine, fentanyl, and midazolam infusion for uncontrolled terminal pain and agitation. *American Journal of Hospice and Palliative Care.* **17**:76–7.

143 Haines D and Gaines S (1999) N of 1 randomised controlled trials of oral ketamine in patients with chronic pain. *Pain.* **83**:283–7.

144 Luczak J *et al.* (1995) The role of ketamine, an NMDA receptor antagonist, in the management of pain. *Progress in Palliative Care.* **3**:127–34.

145 Broadley K *et al.* (1996) Ketamine injection used orally. *Palliative Medicine.* **10**:247–50.

146 Vielvoye-Kerkmeer A *et al.* (2000) The need for ketamine. Comment. *Journal of Pain and Symptom Management.* **19**:1–3.

147 Mercadante S (1996) Ketamine in cancer pain: an update. *Palliative Medicine.* **10**:225–30.

148 Oshima E *et al.* (1990) Continuous subcutaneous injection of ketamine for cancer pain. *Canadian Journal of Anaesthetics.* **37**:385–92.

149 Hughes A *et al.* (1999) Ketamine. *CME Bulletin Palliative Medicine.* **1**:53.

150 Clark JL and Kalan GE (1995) Effective treatment of severe cancer pain of the head using low-dose ketamine in an opioid-tolerant patient. *Journal of Pain and Symptom Management.* **10**:310–14.

151 Coluzzi P (1998) Sublingual morphine: efficacy reviewed. *Journal of Pain and Symptom Management.* **16**:184–92.

152 Bruera E *et al.* (1999) Twice-daily versus once-daily morphine sulphate controlled-release suppositories for the treatment of cancer pain. *Supportive Care in Cancer.* **7**:280–3.

153 Krajnik M and Zylicz Z (1997) Topical opioids – fact or fiction? *Progress in Palliative Care.* **5**:101–6.

154 Krajnik M *et al.* (1998) Opioids affect inflammation and the immune system. *Pain Reviews.* **5**:147–54.

155 Likar R *et al.* (1999) Dose-dependency of intra-articular morphine analgesia. *British Journal of Anaesthesia.* **83**:241–4.

156 Back NI and Finlay I (1995) Analgesic effect of topical opioids on painful skin ulcers. *Journal of Pain and Symptom Management.* **10**:493.

157 Krajnik M *et al.* (1999) Potential uses of topical opioids in palliative care – report of 6 cases. *Pain.* **80**:121–5.

158 Twillman R *et al.* (1999) Treatment of painful skin ulcers with topical opioids. *Journal of Pain and Symptom Management.* **17**:288–92.

3 Alimentary symptoms

Halitosis · Dry mouth · Drooling · Stomatitis · Oral candidiasis · Abnormal taste · Anorexia · Dehydration Cachexia · Dysphagia · Endo-oesophageal intubation Heartburn · Dyspepsia · Gastric stasis · Nausea and vomiting · Obstruction · Constipation · Faecal impaction Diarrhoea · Rectal discharge · Ascites

Halitosis

Halitosis means unpleasant or foul-smelling breath.

Causes

- poor dental and oral hygiene
- necrosis and sepsis in the mouth, pharynx, nose, nasal sinuses or lungs
- severe infection
- gastric stagnation associated with gastric outflow obstruction
- ingestion of substances whose volatile products are excreted by the lungs or saliva, e.g. garlic, onions, alcohol
- smoking.

Management

Correct the correctable

Dental and oral hygiene

- clean teeth with toothbrush and toothpaste b.d.
- consider use of dental floss
- encourage fluid intake
- offer refreshing mouthwashes (*see* p.72).

- gargles and/or mouthwashes on waking, after meals and at bedtime, particularly if there is a heavily furred tongue or necrotic tumour
    cider and soda water in equal parts *or*
    hydrogen peroxide 6% BP *or*
    povidone-iodine 1%.

- modify diet, e.g. exclude garlic and onions

- stop smoking

- consider artificial saliva if the mouth is very dry (*see* p.73).

Infection

- treat oral candidiasis (*see* p.79)

- send sputum for culture and prescribe the appropriate antibiotic

- if suspect necrotic cancer and anaerobic infection, prescribe metro-nidazole 400mg PO b.d.–t.d.s. for 10 days

- if pulmonary candidiasis (rare), prescribe ketoconazole 200mg b.d. or fluconazole 100mg PO for 7 days.

Stagnant gastric contents

Prescribe a prokinetic, e.g. metoclopramide10mg SC stat and 40–100mg/24h by CSCI. If beneficial, convert to metoclopramide 10–20mg PO q.d.s.

Dry mouth

Saliva is a complex biological fluid which is directly essential for oral and dental hygiene and indirectly essential for general health by reducing the risk of infection and malnutrition. The principal functions of saliva are:

- lubrication and cleansing of the mouth

- antimicrobial activity

- remineralization of teeth

- digestion of food.

Normally about 1.5L of saliva is produced in 24h. This is often reduced in advanced disease and is the main cause of dry mouth. It affects >75% of patients,[1] and is sometimes described as a burning mouth.[2]

Poor oral lubrication makes chewing and swallowing difficult and painful, and taste is impaired. These are all factors which will contribute to anorexia.

Dentures may become problematic and speech adversely affected, compounded by frustration and embarrassment. If dry mouth continues for a prolonged period, dental erosion and dental decay (caries) are increasingly likely.

Causes

Dryness of the mouth may be caused by:

- diminished secretion of saliva

- diseased buccal mucosa

- excessive evaporation of fluid from the mouth (Box 3.A).

Box 3.A   Causes of dry mouth in advanced cancer

Cancer
Erosion of buccal mucosa
Replacement of salivary
  glands by cancer
Hypercalcaemia
  ($\rightarrow$ dehydration)

Debility
Anxiety
Depression
Mouth breathing
Dehydration
Infection

Treatment
Local radiotherapy ⎫
Local radical surgery ⎬ affecting salivary glands
Stomatitis associated ⎭
  with neutropenia
Drugs
  antimuscarinics
  opioids
  diuretics
Oxygen without humidification

Concurrent
Uncontrolled diabetes mellitus
  ($\rightarrow$ dehydration)
Hypothyroidism
Auto-immune disease
Amyloid
Sarcoid

Management

Correct the correctable

- review the drug regimen and reduce the dose of antimuscarinic drugs if possible

- substitute a drug with less or no antimuscarinic effects, e.g. an SSRI instead of amitriptyline, and haloperidol instead of prochlorperazine or chlorpromazine
- treat oral candidiasis (*see* p.79).

Non-drug treatment

Encourage the patient to take frequent sips of water, preferably ice-cold, or mineral water. Mix carbonated with plain in equal parts to maintain freshness but decrease excessive gas content, or according to personal preference.

Mouth care

Debride the tongue if furred with, for example:

- a soft toothbrush and cider and soda water in equal parts *or*
- a soft toothbrush and hydrogen peroxide 6% *or*
- one quarter of 1g effervescent ascorbic acid placed on the tongue.

Offer a mouthwash q2h. Effervescent mouthwash tablets (dissolve in 100ml of water) contain peppermint oil, clove oil, spearmint, menthol, thymol and methylsalicylic acid and make a palatable and refreshing mouthwash. Glycerine and thymol tablets are *not* recommended because glycerine produces a rebound drying of the mouth. A small amount (e.g. 0.5ml) of butter, margarine or vegetable oil swished around the mouth with the tongue t.d.s and o.n. may be helpful.[3]

Pineapple chunks can be helpful. They contain ananase, a proteolytic enzyme, which cleans the mouth if sucked like a sweet. Fresh pineapple contains more ananase than tinned pineapple but either can be used.

In moribund patients the mouth should be moistened every 30min with water from a water spray, dropper or sponge stick or ice chips placed in the mouth. In addition:

- smear white soft paraffin ointment (petroleum jelly) on the lips q4h to prevent cracking
- use a room humidifier or air-conditioning when the weather is dry and hot.

Stimulate salivary flow

Solids and acids in the mouth act as salivary stimulants, for example:

- ice chips
- chewing gum

- acid drops, lemon drops, boiled sweets, strong candy
- sips of cold and/or carbonated lemon drinks
- sips of 2% citric acid solution.

Artificial saliva

Artificial saliva can be used p.r.n. Several proprietary artificial salivas are available in the UK including:

- pastilles containing acacia, malic acid etc. (Salivix)
- tablets containing fruit acids, calcium salts and sorbitol (SST)
- porcine gastric mucin spray and lozenges (Saliva Orthana)
- carmellose-based sprays (Glandosane, Luborant, Salivace)
- hydroxyethylcellulose-based gel (Oralbalance); contains salivary peroxidase which enhances the production of hypothiocyanite, an antibacterial ion.

Alternatively, a locally-produced preparation comprising methylcellulose 10g and lemon essence 0.2ml in 1L of water can be used.

Drug treatment

Pilocarpine is a parasympathomimetic agent (predominantly muscarinic) with mild β-adrenergic activity which stimulates secretion from exocrine glands, including radiation-damaged salivary glands.[4] Pilocarpine also increases the concentration of mucins in saliva; these protect the oral mucosa from trauma and dryness.

About 50% of patients with dry mouth are helped by pilocarpine. Start with 5mg t.d.s. and increase if necessary to 10mg t.d.s. *Bowel obstruction, asthma and COPD are contra-indications to its use.* The most common adverse effect is sweating; others include nausea, flushing, urinary frequency, intestinal colic and weakness. Pilocarpine is rarely prescribed by the authors.

Drooling

Drooling is a term used to describe the leakage of saliva from the mouth.[5] Although drooling most commonly occurs with a normal production of saliva, sialorrhoea (excessive saliva) is sometimes a causal factor.

Causes

Most cases of drooling are associated with neuromuscular dysfunction (Box 3.B). The incidence in motor neurone disease is about 40%.[6] Apart from cancers of the head and neck, it is uncommon in advanced cancer.

Box 3.B Causes of drooling

Oral factors
Ill-fitting dentures
Oral cancer ± surgery → deformity
Dysphagia, e.g. cancer of the larynx or oesophagus
Episodic salivation associated with gastro-oesophageal reflux[7]
Idiopathic paroxysmal sialorrhoea[8]

Psychiatric[9]
Psychosis
Depression

Neurological disorders
Motor neurone disease
Cancer of the pharynx
Cancer involving the base of the skull
Cerebrovascular accident
Parkinson's disease
Cerebral palsy

Drugs
Cholinesterase inhibitors
Cholinergic agents
Lithium

Management

Correct the correctable

There is generally little which can be done to correct the causes of drooling in advanced disease. Modification of dentures may help.

Non-drug treatment

Head positioning ± suctioning may help. Irradiating the salivary glands with 4–10Gy also corrects the problem but is rarely indicated in palliative care.

Drug treatment

Prescribe an antimuscarinic drug:

- propantheline
- tricyclic antidepressant

- phenothiazine
- belladonna alkaloid, i.e. hyoscine or atropine
- glycopyrrolate.

The sensitivity of the muscarinic receptors in salivary glands is such that inhibition of salivation occurs with lower doses of antimuscarinic drugs than is needed for other antimuscarinic effects.[10] This reduces the likelihood of adverse effects.

Hyoscine *hydrobromide* is a tertiary amine and readily crosses biological membranes. It is effective orally as well as transdermally, and a local effect on the salivary glands has been postulated.[11–14] It is available as SL tablets 300µg and TD patches which release about 1mg of hyoscine over 72h, i.e. some 300µg/24h compared with 1.2–2.4mg/24h by CSCI for 'death rattle'. Adverse effects with these patches are uncommon, although some have been reported, notably confusion.[15–17]

Hyoscine hydrobromide has also been given by nebulizer, 200–800µg q.d.s.[18,19] The rationale for this is unclear and it is not recommended.

Glycopyrrolate is a highly ionized quaternary ammonium compound and penetrates biological membranes slowly and erratically.[20] In consequence it is unlikely to cause central effects such as confusion.[21,22] Enteral absorption is also poor but 200–400µg PO t.d.s. produces detectable plasma concentrations associated with an antisialogogic effect lasting ≤8h.[23–25] In addition to injections, glycopyrrolate is available as tablets and as a liquid, both of which can be administered via a percutaneous gastrostomy.[26]

Stomatitis

Stomatitis is a general term applied to diffuse inflammatory, erosive and ulcerative conditions affecting the mucous membranes lining the mouth (synonym: sore mouth). Aphthous ulcers are small, round or ovoid ulcers with a definite margin, an erythematous halo and a yellow or grey floor.

Causes

Stomatitis is caused by dry mouth, superadded infection, mucositis and various deficiency states (Box 3.C). There may be a genetic component to aphthous ulcers but stress, haematinic deficiency, neutropenia and immunosuppression may all be precipitants.

Box 3.C   Causes of stomatitis

Dry mouth (see p.70)

Drugs
Corticosteroids ⎫
                ⎬ candidiasis
Antibiotics   ⎭

Infection (associated with altered immunity)
Candidiasis
Aphthous ulcers

Mucositis
Local radiotherapy
Chemotherapy

Malnutrition
Hypovitaminosis
Anaemia
Protein deficiency

Evaluation

Generally there will be an obvious cause of diffuse stomatitis. Because the natural history differs, it is useful to differentiate between:

- minor aphthous ulcers (80% of all aphthae) are less than 5mm in diameter and heal in 7–14 days
- major aphthous ulcers are large ulcers that heal slowly over weeks or months with scarring
- herpetiform ulcers are multiple pinpoint ulcers that heal within about a month.[27]

Management

Correct the correctable

- modify drug regimen, i.e. stop or reduce the dose of antimuscarinic drugs
- treat dry mouth (see p.71).

Non-drug treatment

The following help to reduce pain when ulcers are present:

- avoid spicy foods and acidic fruit juices or carbonated drinks
- drink through a straw to bypass the mouth
- avoid sharp foods such as crisps.

Drug treatment

- treat candidiasis (*see* p.79)

- treat aphthous ulcers, caused by auto-immunity and opportunistic infection, with tetracycline and a corticosteroid topically (Box 3.D)

- coating agents, e.g. carbenoxolone sodium (Bioral gel, Bioplex granules), the granules are dissolved 2g in 30–50ml of warm water and used q.d.s. as a mouthwash

- topical analgesics, e.g.
  choline salicylate oral gel 8.7% (Bonjela), 1–2cm q3h p.r.n.
  benzydamine oral rinse 0.15% (Difflam), a NSAID and a mild local anaesthetic, 15ml q1h p.r.n.; dilute if causes stinging[28]
  flurbiprofen lozenge, 8.75mg q4h p.r.n.
  diphenhydramine (Box 3.E)[29]

- local anaesthetics, e.g.
  lidocaine viscous 2%, applied before meals and as needed
  cocaine hydrochloride 2% solution 10ml (200mg) q4h p.r.n. (prepared extemporaneously); swish around the mouth for several minutes and then spit out (swallowing 200mg of cocaine could lead to agitation and hallucinations)

Box 3.D   Treatment of aphthous ulcers[30]

Antiseptic and antibiotic mouthwashes
Useful when ulcers affect a wide range of oral sites not accessible to covering pastes:

  chlorhexidine gluconate 0.2% mouthwash (Corsodyl); rinse the mouth with 10ml
    tetracycline suspension 250mg t.d.s. for 3 days; prepared by mixing the contents
    of a capsule with a small quantity of water; hold in the mouth for 3min and then
    spit out.

Corticosteroids
Corticosteroids are useful for recurrent attacks:

  hydrocortisone 2.5mg lozenges 1 q.d.s.; ulcers must be at sites where the lozenge
    can be left to dissolve, e.g. in the sulci

  triamcinolone 0.1% dental paste (Adcortyl in Orabase); apply a thin layer
    b.d.–q.d.s. for up to 5 days

  aerosols, when a more potent corticosteroid is needed for sites such as the soft
    palate and oropharynx

  corticosteroid mouthwashes, when ulcers are widespread.

- immunomodulator, e.g. thalidomide 100mg o.d.–b.d. for 10 days in resistant cases of mouth ulceration in HIV+ patients.

Thalidomide is not a licensed drug because, when taken in pregnancy, it causes severe congenital abnormalities (absent or shortened limbs). It also causes irreversible peripheral neuropathy. Its use is best restricted to specialist centres.

Box 3.E   The use of diphenhydramine hydrochloride for oral mucositis

Diphenhydramine is an antihistaminic drug with a topical analgesic effect (*not* readily available in the UK). It is generally given as a locally prepared compound mouthwash.[31]

Proprietary solutions of diphenhydramine contain alcohol 5–14%; *use solutions with a low alcohol content* to avoid causing additional discomfort.[32]

The simplest preparation is diphenhydramine hydrochloride (25mg/5ml) and magnesium hydroxide in equal parts, up to 30ml q2h.[33] Spread around the mouth with the tongue and then swallow or spit out.

Alternative formulations include:

diphenhydramine in kaopectate (equal parts of diphenhydramine elixir 12.5mg/ 5ml and kaopectate); the pectin in the kaopectate helps the diphenhydramine adhere to the mucosa

stomatitis cocktail, National Cancer Institute, USA (equal parts of lidocaine viscous 2%, diphenhydramine elixir 12.5mg/5ml and Maalox, a proprietary antacid). Spit out the mouthwash after 2min.

Oral candidiasis

About 40% of healthy adults carry yeasts in their mouths as commensals.[34] The density of yeasts is greater in those who smoke and/or wear dentures. The proportion of carriers is higher in terminally ill patients.[35,36]

Candida albicans is one of several species which can be isolated from the oral cavity and is responsible for most oral candidal infections. Some infections are caused by one of many other species, e.g. *C. glabrata, C. tropicalis, C. parapsilosis, C. krusei.*[37]

Clinical features

Oral candidiasis generally manifests as:

- white plaques on the mucosa (thin and discrete) and/or tongue (thick and confluent) *or*
- a smooth red painful tongue *or*
- angular stomatitis.

Causes

In advanced cancer, most cases are associated with:

- corticosteroids[38]
- bacterial antibiotics
- diabetes mellitus.

Management

Fungal antibiotics are used to treat oral candidiasis.

Topical agents

- nystatin q.d.s.–q4h
  suspension (100 000 units/ml) 1–5ml
  pastilles (100 000 units)
  popsicles (locally prepared) 5ml of nystatin suspension mixed with blackcurrant or other fruit juice concentrate and frozen in an ice tray with small rounded cups.

Most patients respond to a 10-day course but some need continuous treatment. Patients must remove their dentures before each dose and clean them before re-insertion. Failure to do this leads to treatment failure. At night dentures should be soaked in water containing nystatin 5ml or in dilute sodium hypochlorite solution (Milton).

Systemic agents

Generally these are more convenient than nystatin and obviate the need for denture removal at each administration. Even so, *it is important to remove and clean the underside of the dentures everyday to remove any adherent infected debris.* Any of the imidazole antibiotics can be used:

- ketoconazole 200mg tablet o.d. for 5 days; take after food to reduce gastric irritation. Most patients respond but 1/3 relapse and need retreatment; with a course of >10 days there is risk of liver damage[39]

- fluconazole 150mg capsule stat; response and relapse rates similar to ketoconazole but it is more expensive.[39] Immunosuppressed patients may need 100–200mg o.d. indefinitely; at some centres extended courses of 50mg o.d. are given for patients with a major risk factor (*see* p.79)

- miconazole 125mg/5ml gel q.d.s. is administered by teaspoon and the patient spreads it around the mouth with the tongue; the effect is mainly systemic. Tablets are also available; it is more expensive and less convenient than ketoconazole.

Ketoconazole has an inhibitory effect on cytochrome P450-mediated enzymes. This results in inhibition of adrenal steroid synthesis (corticosteroids, testosterone, oestrogens and progesterone) and of the metabolism of certain drugs. Miconazole and itraconazole have the same effect; fluconazole less so.

Abnormal taste

There are four basic tastes:

- sour (acid)
- bitter (urea)
- sweet (sucrose)
- salt.

About 50% of patients with advanced cancer experience a change in taste sensation. This is not related to primary site, other alimentary symptoms or prognosis. Taste alteration may be:

- a general reduction in sensitivity (hypogeusia, ageusia)
- a specific reduction or increase in sensitivity (dysgeusia), e.g. in relation to sweetness but not to other tastes.

Pathogenesis

The mechanisms underlying taste abnormalities in advanced cancer are largely speculative:

- paraneoplastic
    decreased sensitivity of taste buds
    decreased number of taste buds
- nutritional deficiencies
- drugs (Table 3.1).

Hypogeusia is generally made worse by poor hygiene and oral candidiasis. Older people have a reduced sense of smell which also decreases the enjoyment of food.

Table 3.1 Taste and drugs

Drug	Effect
Phenytoin	Decreases sensitivity
Insulin	Decreased sweet and salt sensitivity after prolonged use
Lidocaine	Decreased sweet and salt sensitivity
Benzocaine	Increased sour sensitivity
5-fluoro-uracil	Alteration in bitter and sour sensitivity
Doxorubicin ⎫ Flurazepam ⎬ Levodopa ⎭	Metallic taste
Lithium	Dairy products taste rancid; celery intolerable

Clinical features

Vague complaints that:

'Food does not taste right'

'Everything tastes like cotton wool'.

Specific complaints that:

'I can't take sweet things anymore'

'I've given up eating meat, it tastes so bitter'

'I find I have to add spoonfuls of sugar to everything'

'I have a metallic taste in my mouth'.

Management

Correct the correctable

Mouth care:

- discontinue causal drugs
- improve mouth care and dental hygiene
- treat oral candidiasis.

Non-drug treatment

The advice of a dietician should be obtained and an appropriate recipe book supplied. General advice includes:

- encourage tart foods, e.g. pickles, lemon juice, vinegar
- recommend food which leaves its own taste like fresh fruit, hard candy
- add or reduce sugar as appropriate
- reduce the urea content of diet by eating white meats, eggs, dairy products
- mask the bitter taste of food containing urea, e.g.
      add wine and beer to soups and sauces
      marinate chicken, fish, meat
      use more and stronger seasonings
      eat food cold or at room temperature
      drink more liquids.

Anorexia

Anorexia (poor appetite) is common in advanced cancer. Anorexia may be primary as in the cachexia-anorexia syndrome (see p.86) or secondary to one or more other conditions (Table 3.2).

Table 3.2   Causes of poor appetite in advanced cancer

Causes	Management possibilities
Unappetizing food	Choice of food by patient
Too much food provided	Small meals
Altered taste	Adjust diet to counter taste change
Dyspepsia	Antacid, antiflatulent, prokinetic drug
Nausea and vomiting	Anti-emetics
Early satiety Fatigue	'Small and often', snacks rather than meals
Gastric stasis	Prokinetic drug
Constipation	Laxatives
Sore mouth	Mouth care
Pain	Analgesics
Malodour	Treatment of malodour
Biochemical	
hypercalcaemia	Correction of hypercalcaemia (see p.218)
hyponatraemia	Demeclocycline 300mg b.d.–q.d.s. if caused by SIADH (see p.224)
uraemia	Anti-emetic
Secondary to treatment	
drugs	Modify drug regimen
radiotherapy chemotherapy	Anti-emetics
Disease process	Appetite stimulant
Anxiety	Anxiolytic
Depression	Antidepressant

Although anorexia and early satiety are often linked, early satiety can also occur without concomitant anorexia ('I look forward to my meals but, then, after a few mouthfuls I feel full up and can't eat any more'). Early satiety without anorexia is associated with various conditions, including:

- a small stomach (postgastrectomy)
- hepatomegaly
- gross ascites.

Management

Non-drug treatment

Whose problem is it? The patient's or the family's?

Helping the patient and family accept and adjust to the reduced appetite is often the focus of management:

- listen to the family's fears
- explain to the family that
    in the circumstances it is normal to be satisfied with less food
    they can assist a fickle appetite by providing food when the patient is hungry (a microwave oven helps with this)
- a small helping looks better on a smaller plate
- offer specific dietary advice, particularly with early satiety
- discourage the 'he must eat or he will die' syndrome by emphasizing that a balanced diet is unnecessary at this stage in the illness
    'Just give him a little of what he fancies'
    'I shall be happy even if he just takes fluids'
- recognize the 'food as love' and 'feeding him is my job' syndromes and use them as an opportunity to discuss the progressive impact of the illness with the spouse/partner
- remember that eating is a social habit; people generally eat better at a table and when dressed.

Drug treatment

Appetite stimulants are appropriate in only a minority of anorexic patients. If used, they should be closely monitored and stopped if no benefit is perceived after 1–2 weeks:

- corticosteroid, e.g. prednisolone 15–30mg o.m. or dexamethasone 2–4mg o.m.; useful in about 50% of patients but the effect generally lasts for only a few weeks[40–42]
- progestogen, e.g. megesterol 160–800mg o.m.; the effect may last for months and generally is associated with weight gain.[43–45]

Appetite stimulants are contra-indicated for early satiety without concomitant anorexia.

Dehydration

Terminally ill patients often lose interest in food as they physically deteriorate. Moribund patients often lose interest in hydration as well but are not distressed provided the mouth is cleaned and moistened regularly.[46,47]

On the other hand, patients who develop acute dehydration, for example as a result of vomiting, diarrhoea or polyuria, experience distressing thirst and generally need parenteral rehydration.[48] However, some patients prefer not to have an infusion even in these circumstances and generally their disinclination should be respected. Remember: the aim is comfort, not a perfect fluid balance chart with normal electrolytes (Box 3.F).

Box 3.F   Parenteral hydration in palliative care

Indications

Generally all the following criteria should be met:

The patient is experiencing symptoms (e.g. thirst, malaise, delirium) for which dehydration is the most likely cause.

Increased oral intake not feasible.

Anticipation that parenteral hydration will relieve the symptoms (e.g. in patients with severe dysphagia, vomiting or diarrhoea).

The patient's general physical condition is relatively good (e.g. some patients with head and neck cancer).

The patient is willing to have parenteral hydration.

The patient and relatives understand that the purpose is to relieve symptoms and not to cure.

It is advisable initially to give a provisional time limit for parenteral hydration, e.g. 2–3 days, after which it will be discontinued if not helpful.

Contra-indications

The patient requests not to have an invasive procedure.

The burdens of parenteral hydration outweigh the likely benefits.

The patient is moribund for reasons other than dehydration.

If it is not in the patient's best interests, parenteral hydration should not be introduced simply to satisfy relatives who insist that something must be done.

For some patients, intermittent SC infusion (hypodermoclysis) is preferable to continuous IV infusion. Either 5% glucose-saline or 0.9% saline can be infused. Amounts vary between 500ml and 2L/24h, given over 3–12h through a 25 gauge needle.[49] Fluid can be administered by this route for several months in patients with, for example, head and neck cancer.

Hyaluronidase is sometimes added to the infusate.[49] This is unnecessary; it does not increase comfort or absorption.[50] In patients with delirium, improved hydration may lead to improved mentation, although not invariably.[51]

Cachexia

Cachexia (marked weight loss and muscle wasting) is often associated with anorexia as the cachexia-anorexia syndrome.

Pathogenesis

Cachexia occurs in over 50% of patients with advanced cancer.[52] The incidence is highest in gastro-intestinal and lung cancers. Unlike starvation where muscle mass is largely preserved, in cachexia there is a marked reduction in both muscle mass and body fat.[53,54] The loss of muscle relates to increased levels of proteolysis-inducing factor.[55]

Cachexia is not correlated with food intake or the stage of the tumour. It may antedate the clinical diagnosis and can occur with a small primary neoplasm.[56] The cachexia-anorexia syndrome is a paraneoplastic phenomenon which may be exacerbated by various factors (Box 3.G). Cytokine production suggests a chronic inflammatory component, which explains the beneficial effect of ibuprofen in some patients.[57,58]

Clinical features

The principal features of the cachexia-anorexia syndrome are:

- marked weight loss
- anorexia
- weakness
- fatigue.

Box 3.G   Causes of cachexia in advanced cancer

Paraneoplastic
Cytokines produced by host cells and
   tumour, e.g.
      tumour necrosis factor
      interleukin-6
      interleukin-1
Proteolysis-inducing factor → abnormal
   metabolism of
      protein
      carbohydrate
Altered fat metabolism
Increased metabolic rate → increased
   energy expenditure
Nitrogen trap by the tumour

Concurrent
Anorexia → deficient food intake
Vomiting
Diarrhoea
Malabsorption
Bowel obstruction
Debilitating effect of treatment
   surgery
   radiotherapy
   chemotherapy
Ulceration ⎫ excessive loss of body
Haemorrhage ⎭ protein

Associated physical features include:

- altered taste sensation

- loose dentures causing pain and difficulty with eating

- pallor (anaemia)

- oedema (hypo-albuminaemia)

- pressure sores.

Psychosocial ramifications extend to:

- ill-fitting clothes which increase the sense of loss and displacement

- altered appearance which engenders fear and isolation

- difficulties in social and family relationships.

Management

Non-drug treatment

Because of abnormal metabolism, aggressive dietary supplementation via a nasogastric tube or IV hyperalimentation is of minimal value in cachexia in advanced cancer.[59] Even so, dietary advice is important, particularly if there are associated changes in taste sensation. Some patients benefit psychologically from powdered or liquid nutritional supplements, and a few gain weight.[60]

Efforts should be directed towards ameliorating the social consequences and physical complications:

- do not weigh the patient routinely

- educate the patient and family about the risk of decubitus ulcers and the importance of skin care

- if affordable, buy new clothes to enhance self-esteem

- reline dentures to improve chewing and facial appearance; as a temporary measure, this can be done at the bedside and lasts about 3 months

- supply equipment to help maintain personal independence, e.g. raised toilet seat, commode, walking frame, wheelchair.

Drug treatment

Megestrol acetate, a progestogen may help.[61,62] However, it is expensive and should be used selectively. The optimum dose is 800mg o.d.[44] but, given the cost, it would be sensible to start with a lower dose, e.g. 160–320mg o.d.[45] The effect of progestogens may be enhanced by the concurrent use of ibuprofen 1200mg/day or other NSAID.[63]

Thalidomide, which inhibits tumour necrosis factor-α and other cytokines, stops weight loss in cachectic patients in a dose of 100–200mg o.n.[64] Eicosapentaenoic acid, present in oily fish, has been shown to protect muscle against proteolysis-inducing factor.[55,65] The use of both agents is developmental.

Dysphagia

Dysphagia (difficulty in swallowing) is the presenting symptom in most pharyngeal and oesophageal cancers. At some stage, dysphagia occurs in almost all patients with head and neck cancer. It is a feature of other cancers which spread to the mediastinum, neck, or base of the skull, e.g. lung cancer and lymphoma. Non-obstructive dysphagia associated with extreme weakness and/or cachexia is also common.

Physiology

Swallowing is a complex phenomenon, involving the brain stem, five cranial nerves, and 34 skeletal muscles.[66] It comprises four distinct phases, two voluntary and two reflexive:

- oral preparatory phase, food is mixed with saliva and chewed to reduce particle size
- oral swallowing phase, the lips are closed to prevent leakage and the anterior tongue retracts and elevates in a wave which pushes the bolus into the oropharynx
- pharyngeal phase, this is triggered by the bolus reaching the posterior tongue. The larynx closes, breathing stops, and a peristaltic wave moves the bolus into the oesophagus in less than 1 second. These complex actions are necessary to protect the airway because the pharynx is a shared passage for air and food
- oesophageal phase, reflex peristalsis carries the bolus into the stomach.

Causes

There are many causes of dysphagia in advanced cancer (Box 3.H). Two basic processes are involved:

- mechanical obstruction
- neuromuscular defects.

Dysphagia with severe odynophagia (painful swallowing) is occasionally caused by oesophageal spasm provoked by oesophagitis, e.g. radiation-induced or acid reflux.[67]

Evaluation

With organic obstruction, patients almost always can identify the site of the problem.[66] The patient's description and personal observation by the physician or nurse provide additional information (Table 3.3):

- distinguish between dysphagia and odynophagia (painful swallowing)
- obstructing lesions cause dysphagia for solids initially with later progression to liquids
- neuromuscular disorders cause dysphagia for both solids and liquids about the same time.[68]

Box 3.H   Causes of dysphagia in advanced cancer

Cancer
Mass lesion in mouth, pharynx or oesophagus
Infiltration of pharyngo-oesophageal wall
  → damage to nerve plexus
External compression (mediastinal mass)
Perineural tumour spread (vagus and
  sympathetic)
Tumour spread across base of skull
  → cranial nerve palsies
Metastases in base of skull
  → cranial nerve palsies
Leptomeningeal infiltration
  → cranial nerve palsies
Cerebral metastatic disease
  → bulbar palsy
Paraneoplastic

Debility
Dry mouth
Pharyngo-oesophageal candidiasis
Pharyngeal bacterial infection
Anxiety → oesophageal spasm
Drowsiness and disinterest
Extreme weakness (patient moribund)
Hypercalcaemia (rare)

Treatment
Surgery
  lingual
  buccal
Postradiation fibrosis
  difficulty in opening mouth and
    moving tongue
  prolonged oesophageal transit
  oesphageal stricture
Displacement of
  endo-oesophageal tube
Drugs (dystonic reaction)
  neuroleptics
  metoclopramide

Concurrent
Reflux oesophagitis
Benign stricture
Iron deficiency

Management

Correct the correctable

Possible ways of maintaining the lumen include:

* trial of corticosteroids[69]

* intermittent bouginage with blunt-tipped bougie (rarely used in UK)

* endoscopic dilation, benefits >50% of patients but often for only 1–2 weeks

* radiotherapy (teletherapy or brachytherapy), benefits >50% of patients for a median of 4 months

Table 3.3   Evaluation of dysphagia[68]

Information provided	Possible interpretation
Leakage from mouth, drooling	Poor lip closure, reduced lip sensation, abnormal tongue movement or reduced/absent swallowing reflex
Bites cheeks or tongue	Reduced lip or tongue sensation
Frequent nasal regurgitation	Palatal dysfunction
Food collecting	
in mouth	Poor lip, buccal or tongue control
in vallecula/pyriform fossae	Reduced/absent swallowing reflex
Patient washes food down with a drink or pushes food in with finger	Reduced tongue control
Patient tilts head down during swallowing	Delayed swallowing reflex or poor laryngeal closure
Difficulty with solids	
in triggering swallowing	Poor tongue control
food sticks	Obstruction
Lack of awareness where food is during swallowing	Sensory loss
Difficulty with liquids	Poor tongue control, reduced/absent swallowing reflex, muscular incoordination, soft palate, paralysis or fixation, severe obstruction
Coughing, choking	Aspiration due to
before swallowing	poor tongue control or delayed or absent swallowing reflex
during swallowing	reduced airway protection
after swallowing	reduced pharyngeal emptying, reduced laryngeal elevation, cricopharyngeus dysfunction, pharyngeal or oesophageal obstruction or tracheo-oesophageal fistula
Voice changes	
inability to say 'pa'	Poor lip closure
inability to say 'ka'	Poor movement of posterior tongue
'gargle' type voice	Aspiration
'hot potato' voice	Vallecular tumours
'breathy' voice/hoarseness	Recurrent laryngeal nerve palsy

- LASER treatment[70]
- intubation (see p.95).[71]

Endoscopic LASER therapy produces better relief of dysphagia than intubation.[70,72,73] Several treatments are generally required – more so with prograde resections. In about 1/4 of the patients, restoration of the lumen does not result in an adequate oral intake.[70]

Alcohol injection of the malignant obstructions produces similar results to LASER therapy and is an alternative when LASER therapy is not available.[70,74,75]

Non-drug treatment

Seek agreement between the patient, family and staff about feeding goals and treatment plans; this stems from an adequate explanation of what can and cannot be done or expected. Specific dietary advice should be given:

- maximize calorie intake in small volume meals, e.g.
    adding cream to soup etc.
    eating cold sour cream by the spoonful
- recommend suitable soft food cookbooks
- use liquidizer/blender
- offer general advice about mealtimes (Box 3.I).

Many speech therapists have an interest in neuromuscular dysphagia and will offer advice about swallowing techniques and communication. For example:

- if necessary, stabilize the head with pillows/cushions so that the chin tilts slightly down towards the chest; aspiration is often prevented in this position because the trachea is more likely to be closed when swallowing[76]
- liquids may be harder for a patient to swallow than soft solids
- because the oropharynx may continue to function relatively normally even when the lips and tongue are significantly affected, small amounts of food placed carefully with a spoon towards the back of the mouth may be swallowed more easily
- neostigmine 15mg PO 30–45min before meals may temporarily improve swallowing (not used by the authors).

Box 3.1 Helpful hints to aid feeding in patients with dysphagia (adapted from Speech and Language Therapy, Frenchay Hospital, Bristol, UK)

Posture
Make sure that you are sitting comfortably, head upright.

Relax
Ensure you are in a calm frame of mind before eating or drinking.

Do not talk
Be quiet before and while you eat and drink.

Yawn
Before the meal, if your throat feels tight, try to yawn to ease the constriction.

Feeding routine
Small amount → close lips → chew → pause → purposeful swallow → pause.

Texture
Try to avoid mixing fluids and solids.

Take time
Do not hurry. Always stop eating if you feel tired. Have small regular meals, not one large one.

After the meal
Drink a small amount of water to rinse your mouth out, also cough to make sure throat is clear.

Sit
Remain sitting for at least half an hour after eating or drinking.

Feeding tubes

Sometimes artificial nutrition is necessary and appropriate:

- endo-oesophageal intubation (*see below*)

- Clinifeed enteric tube; transnasal placement by a doctor on the ward is possible if the oesophageal lumen >1cm

- a feeding gastrostomy.[77]

A Clinifeed enteric tube or a feeding gastrostomy is generally contra-indicated in advanced cancers. The question arises more in patients with neurological disorders, e.g. poststroke and motor neurone disease (Figure 3.1).[78]

Patients with MND frequently do not want their dying prolonged by artificial feeding and are relieved when a doctor sensitively confirms that they will not be forced to have a nasogastric tube or gastrostomy. A few, generally those with dysphagia and dysarthria but little limb disability, request and benefit from artificial feeding.[79]

Much depends on both the speed of deterioration and the opinion of the patient and family, together with those of the professional carers. If in doubt, it is better to delay several days, or even weeks, before deciding to go ahead. It is easier not to start a treatment than to stop it. Ethical and practical guidelines on artificial nutrition in terminal cancer patients are available.[80–82]

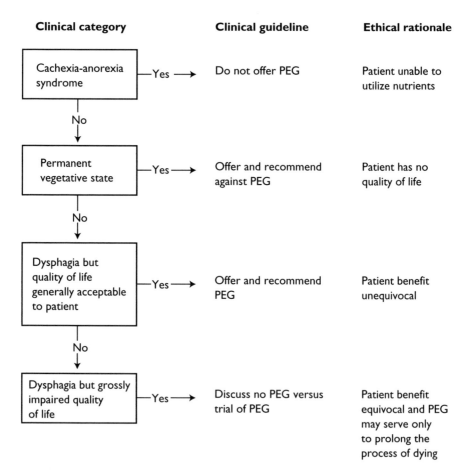

Figure 3.1   Decision-making algorithm for percutaneous endoscopic gastrostomy (PEG) tube placement.[78]

Drug treatment

Dysphagia and odynophagia caused by oesophagitis and oesophageal spasm has been treated successfully with glyceryl trinitrate 400μg SL 15min a.c.[67] If total obstruction leads to drooling, prescribe an antisecretory drug (*see* p.74).

Endo-oesophageal intubation

An indwelling flexible endo-oesophageal tube (e.g. Celestin) or an expandable stent[83] can be used to maintain a passage for fluid and food through a narrowed portion of the oesophagus or gastro-oesophageal junction. Expandable metal stents are 20–30 times more expensive and functional superiority is unproven.[84] However, they have been used success-fully in patients with a tracheo-oesophageal fistula.[85]

The upper end of a flexible tube is wider than the rest of the tube. This impedes downwards displacement and acts as a funnel for ingested food. The tube is introduced by a surgeon through an upper abdominal incision or via a fibre-optic gastroscope. Radiotherapy does not affect the tube.

Indications for use

- marked dysphagia for semisolids including liquidized/blenderized foods
- patient relatively independent and active.

An endo-oesophageal tube is *contra-indicated* in moribund patients.

Postoperative management

- elevate on 2–3 pillows to prevent reflux of gastric contents
- begin with a fluid diet but change after 1–2 days to a semisolid one
- confirm the position of the tube with a Gastrografin swallow after 3–4 days
- introduce solids after 5–7 days; the patient must chew food twice as long as normal (Box 3.J)

Box 3.J   Dietary recommendations for patients with an endo-oesophageal tube

Protein-rich food

Eat	Avoid
Tender meat in gravy	Tough or dry meats
Flaked fish in sauce	Any fish with bones or without sauce
Grated cheese/cheese in sauce	Lumps of hard cheese
Soft cheese – cottage/cream	Fried or hard boiled eggs
Soft boiled and scrambled eggs	
Milk – full cream, evaporated/condensed	

Fruit and vegetables

Include	Exclude
Fruit juices	Dried fruit, e.g. raisins, sultanas etc.
Peeled soft or stewed fruits (no pips)	Nuts
Puréed tinned fruit	Raw vegetables or salads, e.g. lettuce, tomato
Yoghurts/mousses	Stringy vegetables, e.g. beans, sweetcorn, peas, cauliflower stalks, cabbage stalks
Soft well-cooked mashed vegetables	Fibrous or pithy fruits, e.g. grapefruit, orange, pineapple, grapes
	Fruit skins/pips, e.g. damson jam, peach, pear or apple skin

Starches

Eat	Avoid
Potato, mashed with butter	Chips or roast potatoes
Boiled white rice or spaghetti	Potato crisps/snacks
Tinned spaghetti, macaroni, milk puddings	Wholegrain rice
Day-old wholemeal bread with plenty of butter/margarine	Granary bread
Soft crumbly biscuits, e.g. digestive, shortbread, chocolate-coated biscuits	French sticks, new white bread or bread crusts
Semisolid smooth breakfast cereals, e.g. porridge, Ready Brek, All Bran, Weetabix	Hard flaky biscuits, e.g. water biscuits
	Doughy cakes and fruit cake
	Puff pastry and Danish pastry
	Muesli, nutty cereals
	Shredded Wheat

- avoid the following completely
    fish, bony or without sauce
    hard boiled eggs
    oranges and other pithy fruit

- sips of a carbonated drink are taken frequently during and after every meal; but less so in patients with a small stomach capacity.

The tube rarely gets blocked if advice is carefully followed by the patient (Box 3.K).

Box 3.K   General advice to patients with an endo-oesophageal tube

A plastic tube has been put into your food pipe to help you eat and drink more easily.

Because this has an internal opening about the size of your index finger, you need to be careful with what you swallow; hard or lumpy food may block the tube.

Never take tablets unless crushed or dissolved.

Take small mouthfuls of food and chew well.

Always sip a fizzy/carbonated drink with your meal.

Eat 'little and often', e.g. 6 snacks rather than 2–3 big meals.

Food should never be eaten dry; lubricate with butter, margarine, milk, ice cream, gravy, sauce etc.

Don't use baby foods; they are designed for a baby and are low in protein and calories.

Drink more nourishing fluid and less tea, coffee, squash, water.

Continue to drink alcohol in moderation; preferably adding a fizzy/carbonated mixer to your favourite tipple and sip it with your meals, e.g. gin and tonic, beer shandy, Bucks Fizz.

If your tube becomes blocked, try:

    sipping a fizzy drink
    jumping
    standing up
    sipping another drink.

If this doesn't work, contact your doctor for further advice and help.

Although a blocked tube is distressing, it is not a serious medical problem.

Heartburn

Heartburn is a burning retrosternal discomfort which is generally caused by the reflux of acidic gastric contents into the oesophagus. Heartburn is associated with:

- regurgitation of stomach acid or bile salts
- painful swallowing
- transient dysphagia for solid foods only
- water brash (episodic hypersalivation)[7]
- intermittent cough or wheezing
- weakness secondary to anaemia caused by bleeding from oesophageal ulceration.

Pathogenesis

The distal 5cm of the oesophagus is a high pressure zone (normally 10–12mmHg) which prevents reflux. This lower oesophageal sphincter relaxes with swallowing and its tone increases when the stomach is filled. Reflux occurs when the lower oesophageal sphincter becomes dysfunctional (Box 3.L).

Many drugs have an adverse effect on lower oesophageal sphincter tone (Box 3.L). The onset of heartburn within 1–2 days of commencing a new drug should alert the doctor to this possibility. The use of morphine and other opioids can cause reflux secondary to delayed gastric emptying.

Management

Correct the correctable

- stop or reduce the dose of causal drugs if possible
- change to a drug with less or no antimuscarinic effects, e.g. an SSRI instead of a tricyclic antidepressant
- modify diet (Box 3.L)
- stop smoking
- abdominal paracentesis if marked ascites present
- weight reduction if obese (generally not applicable in advanced cancer).

Box 3.L Factors which decrease the competence of the lower oesophageal sphincter

Dietary	**Drugs**
Alcohol	Nicotine
Chocolate	Antimuscarinics
Fat	Benzodiazepines
Carminatives	Calcium-channel blockers
mint, anise, dill	Nitrates and nitrites
Carbonated beverages	Oestrogens
Aerophagic habits	Pethidine/meperidine
chewing gum	Theophylline
sucking hard candy	
Very big meals	

Mechanical
Constricting abdominal garments
Obesity
Ascites
Lying flat

Non-drug treatment

- avoid constricting garments and lying flat after meals

- elevate the head of the bed by 10cm.

Drug treatment

- occasional heartburn responds to antacids p.r.n.

- prescribe a prokinetic to increase lower oesophageal pressure, e.g. metoclopramide

- reduce gastric acid by prescribing an H_2-receptor antagonist or a PPI.

For severe heartburn, a PPI and a prokinetic may both be needed.

Dyspepsia

Dyspepsia is discomfort or pain in the upper abdomen, particularly after meals, generally related to a functional or an organic disorder of the stomach or duodenum (synonym: indigestion).

Pathogenesis

There are many causes of dyspepsia (Box 3.M). From a therapeutic perspective in advanced cancer, dyspepsia can be divided into four categories:

- small stomach capacity
- gassy
- acid
- dysmotility.

Box 3.M   Causes of dyspepsia in advanced cancer

Cancer
Small stomach capacity
  large unresected stomach cancer
  massive ascites
Gatroparesis (paraneoplastic
  visceral neuropathy)

Treatment
Postsurgical
  postgastrectomy
  reflux oesophagitis
Radiotherapy
  lumbar spine
  epigastrium
Drugs
  physical irritant → gastritis, e.g.
    iron, tranexamic acid
  acid stimulant → gastritis, e.g.
    NSAIDs, corticosteroids
  delayed gastric emptying, e.g.
    antimuscarinics, opioids, cisplatin

Debility
Oesophageal candidiasis
Minimal food and fluid intake
Anxiety → aerophagia

Concurrent
Organic dyspepsia
  peptic ulcer
  reflux oesophagitis
  cholelithiasis
  renal failure
Non-ulcer dyspepsia
  dysmotility
  aerophagia

Functional dyspepsia (dyspepsia without apparent organic cause) is generally caused by dysmotility. It is seen in about 25% of the general population and therefore is common in patients with cancer.

Many cases of 'squashed stomach syndrome'[86] and 'cancer-associated dyspepsia syndrome'[87] are probably cases of functional dyspepsia and/or gastric stasis (see p.102) exacerbated by:

- hepatomegaly
- gross ascites.

Evaluation

It is important to differentiate between the four types of dyspepsia because the treatment differs. Careful history taking generally indicates which type is predominant. Patients with dysmotility may also have symptoms or a history of irritable bowel syndrome.

Management

Small stomach capacity

If dyspepsia is associated with a small stomach capacity, patients should be advised to separate their main fluid from their solid intake, and to eat 'small and often', i.e. take 5–6 small meals/snacks during the day rather than 2–3 big meals.

Patients with a small stomach capacity may benefit from an antiflatulent after meals, to help clear space in an overfull stomach (see below).

Gassy dyspepsia

Prescribe an antiflatulent, e.g. dimeticone. This is available on its own but may conveniently be given in the form of Asilone, a proprietary antacid. Depending on a patient's individual needs, this can be given p.r.n., q.d.s., or both.

Acid dyspepsia

Prescribe an antacid, an H_2-receptor antagonist (e.g. cimetidine, ranitidine) or a PPI (e.g. lansoprazole, omeprazole). A PPI should also be used in cases of NSAID-related gastritis.[87–89]

Dysmotility dyspepsia

This is not helped by gastric acid reduction. Prescribe metoclopramide to normalize disordered gastric motility.

Gastric stasis

Gastric stasis (delayed gastric emptying) is common in advanced cancer. It accounts for about 25% of cases of nausea and vomiting.[90]

Clinical features

The clinical features of gastric stasis range from mild dyspepsia and anorexia to persistent severe nausea and large-volume vomiting (Box 3.N). Gastric stasis is normally functional and is associated with one or more of the following conditions:

- dysmotility dyspepsia (often longstanding)
- constipation[91]
- drugs (opioids, antimuscarinics, aluminium hydroxide, levodopa)
- cancer of the head of the pancreas (disrupts duodenal transit)[92]
- paraneoplastic autonomic neuropathy
- retroperitoneal disease (→ nerve dysfunction)
- spinal cord compression
- diabetic autonomic neuropathy.

Management

Management comprises explanation and the use of a prokinetic drug, e.g. metoclopramide (Figure 3.2). As a general rule, *prokinetic and antimuscarinic drugs should not be prescribed concurrently*. Antimuscarinic drugs block cholinergic receptors on intestinal muscle fibres,[93] and thereby competitively block the effect of prokinetic drugs. However, domperidone and metoclopramide will still exert an antagonistic effect at the dopamine-type 2 receptors in the chemoreceptor trigger zone (area postrema) in the brain stem.

Metoclopramide, with its dual mode of action, is generally preferable; it is available both in oral formulations and injections. However, because it does not cross the blood-brain barrier, domperidone should be used in patients with parkinsonism in whom central dopamine type-2 receptor antagonism is likely to be detrimental.

Box 3.N   Clinical features of gastric stasis

Symptoms

Early satiety	Belching
Postprandial fullness	Hiccup
Epigastric bloating	Nausea
Epigastric discomfort	Retching
Heartburn	Vomiting

Signs

Epigastric distension ⎫
Succussion splash   ⎬ not invariable

A succussion splash requires >400–500ml of fluid in the stomach and plenty of gas.

Bowel sounds, generally normal but may be decreased if the stasis is drug-induced.

If associated with autonomic neuropathy, there is often evidence of other autonomic abnormalities, e.g. orthostatic hypotension without a compensatory tachycardia.

Drug treatment
The use of metoclopramide generally leads to improvement and the resolution of the succussion splash.

Gastric outflow obstruction

Gastric stasis is occasionally associated with an organic obstruction:

- cancer of the gastric antrum

- external compression of the gastric antrum or duodenum by a tumour.

If severe, this causes major difficulties in management. Each case needs individual evaluation and treatment. In most cases, the obstruction is not complete. Even with no oral intake, the stomach needs to clear:

- swallowed saliva (normally 1500ml/24h)

- basal gastric juices (1500ml/24h).

Thus, if a patient is vomiting less than 2–3L/24h, something is getting past the obstruction.

An antimuscarinic drug with both antisecretory and antispasmodic properties should be prescribed, e.g. hyoscine *butylbromide* 80–120mg/24h by CSCI.

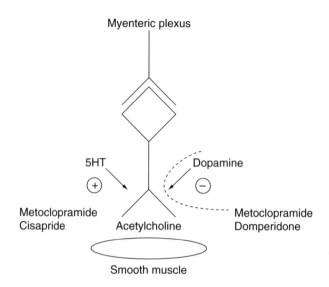

Myenteric plexus

5HT — Dopamine

Metoclopramide
Cisapride

Acetylcholine

Metoclopramide
Domperidone

Smooth muscle

Figure 3.2 Schematic representation of drug effects on antroduodenal coordination via a postganglionic effect on the cholinergic nerves from the myenteric plexus.

⊕ stimulatory effect of 5HT triggered by metoclopramide and cisapride; ⊖ inhibitory effect of dopamine; ---- blockade of dopamine inhibition by metoclopramide and domperidone. (The licence for cisapride has been suspended.)

This approximately halves gastric secretions and will also reduce salivary volume.[94] In countries where parenteral hyoscine *butylbromide* is not available, glycopyrrolate 600–1200µg/24h can be substituted. Somatostatin analogues which are antisecretory but not antispasmodic are used at some centres e.g. octreotide 300–600µg/24h. Their cost is a potentially limiting factor. A venting procedure is occasionally necessary, e.g. nasogastric tube or gastrostomy.

Nausea and vomiting

Nausea is an unpleasant feeling of the need to vomit, often accompanied by autonomic symptoms, e.g. pallor, cold sweat, salivation, tachycardia and diarrhoea.

Retching is rhythmic, laboured, spasmodic movements of the diaphragm and abdominal muscles, generally occurring in the presence of nausea and often culminating in vomiting.

Vomiting is the forceful expulsion of gastric contents through the mouth.

Neuro-anatomy

The area postrema is in the floor of the 4th ventricle in the brain stem (Figure 3.3).[96] It includes a functional entity called the chemoreceptor trigger zone. Because the area postrema lies outside the blood-brain barrier it is 'bathed' in the systemic circulation. Dopamine receptors in the area postrema are stimulated by high concentrations of emetogenic substances such as calcium ions, urea, morphine and digoxin. The area postrema also receives input from the vestibular apparatus and the vagus.

The nucleus tractus solitarius is the main central connection of the vagus and lies partly in the deeper layers of the area postrema (Figure 3.3).[96] It contains the greatest concentration of $5HT_3$-receptors in the brain stem. The emetic pattern generator is close to the area postrema but lies fully within the blood-brain barrier. It comprises a collection of motor nuclei, including the nucleus ambiguus, ventral and dorsal respiratory groups, and the dorsal motor nucleus of the vagus.

Vomiting is a complex reflex process involving coordinated activities of the gastro-intestinal tract, diaphragm and abdominal muscles. Nausea is an expression of autonomic stimulation; retching and vomiting are mediated via somatic nerves. Atony of the stomach, lower oesophageal sphincter and pylorus is associated with retroperistalsis. The expulsive effort of vomiting is produced by the primary and accessory muscles of respiration, notably the abdominal muscles. The emetic pattern generator (vomiting centre) coordinates the process, receiving and integrating input from several sources (Figure 3.4).[97]

Causes

Although there are many causes of nausea and vomiting in advanced cancer (Box 3.O), four account for most cases (Figure 3.5).[91] Although in physically fit people constipation rarely causes vomiting, in advanced cancer it is probably a common contributory factor, particularly if it has progressed to faecal impaction.

Evaluation

- clarify whether it is vomiting, and not just expectoration or regurgitation
- examine the abdomen
- do a rectal examination if faecal impaction is a possibility

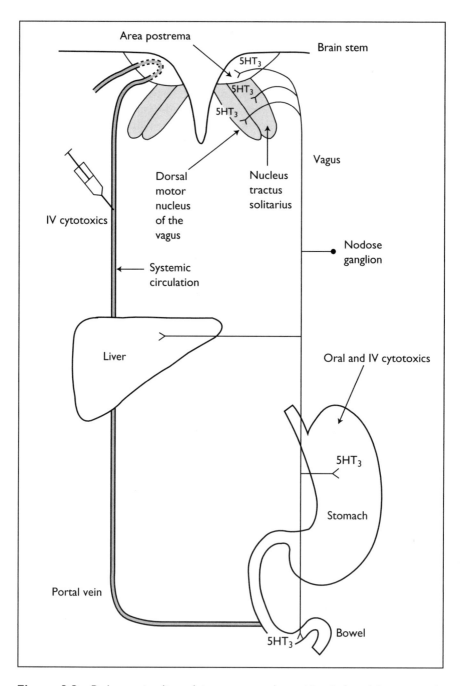

Figure 3.3 Pathways implicated in nausea and vomiting induced by cytotoxic drugs and the sites of action of 5HT$_3$-receptor antagonists. Modified from Barnes and Barnes, 1991.[96]

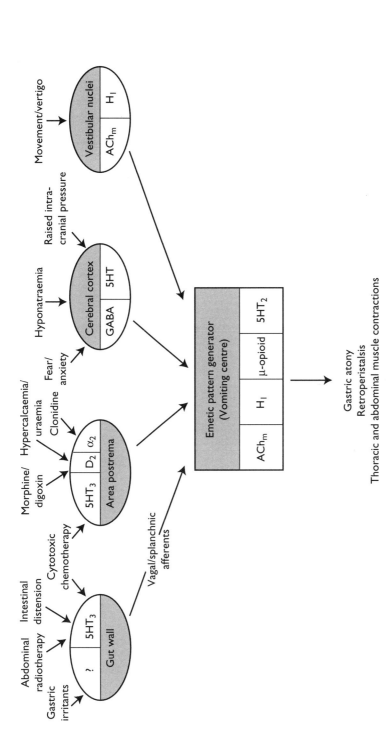

Figure 3.4   Diagram of the neural mechanisms controlling vomiting. Modified from Twycross et al., 1997.[97] Abbreviations refer to receptor types: Ach_m = muscarinic cholinergic; α_2 = α_2-adrenergic; D_2 = dopamine type 2; GABA = gamma-aminobutyric acid; 5HT, $5HT_2$, $5HT_3$ = 5-hydroxytryptamine (serotonin) type undefined, type 2, type 3; H_1 = histamine type 1. Anti-emetics act as antagonists at these receptors, whereas the central anti-emetic effects of clonidine and opioids are agonistic.

Box 3.0   Causes of nausea and vomiting in advanced cancer

Cancer
Gastroparesis (paraneoplastic
   visceral neuropathy)
Blood in stomach
Constipation
Faecal impaction
Bowel obstruction
Hepatomegaly
Gross ascites
Brain metastases
Raised intracranial pressure
Cough
Pain
Anxiety
Hypercalcaemia
Hyponatraemia
Renal failure

Debility
Constipation
Cough
Infection

Treatment
Radiotherapy
Chemotherapy
Drugs
   antibiotics
   aspirin
   carbamazepine
   corticosteroids
   digoxin
   iron
   irritant mucolytics
   lithium
   NSAIDs
   oestrogens
   opioids
   theophyllines

Concurrent
Functional dyspepsia
Peptic ulcer
Alcohol gastritis
Renal failure
Ketosis

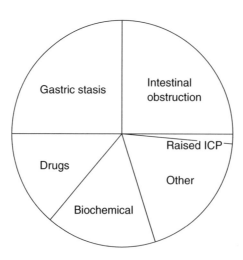

Figure 3.5   Common causes of nausea and vomiting in advanced cancer.[90]
ICP = intracranial pressure.

- if the cause is not apparent, examine the CNS for signs of brain metastases or raised intracranial pressure
- consider checking the plasma concentrations of
  creatinine
  calcium and albumin
  carbamazepine
  digoxin
- review the drug regimen; could a recently prescribed drug be the cause, e.g. NSAID or opioid?

Management

Correct the correctable

- cough → antitussive
- gastritis → reduction of gastric acid
  antacid
  H_2-receptor antagonist
  PPI
- consider stopping gastric irritant drugs
  antibiotic
  corticosteroid
  irritant mucolytic
  NSAID
- constipation → laxative
- raised intracranial pressure → corticosteroid
- hypercalcaemia → bisphosphonate (see p.219).

Non-drug treatment

- a calm environment away from the sight and smell of food, which can both be nauseating
- snacks, e.g. a few mouthfuls, and not big meals
- if the patient is the household cook, someone else may need to take on this role.

Drug treatment

Guidelines 3.1: Nausea and vomiting in palliative care (p.386).

On the basis of putative sites of action it is possible to derive anti-emetic drugs of choice for different situations (Table 3.4). The initial choice is often:

- metoclopramide (50%)
- haloperidol (25%).

Other commonly used drugs are:

- hyoscine *butylbromide* or glycopyrrolate
- cyclizine
- levomepromazine.

Table 3.4   Anti-emetic classification

Putative site of action	Class	Example
Central nervous system		
Emetic pattern generator (vomiting centre)	Antimuscarinic	Hyoscine hydrobromide
	Antihistaminic antimuscarinic	Cyclizine, dimenhydrinate, phenothiazines[a]
	5HT$_2$-receptor antagonist	Levomepromazine[b]
Area postrema (chemoreceptor trigger zone)	D$_2$-receptor antagonist	Haloperidol, phenothiazines, metoclopramide, domperidone
	5HT$_3$-receptor antagonist	Granisetron, ondansetron tropisetron
Cerebral cortex	Benzodiazepine	Lorazepam
	Cannabinoid	Nabilone
	Corticosteroid	Dexamethasone[c]
Gastro-intestinal tract		
Prokinetic	5HT$_4$-receptor agonist	Metoclopramide
	D$_2$-receptor antagonist	Metoclopramide, domperidone
Vagal 5HT$_3$-receptor	5HT$_3$-receptor antagonist	Granisetron, ondansetron tropisetron
Anti-inflammatory effect	Corticosteroid	Dexamethasone[c]

a the antihistaminic and antimuscarinic properties of phenothiazines vary
b levomepromazine is a phenothiazine with 5HT$_2$ antagonist properties; this makes it a potent anti-emetic; its main disadvantages are sedation and postural hypotension
c the mode of action of dexamethasone as an anti-emetic is still conjecture.

$5HT_3$-receptor antagonists are of particular benefit in situations where there is a massive release of serotonin (5HT) from enterochromaffin cells or platelets, e.g. chemotherapy, abdominal radiation, obstruction (distension), renal failure.

Dexamethasone is often used as an 'add-on' anti-emetic when all else fails. It is also widely used for chemotherapeutic vomiting and may help in intestinal obstruction.[98,99] Dexamethasone possibly acts by reducing the permeability of the chemoreceptor trigger zone and of the blood-brain barrier to emetogenic substances, and by reducing the neuronal content of gamma-aminobutyric acid (GABA) in the brain stem. In obstruction, dexamethasone will also help by reducing inflammation at the site of the block, thereby increasing the lumen.

Obstruction

The focus here is on patients for whom available anticancer treatments have been exhausted. Obstruction of the alimentary tract can occur at any level. It is useful to think in terms of four syndromes:

- oesophageal, commonly the gastro-oesophageal junction
- gastric outlet and proximal small bowel
- distal small bowel
- large bowel.

At each level, the obstruction can be functional (paralytic) or organic (mechanical), or both. It can also be:

- partial or complete
- transient (acute) or persistent (chronic).

Organic oesophageal obstruction, manifesting as dysphagia for solids first and liquids subsequently, is generally managed by palliative surgery (e.g. LASER therapy), insertion of an endo-oesophageal tube or palliative radiotherapy.

Gastric outlet and proximal small bowel obstruction share many clinical features, whereas the features of a distal ileal obstruction shade into those of a colonic obstruction. In advanced cancer, patients commonly have multiple sites of obstruction involving both small and large bowel.

Causes

Bowel obstruction in advanced cancer may be caused by one or more of the following:

- the cancer itself
- past treatment, e.g. adhesions, postradiation ischaemic fibrosis
- drugs, e.g. opioids, antimuscarinics
- debility, e.g. faecal impaction
- an unrelated benign condition, e.g. strangulated hernia.

Clinical features of intestinal obstruction

Abdominal pain associated with the underlying cancer is present in >90% of cases. Vomiting is invariable and intestinal colic is common.[100] Distension is variable and bowel habit ranges from absolute constipation to diarrhoea secondary to bacterial liquefaction of retained faeces. Bowel sounds vary from absent in functional obstructions to hyperactive and audible (borborygmi) in some organic obstructions. *Tinkling bowel sounds are uncommon.*

Surgical management

Surgical intervention is contra-indicated in each of the following circumstances:

- previous laparotomy findings preclude the prospect of a successful intervention
- diffuse intra-abdominal carcinomatosis as evidenced by diffuse palpable intra-abdominal tumours
- massive ascites which re-accumulates rapidly after paracentesis.[101]

Surgical intervention should be considered if the following criteria are all fulfilled:

- a single discrete organic obstruction seems likely, e.g. postoperative adhesions or an isolated neoplasm

- the patient's general condition is good, i.e. he does not have widely disseminated disease and has been independent and active

- the patient is willing to undergo surgery.

Medical management

In patients in whom an operative approach is contra-indicated, it is generally possible to relieve symptoms adequately with drugs. *A nasogastric tube and IV fluid are rarely necessary.*

Management focuses primarily on the relief of nausea and vomiting. For those without colic and who are still passing flatus, a prokinetic drug is the initial drug of choice. For patients with severe colic, prokinetic drugs are contra-indicated. Instead prescribe an antisecretory and antispasmodic drug, e.g. hyoscine butylbromide (*see* p.387).

Bulk-forming, osmotic and stimulant laxatives should also be stopped. A series of drug changes over several days may be necessary before optimum relief is achieved. For the constant background cancer pain, morphine or diamorphine should be given regularly. If the patient is receiving parenteral metoclopramide or hyoscine butylbromide, the opioid can also be given by CSCI.

A phosphate enema should be given if constipation is a probable contributory factor and a faecal softener prescribed, i.e. docusate sodium tablets 100–200mg b.d.

Corticosteroids benefit some patients with inoperable intestinal obstruction.[98] Because spontaneous resolution occurs in at least 1/3 of patients, it is important not to prescribe a corticosteroid too soon. Treat the symptoms as suggested above and then, after 7–10 days, if the obstruction has not settled, a trial of corticosteroid for 3 days should be considered, e.g.:

- dexamethasone 10mg SC

- methylprednisolone 40mg IV over 1h.[99]

If there is improvement, either continue with the corticosteroid at a lower dose PO or stop and review the need for long-term treatment.

Corticosteroids probably act by reducing local oedema and improving the patency of the bowel lumen. They may also reduce pressure on intestinal nerves, thereby correcting neural dysfunction (and the associated functional obstruction). These actions are distinct from the specific anti-emetic effect of corticosteroids.[102]

A persistent complete inoperable obstruction is a challenging prospect. Occasionally, two classes of drugs may be necessary, namely:

* somatostatin analogues, e.g. octreotide

* 5HT$_3$-receptor antagonists, e.g. granisetron, ondansetron, tropisetron.

Octreotide has an antisecretory effect throughout the alimentary tract. Despite its cost, it is the preferred antisecretory drug at some centres. Octreotide is generally given by CSCI; typical doses are 250–500µg/24h, occasionally more.

Maximum benefit is achieved more quickly with octreotide (24h), compared with hyoscine butylbromide (72h).[95] A reduction in intestinal contents reduces distension and thereby the likelihood of colic and vomiting. Some centres convert to the long-acting lanreotide which is given IM every 2 weeks; each injection costs over £300.

Generally, consider using octreotide when hyoscine butylbromide 200mg by CSCI fails to relieve the vomiting. However, it is not antispasmodic and if colic persists, it should be used concurrently with hyoscine butylbromide (or glycopyrrolate).

Because raised intraluminal pressure results in the release of 5HT (serotonin) from the enterochromaffin cells in the bowel wall, some patients benefit from a 5HT$_3$-receptor antagonist. *A venting gastrostomy is rarely necessary for symptom relief in advanced cancer.*[103]

Inoperable patients managed by drug therapy should be encouraged to drink and eat small amounts of their favourite beverages and food. Some patients find that they can manage food best in the morning.

Antimuscarinic drugs and diminished fluid intake often result in a dry mouth and thirst. These are generally relieved by conscientious mouth care. A few ml of fluid every 30min, possibly administered as a small ice cube, often brings relief. *IV hydration is rarely needed.*

Duodenum

Obstruction here is generally caused by cancer of the head of the pancreas. Most are functional and caused by disruption of duodenal peristalsis:

* try metoclopramide 60mg/24h by CSCI

- if beneficial, optimize the dose up to 100mg/24h; higher doses generally mean that the syringe will have to be changed q12h which may be impractical

- if the vomiting is made worse, it indicates mechanical obstruction; discontinue metoclopramide and prescribe an antihistaminic anti-emetic or hyoscine butylbromide instead (*see* p.113)

- if metoclopramide is of partial benefit, add dexamethasone 10–20mg PO/SC o.d. for 3 days; if improvement occurs it suggests that local tumour-induced inflammation was a causal factor

- if none of the above is of benefit, discuss the use of a nasogastric tube or a venting gastrostomy with the patient.

With a high bowel obstruction, it is generally not possible to stop vomiting completely; a practical goal is reducing the frequency to 2–3 times/24h.

Pylorus

Gastric cancer may obstruct the pylorus. If surgery is contra-indicated:

- prescribe an antisecretory drug, e.g. hyoscine butylbromide 60–120mg/24h or octreotide 250–500µg/24h by CSCI

- try dexamethasone 10–20mg SC o.d. for 3 days

- discuss the use of a nasogastric tube or a venting gastrostomy with the patient.

Constipation

Constipation (difficulty in defaecation) is common in advanced cancer. Diminished food and fibre intake, lack of exercise and drugs are all contributory (Box 3.P). Because of the patient's physical limitations and associated anorexia, laxatives are generally the mainstay of treatment.

Box 3.P   Causes of constipation in advanced cancer

Cancer
Hypercalcaemia
Paraneoplastic visceral neuropathy

Drugs
Opioids
NSAIDs
Antimuscarinics
   antihistaminic anti-emetics
   phenothiazines
   tricyclics
5HT$_3$-receptor antagonists

Vincristine
Diuretics
   dehydration
   hypokalaemia

Debility
Inactivity
Poor nutrition
   decreased intake
   low residue diet
Poor fluid intake
Dehydration
   vomiting
   polyuria
   fever
Weakness
Inability to reach toilet when
   there is an urge to defaecate

Management

General measures

- stop or reduce the dose of constipating drugs

- mobilize the patient if possible

- a prompt response to the patient's request for a commode or for help to get to the toilet

- use of a commode rather than a bedpan

- support the patient's feet on a foot stool to help brace the abdominal muscles

- raise the toilet seat and install hand rails in the patient's home to increase toilet independence.

Diet

- increase food intake

- add bran to diet

- increase fluid intake

- encourage fruit juices.

Drug treatment

Guidelines 3.2: Opioid-induced constipation (p.388).

Knowledge of the different classes of laxatives (Box 3.Q) and the composition of various preparations (Box 3.R) permits rational combinations to be used (Figures 3.6 and 3.7). Surface wetting agents are commonly called faecal softeners; osmotic laxatives act primarily on the small bowel ('small bowel laxatives'); contact laxatives generally act exclusively on the large bowel ('large bowel laxatives'). The best starting point varies from patient to patient. Sometimes it is appropriate to begin and continue with rectal measures or just to use a faecal softener, as in most patients with inoperable bowel obstruction.

About 90% of patients receiving morphine require a laxative.[104] Opioids induce constipation principally by enhancing intestinal ring contractions. This results in hypersegmentation, which impedes peristalsis. A contact (stimulant) laxative which *relaxes* ring contractions is the logical management option.

Box 3.Q Classification of laxatives

Bulk-forming drugs (fibre)
Ispaghula husk (e.g. Fybogel, Regulan)
Methylcellulose
Sterculia (e.g. Normacol)

Lubricants
Liquid paraffin/mineral oil

Surface-wetting agents
Docusate sodium
Poloxamer

Osmotic laxatives
Lactulose syrup
Macrogols (polyethylene glycols) 3350
Liquid paraffin and magnesium hydroxide emulsion BP
Magnesium hydroxide suspension (Milk of magnesia)
Magnesium sulphate (Epsom salts)

Contact (stimulant) laxatives
Bisacodyl
Dantron
Senna
Sodium picosulphate

Box 3.R Composition of laxatives (UK)

Bulk-forming drugs

Fybogel (sachet) ⎫
Regulan (sachet) ⎭   Ispaghula husk 3.4–6.4g

Normacol granules   Sterculia 6.2g/10g

Normacol plus granules   Sterculia 6.2g/10g + frangula 800mg/10g

Celevac tablet   Methylcellulose 500mg

Surface-wetting agents

Docusate sodium syrup 50mg/5ml[a]

Docusate sodium tablet 100mg[a]

Osmotic laxatives

Lactulose syrup 3.35g/5ml

Movicol sachet   Macrogols (polyethylene glycols) 3350

Liquid paraffin and magnesium   Magnesium hydroxide mixture BP
  hydroxide emulsion BP (10ml)   7.5ml + liquid paraffin 2.5ml

Milk of magnesia suspension (5ml)   Magnesium hydroxide 350mg

Epsom salts   crystals (5ml) ⎫
           solution (10ml) ⎭   Magnesium sulphate 4g

Contact (stimulant) laxatives

Standardized senna tablet 7.5mg

Bisacodyl tablet 5mg

Bisacodyl suppository 5mg, 10mg

Sodium picosulphate syrup 5mg/5ml

Co-danthrusate suspension (5ml)/capsule   Dantron 50mg + docusate sodium 60mg

Co-danthramer suspension (5ml)/capsule   Dantron 25mg + poloxamer 200mg

Co-danthramer strong capsule   Dantron 37.5mg + poloxamer 500mg

Co-danthramer strong suspension (5ml)   Dantron 75mg + poloxamer 1g

---

a   docusate enhances the absorption of liquid paraffin; combined preparations of these substances are prohibited in some countries.

Contact laxatives

Patients receiving an opioid often need a higher dose of a contact (stimulant) laxative than that recommended by the manufacturers. Many benefit from the addition of a faecal softener. In the UK, most palliative care units use co-danthrusate or co-danthramer, i.e. a combination of a contact laxative (dantron) and a faecal softener (Box 3.Q). Because of concern about possible carcinogenicity,[105,106] the licence for dantron-containing laxatives in the UK is

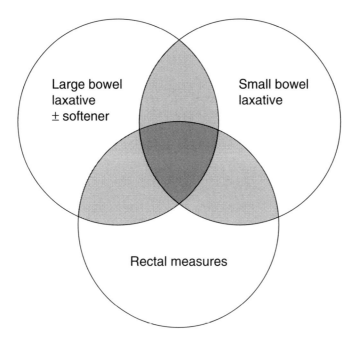

Figure 3.6   A 3-component approach to drug treatment for constipation.

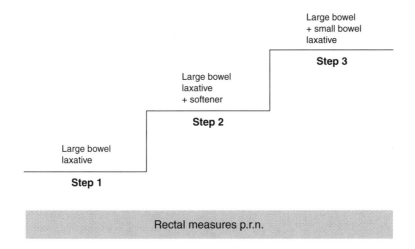

Figure 3.7   A therapeutic step-ladder with safety net (rectal measures) for drug-induced constipation. Doses should be titrated upwards as necessary, e.g. bisacodyl 10mg o.n.–t.d.s. PO on Step 1. Many centres begin on Step 2 (*see* p.388).

now restricted to terminally ill patients. Alternatives include senna or bisacodyl + docusate sodium.

Although the laxative requirement increases as the dose of morphine is increased in any given individual, there is no correlation between the dose of morphine and the effective dose of laxatives in patients as a whole.[107,108] Even so, knowledge of modal doses is helpful in targeting an appropriate starting dose:

- the modal dose of co-danthrusate for patients *not* taking morphine is 1–2 capsules o.n.

- the modal dose of co-danthrusate for patients taking morphine is 2 capsules b.d.

Some opioids are less constipating than equi-analgesic doses of morphine:

- fentanyl[109]

- methadone[110]

- tramadol.[111]

Opioid antagonists

Other options include opioid antagonists given PO in a dose that reverses constipation but does not reverse analgesia. At present the use of opioid antagonists in this way is still mainly experimental.[112,113] However, one centre has a straightforward regimen for PO naloxone.[113] The dose is escalated daily if necessary over 4 days from 3mg t.d.s. to 12mg t.d.s. The median effective dose is 6mg t.d.s. (0800, 1200, 1600h). Mild–moderate abdominal cramps are common and represent an urge to defaecate. Most patients find naloxone better than traditional laxatives because of its rapid action and the ease of defaecation. The effective dose does not correlate with the dose of morphine; some patients need less than the standard starting dose.

Bulk-forming drugs

Bulk-forming drugs have little to offer in the management of opioid-induced constipation, and sometimes make matters worse. Many patients prescribed lactulose for opioid-induced constipation remain constipated, probably because of a failure to titrate the dose upwards. Examination may reveal palpable 'faecal porridge' in the caecum but 'faecal rock cakes' in the descending colon, thereby emphasizing the importance of reversing colonic hypersegmentation with a contact laxative.

Herbal preparations

There are many over-the-counter (OTC) laxatives available, including herbal remedies. An Ayurvedic liquid herbal preparation *Misrakasneham*, containing

21 herbs, castor oil, ghee and milk, is as effective as senna 15–20mg, has a tolerable taste, requires only a small volume to be taken o.d. (2.5–10ml) and is cheaper.[114] Fresh baker's yeast can also be used to good effect.[114]

Rectal measures

One third of patients receiving morphine continue to need rectal measures either regularly or intermittently despite oral laxatives.[86,107] These comprise laxative suppositories, enemas and digital evacuation. Sometimes these measures are elective, e.g. in paraplegics and in the very old and debilitated (Box 3.S).

Box 3.S   Rectal measures for the relief of constipation or faecal impaction

Suppositories

Glycerol 4g, has a hygroscopic and lubricant action. Also claimed to be a rectal stimulant but this is unsubstantiated.

Bisacodyl 10mg, after hydrolysis by enteric enzymes, stimulates propulsive activity.[115]

Carbalax, a mixture of sodium bicarbonate and sodium phosphate which reacts in the rectum, releasing 200ml of carbon dioxide and stimulating evacuation by rectal distension.

Enemas

Surface-wetting micro-enemas, containing 90–120mg of docusate sodium/5ml.

Lubricant enema, arachis/peanut oil (130ml), generally instilled and left overnight before giving stimulant laxative suppository or other enema.

Osmotic micro-enemas, small volume (5ml) containing sodium citrate, glycerol and sorbitol.

Osmotic standard enemas, large volume (120–130ml) phosphate enemas.

Suppositories take about 30min to dissolve after insertion. In patients who defaecate within 5min of the insertion of a bisacodyl suppository, the mechanism of action is ano-rectal stimulation and not pharmacological. A response after 20–30min reflects systemic absorption and subsequent hydrolysis to the active metabolite.

In the UK, most patients needing laxative suppositories receive both glycerol and bisacodyl. Bisacodyl may result in some delayed rectal discharge or faecal incontinence. Carbalax is often used by patients with chronic neurological dysfunction, e.g. paraplegia. It is in effect a gas enema and is safer than a large-volume phosphate enema.[116]

Osmotic micro-enemas contain mainly sodium citrate and sodium lauryl sulpho-acetate together with several excipients, including glycerol and sorbitol. Sodium-lauryl sulpho-acetate is a wetting agent (similar to docusate) whereas sodium citrate draws fluid into the bowel by osmosis, an action enhanced by sorbitol, and displaces bound water from the faeces.

Digital evacuation is the ultimate approach to faecal impaction. However, the need for this can be reduced by using macrogols (polyethylene glycols) 3350.[117,118] This comes in sachets, and each sachet is taken in 125ml of water. The recommended dose is 8 sachets (1L) on day 1 and repeat on day 2 p.r.n. Most patients do not need a full second day's dose.

Some patients use macrogols 3350 as their normal regular laxative in a dose of 1–3 sachets/day. Although it is more expensive than lactulose, another osmotic laxative, it is more effective and better tolerated.[119]

Faecal impaction

Faecal impaction means the lodging of faeces in the rectum (90%) or in the colon, occasionally as far back as the caecum.

Pathogenesis

Incomplete evacuation leads to cumulation of faeces in the rectum. The faeces become very firm because fluid is absorbed from them while they remain in contact with the bowel mucosa. Additional faecal material increases the size of the mass so that it becomes physically impossible for it to be evacuated. Bacterial liquefaction of more proximal faeces may result in overflow diarrhoea and faecal leakage.

Sometimes a soft impaction occurs. This is more likely if the impaction occurs despite the use of a bulk-forming drug or a faecal softener.

Causes

The causes of faecal impaction are similar to those of constipation (Box 3.T).

Box 3.T Causes of faecal impaction in advanced cancer

Cancer Tumour blocking passage of solid faeces	**Debility** Weakness Being bedbound
Drugs Aluminium antacids Barium Antimuscarinics Opioids	Mental impairment **Concurrent** Anal stricture Anal fissure

---

Clinical features

The patient complains of constipation or of the frequent passage of small quantities of fluid faeces together with some or all of the following:

- rectal discharge

- spasmodic rectal pain; may be agonizing

- abdominal colic

- abdominal distension

- nausea and vomiting.

A very ill or elderly patient may develop an agitated delirium.

Evaluation

A high level of suspicion is helpful in the diagnosis of faecal impaction and overflow. The patient may indicate that he has become progressively more constipated but then, 'They suddenly became loose. The trouble is I can't tell when my bowels are going to act, sometimes I have no warning.'

Abdominal examination frequently reveals hard faecal material in the descending and sigmoid colon; the transverse and ascending colon may also be involved. A dilated caecum may also be noted. Although rectal examination generally confirms the presence of a large faecal mass, an empty rectum cannot rule out a high impaction.

Management

Soft faeces

- bisacodyl 10–20mg PR o.d. until there is a negative response
- contact with the rectal mucosa is essential for absorption
- give PO if mucosal contact impossible.

Hard faeces

If suppositories and osmotic enemas fail to achieve an evacuation:

- give an arachis oil retention enema (130ml) overnight
- premedicate with IV midazolam, disrupt the faecal mass by finger manipulation and remove piecemeal
- follow with a high phosphate enema the next day; use a 45cm plastic catheter attached to the enema-giving set
- prescribe oral laxatives in order to prevent recurrence.

An alternative approach to softening hard impacted faeces is to give a retention enema of docusate sodium, e.g. 300mg in 100ml (i.e. diluted oral syrup), or a proprietary docusate sodium micro-enema (these contain 90–120mg).

Diarrhoea

Diarrhoea is an increase in the frequency of defaecation and/or fluidity of the faeces. If severe, it may manifest as faecal incontinence.

Causes

There are many potential causes (Box 3.U) but the most common are:

- laxative overdose
- faecal impaction with overflow
- partial bowel obstruction.[86]

Box 3.U   Causes of diarrhoea in advanced cancer ('LOOSED')

**Length of bowel
(shortened)**
Bowel resection, colostomy
Ileostomy, ileocolic fistula

Overflow
Faecal impaction
Obstruction

Osmotic
Non-absorbable sugars, e.g.
  lactulose, sorbitol-
  containing solutions
Magnesium salts

Enhanced motility
Constitutional
Irritable bowel syndrome
Diet, e.g. bran, fruit, curry, alcohol
Steatorrhoea, e.g. pancreatic cancer,
  obstructive jaundice, blind loop
  syndrome
Visceral neuropathy, e.g. diabetic,
  paraneoplastic
Coeliac plexus block[121]
Lumbar sympathectomy
Carcinoid syndrome
Hyperthyroidism

Drugs (see Box 3.V)

Secretory
Infective, e.g. gastro-enteritis, cholera, pseudomembranous colitis
Injury, e.g. ulcerative colitis, radiation, chemotherapy
Cholegenic (non-absorbed bile acids)

Other relatively common causes include:

- gastro-enteritis, mainly viral

- radiation enteritis

- drugs (Box 3.V)

- steatorrhoea.

Diarrhoea is common in AIDS; pathogens are identifiable in about $1/2$ the cases.[120]

Cholegenic diarrhoea

Active absorption of bile acids occurs mainly in the distal ileum. Non-absorbed bile acids are metabolized in the colon by bacterial enzymes to form unconjugated α-dihydroxy bile acids which stimulate fluid and

---

Box 3.V   Drug-induced diarrhoea in advanced cancer

Common	Occasional	Chemotherapy
Laxatives	Cisapride (licence suspended)	5-fluoro-uracil
Misoprostol	NSAIDs	Mitomycin
Antacids	Oestrogens	Methotrexate
magnesium salts	diethylstilboestrol >3mg/day	Cytosine
SSRIs	Theophylline	arabinoside
Antibiotics, e.g.	Anticholinesterases	Doxorubicin
erythromycin	neostigmine	Etoposide
penicillins	Hypoglycaemics	Asparaginase
sulphonamides	sulphonylureas, e.g.	
tetracyclines	chlorpropamide	**Overflow[b]**
Iron	biguanides, e.g. metformin	Opioids
Mefenamic acid	Sorbitol[a]	Antimuscarinics
	Caffeine	Aluminium
		hydroxide

a   a non-absorbable disaccharide used as a sweetener in 'sugar free' liquid medicines
b   all drugs which predispose to constipation may lead to overflow diarrhoea.

electrolyte secretion. This results in cholegenic diarrhoea which is often explosive and watery, and poorly responsive to standard antidiarrhoeals.

Cholegenic diarrhoea is uncommon in cancer patients. However, the loss of the ileocaecal valve may lead to bacterial invasion of the small intestine with consequential severe diarrhoea; this responds to metronidazole.

Pseudomembranous colitis

Pseudomembranous colitis is an uncommon complication of antibiotic therapy (Table 3.5). Symptoms generally begin within 1 week of starting anti-biotic therapy or shortly after stopping, but may occur up to 1 month later. It is caused by colonization of the bowel by *Clostridium difficile* and the production of toxins A and B which cause mucosal damage.

C. difficile is strongly anaerobic and difficult to culture. Treatment is based on the history and clinical features. Faecal tests to detect *C. difficile* toxins serve to confirm. If in doubt, endoscopy and rectal biopsy are of value, although a trial of therapy is more practical:

• metronidazole 400mg t.d.s. PO for 10 days (cheap)

• vancomycin 125mg q.d.s. PO for 10 days (expensive).

Table 3.5   Pseudomembranous colitis

Clinical features	Causal antibiotics	
	Most prevalent	Highest incidence
Explosive foul-smelling watery diarrhoea + mucus ± blood	Ampicillin	Clindamycin
	Amoxycillin	Lincomycin
Abdominal pain	Cephalosporins	
Tenderness	Ciprofloxacin	
Fever		

About 20% of patients relapse, most within 3 weeks. Mild relapses often resolve spontaneously. Repeated relapses require prolonged treatment with slowly decreasing doses of vancomycin.[122]

Evaluation

A carefully elicited history and clinical examination is often sufficient to determine the most likely cause. A careful review of medication is important, and will generally indicate whether too much laxative is the cause. If the history and examination do not point to a likely cause, faecal microscopy and culture is possibly indicated.

Management

Correct the correctable

- review diet, and modify if indicated (Box 3.W)

- consider antibiotic treatment if cause infective or if bacterial overgrowth seems likely

- prescribe specific antidote (Box 3.X).

Box 3.W   Laxative foods

Raw fruit (fresh or dried)   Coleslaw
Nuts   Sauerkraut
Greens   Spicy foods
Beans   Wholegrain cereals
Lentils   Wholemeal foods
Onion

Box 3.X   Drugs for treating diarrhoea

Disease specific   **Non-specific**
Acute radiation enteritis   Absorbants
  NSAID   hydrophilic bulking agents
  octreotide   pectin

Steatorrhoea   Adsorbants
  pancreatin supplements   kaolin
                                                chalk
Cholegenic diarrhoea   activated charcoal
  colestyramine (an anion exchange resin)
                                              Mucosal PG inhibitors
Pseudomembranous colitis   aspirin
  metronidazole   bismuth subsalicylate
  vancomycin
                                              Opioids
Ulcerative colitis   codeine
  sulfasalazine   morphine
  mesalazine   diphenoxylate
  corticosteroids   loperamide

Infection   Somatostatin analogues
  appropriate antibiotic   octreotide

Drug treatment

- review medication, including laxatives, and modify if indicated

- prescribe a non-specific antidiarrhoeal drug (Box 3.X).

Loperamide is about 3 times more potent than diphenoxylate and 50 times more potent than codeine. It is longer acting and generally needs to be given only b.d. The following regimens are approximately equivalent:

loperamide 2mg b.d

diphenoxylate 2.5mg (in Lomotil) q.d.s.

codeine phosphate 60mg t.d.s.–q.d.s.

Kaolin and morphine mixture BP is an alternative.

Loperamide 4mg is the normal initial dose for acute diarrhoea, followed by 2mg after each loose bowel action. It is uncommon to need more than 16mg/24h.[123] In AIDS, PO morphine or diamorphine by CSCI may be necessary to achieve control. These have both peripheral and central constipating effects, whereas loperamide acts only peripherally.

If the response to high-dose loperamide or other opioid is poor, octreotide 250μg/24h by CSCI should be tried. In controlling radiation-induced diarrhoea, octreotide is more effective than diphenoxylate 10mg/24h, although not all patients respond.[124]

Thalidomide 400mg/day has been used for otherwise resistant chemotherapy-induced diarrhoea.[125]

Pancreatic enzyme replacement

Pancreatin is a standardized preparation of animal lipase, protease and amylase. Pancreatin hydrolyses fats to glycerol and fatty acids, changes protein into proteoses and derived substances, and converts starch into dextrin and sugars.

It is given by mouth in pancreatic deficiency in daily doses of $\leq 8g$ in divided doses. Because 90% of administered pancreatin is destroyed in the stomach by gastric acid, pancreatin should be given with an H_2-receptor antagonist or PPI.

Preparations of choice are:

- Creon 10 000 capsules, each contains enteric-coated granules providing, inter alia, lipase 10 000 units. Initially give 1–2 capsules with each meal, either whole or capsule contents added to fluid or soft food which must be swallowed without chewing; titrate dose upwards until a satisfactory response is obtained

- Creon 25 000 capsules, each contains enteric-coated granules providing, inter alia, lipase 25 000 units. Initially 1 capsule with each meal, taken as above.

Fibrotic strictures of the colon have developed in children aged 2–13 years with cystic fibrosis who have used certain high-strength preparations of pancreatin, e.g. Nutrizym 22 and Pancreatin HL. Fibrosing colonopathy has not been reported in adults or in patients without cystic fibrosis. Creon 25 000 has not been implicated.

Non-drug treatment

If the diarrhoea is unresponsive to the above measures and is causing faecal incontinence, an anal plug should be considered (Conveen, UK). When inserted, it is the size of a large suppository but expands over 30 seconds after contact with moisture and forms a self-retaining plug. It can be left in place for up to 12h and is removed by pulling on its cloth tail. Anal plugs are available in two sizes, small and large.

Rectal discharge

This manifests as:

- discharge
- maceration
- pruritus
- malodour.

Causes

- patulous anus
- haemorrhoids
- faecal impaction and overflow
- following bowel evacuation after laxative suppositories (transient)
- rectal tumour
- radiation coloproctitis
- fistula, e.g. ileorectal, rectovesical.

Management

Correct the correctable

- faecal disimpaction (*see* p.124)

- reduce tumour size
    radiation therapy
    fulguration (surgical diathermy)
    transanal resection
    LASER treatment

- reduce peritumour or postradiation inflammation
    prednisolone suppositories 5mg b.d.
    prednisolone retention enema 20mg every 2–3 days.

Non-drug treatment

Protect the skin of the perineum and genitalia:

- do not use toilet paper

- wash anal area with a soft cloth after each bowel movement and as necessary

- use water only; do not use soap

- pat dry with soft cloth

- if above measures do not keep the area dry, protect skin with a barrier ointment, e.g. Morhulin (zinc oxide 38%) or Comfeel barrier cream

- monitor carefully for small blisters suggestive of fungal infection; treat with clotrimazole 1% solution or cream b.d.–t.d.s.

- use cotton underclothes and change at least o.d.

Drug treatment

If anal hygiene fails to relieve pruritus ani, prescribe a systemic antihistamine.

Ascites

Ascites (excessive fluid in the peritoneal cavity) is asymptomatic when mild but distressing when severe (Box 3.Y). Malignant disease accounts for about 10% of all cases of ascites.[126]

Box 3.Y   Clinical features of ascites

Abdominal distension	Acid reflux
Abdominal discomfort/pain	Nausea and vomiting
Inability to sit upright	Leg oedema
Early satiety	Breathlessness
Dyspepsia	Feeling of suffocation

Ovarian cancer is the commonest primary tumour associated with ascites; 30% at presentation and 60% terminally.[127] Ascites is associated with a poor prognosis; mean survival is about 5 months after detection. Survival is worse in patients with an unknown primary and with gastro-intestinal cancers, better with cancer of the ovary and best with lymphoma.[128]

Pathogenesis

Ascites results from an imbalance between fluid influx and efflux in the peritoneal cavity. An increased fluid influx is associated with:

- peritoneal metastases
- increased peritoneal permeability
- increased renin production secondary to raised hepatic vein pressure causing sodium and water retention which further feeds the ascitic process.

A reduced fluid efflux is associated with:

- subphrenic lymphatics blocked by tumour infiltration
- liver metastases leading to hypo-albuminaemia and possibly portal hypertension.

Management

Correct the correctable

If appropriate and successful, chemotherapy will control ascites. This can be either systemic *or* intraperitoneal.

Non-drug treatment

Paracentesis

Paracentesis is appropriate for patients with a tense distended abdomen and for those who cannot tolerate spironolactone tablets. The aim is to remove as much fluid as possible using an IV cannula or suprapubic catheter. Patients obtain short-term relief even after the removal of 2L. Paracentesis can be repeated if diuretics do not prevent re-accumulation. For patients who have had difficulties in the past, a paracentesis with ultrasound guidance should be considered.

Peritoneovenous shunt

This is a possible option in a patient who is relatively fit but has rapidly recurring ascites despite drainage and diuretic therapy.[129] Shunts are not often used in malignant ascites. When used, they may function satisfactorily for only a few weeks.[130]

Drug treatment

Spironolactone is the key to success because it antagonizes aldosterone:

- starting dose 100–200mg o.m.

- increase the dose by 100mg every 3–7 days to achieve a weight loss of 0.5–1kg/24h

- typical maintenance dose is 300mg o.d.

- occasionally 400–600mg o.d. may be necessary.[131,132]

Two thirds of patients are controlled on spironolactone 300mg o.d. or less[133]

If not achieving the desired weight loss with spironolactone 300–400mg/24h, consider adding furosemide 40mg o.n. Elimination of ascites may take 10–28 days. The dose of the loop diuretic should be reduced once a satisfactory result is achieved. Failure with diuretic therapy often relates to:

- gastric intolerance (spironolactone)

- too small a dose of spironolactone

- failure to use concurrent loop diuretic in resistant cases.

References

1   Jobbins J *et al.* (1992) Oral and dental disease in terminally ill cancer patients. *British Medical Journal.* **304**:1612.

2   De-Conno F *et al.* (1989) Oral complications in patients with advanced cancer. *Journal of Palliative Care.* **5**:7–15.

3   Kusler D and Rambur B (1992) Treatment for radiation-induced xerostoma: An innovative study. *Cancer Nursing.* **15**:191–5.

4   Anonymous (1994) Oral pilocarpine for xerostomia. *Medical Letter.* **34**:76.

5   Lucas V and Schofield L (2000) Treatment of drooling. *European Journal of Palliative Care.* **7**:5–7.

6   Newick P and Laughton-Hewer R (1984) Motor neurone disease – can we do better? *British Medical Journal.* **289**:539–42.

7   Mandel L and Tamari K (1995) Sialorrhoea and gastrooesophageal reflux. *Journal of the American Dental Association.* **126**:1537–41.

8   Lieblich S (1989) Episodic supersalivation (idiopathic paroxysmal sialorrhoea). Description of a new clinical syndrome. *Oral Surgery, Oral Medicine and Oral Pathology.* **68**:159–61.

9   Cohen G *et al.* (1990) Salivary complaints; a manifestation of depressive illness. *NY State Dental Journal.* **56**:31–3.

10 Ali-Melkkila T *et al.* (1993) Pharmacokinetics and related pharmacodynamics of anticholinergic drugs. *Acta Anaesthesiologica Scandinavica.* **37**:633–42.

11 Clissold S and Heel R (1985) Transdermal hyoscine (scopolamine). A preliminary review of its pharmacodynamic properties and therapeutic efficacy. *Drugs.* **29**:189–207.

12 Markkanen Y *et al.* (1987) Serum anti-muscarinic activity after a single dose of oral scopolamine hydrobromide solution measured by radioreceptor assay. *Oral Surgery, Oral Medicine and Oral Pathology.* **63**:534–8.

13 Dreyfuss P *et al.* (1991) The use of transdermal scopolamine to control drooling. *American Journal of Physical Medicine and Rehabilitation.* **70**:220–2.

14 Dunlop R and Hockley J (1990) Transdermal hyoscine and drooling (letter). *Palliative Medicine.* **4**:328–9.

15 Wilkinson J (1987) Side-effects of transdermal scopolamine. *Journal of Emergency Medicine.* **5**:389–92.

16 Ziskind A (1988) Transdermal scopolamine-induced psychosis. *Postgraduate Medicine.* **84**:73–6.

17 Tune I *et al.* (1992) Anticholinergic effects of drugs commonly prescribed for the elderly; potential means of assessing risk of delirium. *American Journal of Psychiatry.* **149**:1393–4.

18 Zeppetella G (1999) Nebulised scopolamine in the management of oral dribbling: three case reports. *Journal of Pain and Symptom Management.* **17**:293–5.

19 Doyle J *et al.* (2000) Nebulized scopolamine. *Journal of Pain and Symptom Management.* **19**:327–8.

20 Mirakhur R and Dundee J (1983) Glycopyrrolate pharmacology and clinical use. *Anaesthesia.* **38**:1195–204.

21 Gram D *et al.* (1991) Central anticholinergic syndrome following glycopyrrolate. *Anesthesiology.* **74**:191–3.

22 Wigard D (1991) Glycopyrrolate and the central anticholinergic syndrome (letter). *Anesthesiology.* **75**:1125.

23 Ali-Melkkila T *et al.* (1989) Glycopyrrolate; pharmacokinetics and some pharmacodynamics findings. *Acta Anaesthesiologica Scandinavica.* **33**:513–7.

24 Blasco P (1996) Glycopyrrolate management of chronic drooling. *Archives of Paediatric Adolescent Medicine.* **150**:932–5.

25 Olsen A and Sjogren P (1999) Oral glycopyrrolate alleviates drooling in a patient with tongue cancer. *Journal of Pain and Symptom Management.* **18**:300–2.

26 Lucas V (1998) Use of enteral glycopyrrolate in the management of drooling. *Palliative Medicine.* **12**:207.

27 Scully C and Shotts R (2000) ABC of oral health: mouth ulcers and other causes of orofacial soreness and pain. *British Medical Journal.* **321**:162–5.

28 Kim J *et al.* (1985) A clinical study of benzydamine for the treatment of radiotherapy induced mucositis of the orpharynx. *International Journal of Tissue Reaction.* **7**:215–18.

29 Turhal N *et al.* (2000) Efficacy of treatment to relieve mucositis-induced discomfort. *Supportive Care in Cancer.* **8**:55–8.

30 Odell E *et al.* (2000) Comprehensive review of treatment for recurrent aphthous stomatitis. URL http:www.umds.ac.uk/dental/opath/daphtrt1.htm and daphtrt2.htm 1–10.

31 NIH Consensus Development Conference Statement (1989) Oral complications of cancer therapies, prevention and treatment. *NIH Consensus Statement.* **7**:1–11.

32 Mueller B *et al.* (1995) Mucositis management practices for hospitalized patients: National survey results. *Journal of Pain and Symptom Management.* **10**:510–20.

33 Burgess J *et al.* (1990) Pharmacological management of recurrent oral mucosal ulceration. *Drugs.* **39**:54–65.

34 Arendorf T and Walker D (1979) Oral Candidal populations in health and disease. *British Dental Journal.* **147**:267–72.

35 Finlay I (1986) Oral symptoms and Candida in the terminally ill. *British Medical Journal.* **292**:592–3.

36 Jobbins J *et al.* (1992) Oral carriage of yeasts, coliforms and staphylococci in patients with advanced malignant disease. *Journal of Oral Pathology and Medicine.* **21**:305–8.

37 Samaranayake L and Lamey P (1998) Oral candidosis. 1: clinicopathological aspects. *Dental Update.* **15**:227–31.

38 Hanks GW *et al.* (1983) Corticosteroids in terminal cancer – a prospective analysis of current practice. *Postgraduate Medical Journal.* **59**:702–6.

39 Regnard C (1994) Single dose fluconazole versus five day ketoconazole in oral candidiasis. *Palliative Medicine.* **8**:72–3.

40 Moertel C *et al.* (1974) Corticosteroid therapy for preterminal gastrointestinal cancer. *Cancer.* **33**:1607–9.

41 Bruera E *et al.* (1985) Action of oral methylprednisolone in terminal cancer patients: a prospective randomized double-blind study. *Cancer Treatment Reports.* **69**:751–4.

42 Bruera E *et al.* (1998) Effectiveness of megestrol acetate in patients with advanced cancer: a randomized, double-blind, crossover study. *Cancer Prevention Control.* **2**:74–8.

43 Downer S *et al.* (1993) A double blind placebo controlled trial of medroxyprogesterone acetate (MPA) in cancer cachexia. *British Journal of Cancer.* **67**:1102–5.

44   Loprinzi C *et al.* (1994) Phase III evaluation of 4 doses of megestrol acetate as therapy for patients with cancer anorexia and/or cachexia. *Oncology.* **51**:2–7.

45   Westman G *et al.* (1999) Megestrol acetate in advanced, progressive, hormone-insensitive cancer. Effects on the quality of life: a placebo-controlled, randomised, multicentre trial. *European Journal of Cancer.* **35**:586–95.

46   Burge F (1993) Dehydration symptoms of palliative care cancer patients. *Journal of Pain and Symptom Management.* **8**:454–64.

47   Meares C (1994) Terminal dehydration: A review. *American Journal of Hospice and Palliative Care.* **11**:10–14.

48   Dunphy K *et al.* (1995) Rehydration in palliative and terminal care: if not – why not? *Palliative Medicine.* **9**:221–8.

49   Fainsinger R *et al.* (1994) The use of hypodermoclysis for rehydration in terminally ill cancer patients. *Journal of Pain and Symptom Management.* **9**:298–302.

50   Constans T *et al.* (1991) Hypodermoclysis in dehydrated elderly patients: local effects with and without hyaluronidase. *Journal of Palliative Care.* **7**:10–12.

51   Bruera E *et al.* (1995) Changing pattern of agitated impaired mental status in patients with advanced cancer: association with cognitive monitoring, hydration, and opioid rotation. *Journal of Pain and Symptom Management.* **10**:287–91.

52   Bruera E and Higginson I (1996) *Cachexia-Anorexia in Cancer Patients.* Oxford University Press, Oxford.

53   Nelson K *et al.* (1994) The cancer anorexia-cachexia syndrome. *Journal of Clinical Oncology.* **12**:213–25.

54   Puccio M and Nathanson L (1997) The cancer cachexia syndrome. *Seminars in Oncology.* **24**:277–87.

55   Hussey H and Tisdale M (1999) Effect of cachectic factor on carbohydrate metabolism and attenuation by eicosapentaenoic acid. *British Journal of Cancer.* **80**:1231–5.

56   Jaskowiak N and Alexander H (1997) The pathophysiology of cancer cachexia. In: D Doyle, G Hanks and N MacDonald (eds) *Oxford Textbook of Palliative Medicine.* Oxford University Press, Oxford, pp 534–48.

57   Preston T *et al.* (1995) Effect of ibuprofen on the acute-phase response and protein metabolism in patients with cancer and weight loss. *British Journal of Surgery.* **82**:229–34.

58   McMillan D *et al.* (1998) Longitudinal study of body cell mass depletion and the inflammatory response in cancer patients. *Nutrition and Cancer.* **31**:101–5.

59   Barber M *et al.* (1998) Current controversies in cancer. Should cancer patients with incurable disease receive parenteral or enteral nutritional support? *European Journal of Cancer.* **34**:279–85.

60   Bruera E and MacDonald N (1988) Nutrition in cancer patients: an update and review of our experience. *Journal of Pain and Symptom Management.* **3**:133–40.

61   Strang P (1997) The effect of megestrol acetate on anorexia, weight loss and cachexia in cancer and AIDS patients (review). *Anticancer Research.* **17**:657–62.

62   Vadell C *et al.* (1998) Anticachectic efficacy of megestrol acetate at different doses and versus placebo in patients with neoplastic cachexia. *American Journal of Clinical Oncology.* **21**:347–51.

63   McMillan D *et al.* (1997) A pilot study of megestrol acetate and ibuprofen in the treatment of cachexia in gastrointestinal cancer patients. *British Journal of Cancer.* **76**:788–90.

64 Boasberg P *et al.* (2000) Thalidomide induced cessation of weight loss and improved sleep in advanced cancer patients with cachexia. *ASCO Online.* Visited 21: Abstract 2396.

65 Burns C *et al.* (1999) Phase I clinical study of fish oil fatty acid capsules for patients with cancer cachexia: cancer and leukemia group B study 9473. *Clinical Cancer Research.* **5**:3942–7.

66 Logemann JA (1983) *Evaluation and Treatment of Swallowing Disorders.* College Hill Press, San Diego.

67 McDonnell F and Walsh D (1999) Treatment of odynophagia and dysphagia in advanced cancer with sublingual glyceryl trinitrate. *Palliative Medicine.* **13**:251–2.

68 Twycross R and Regnard C (1997) Dysphagia, dyspepsia, hiccup. In: D Doyle, G Hanks and N MacDonald (eds) *Oxford Textbook of Palliative Medicine.* Oxford University Press, Oxford, pp 499–512.

69 Carter R *et al.* (1982) Pain and dysphagia in patients with squamous carcinomas of the head and neck: the role of perineural spread. *Journal of the Royal Society of Medicine.* **75**:598–606.

70 Murray FE *et al.* (1988) Palliative laser therapy of advanced esophageal carcinoma: an alternative perspective. *American Journal of Gastroenterology.* **83**:816–20.

71 Boyce H (1999) Palliation of dysphagia of esophageal cancer by endoscopic lumen restoration techniques. *Cancer Control.* **6**:73–83.

72 Carter R *et al.* (1992) Laser recanalization versus endoscopic intubation in the palliation of malignant dysphagia: a randomized prospective study. *British Journal of Surgery.* **79**:1167–70.

73 Lewis-Jones CM *et al.* (1995) Laser therapy in the palliation of dysphagia in oesophageal malignancy. *Palliative Medicine.* **9**:327–30.

74 Nwokolo CU *et al.* (1994) Palliation of malignant dysphagia by ethanol induced tumour necrosis. *Gut.* **35**:299–303.

75 Chung SCS *et al.* (1994) Palliation of malignant oesophageal obstruction by endoscopic alcohol injection. *Endoscopy.* **26**:275–7.

76 Shanahan T *et al.* (1993) Chin-down posture effect on aspiration in dysphagic patient. *Archives of Physical Medicine and Rehabilitation.* **74**:736–9.

77 Moran B and Frost R (1992) Percutaneous endoscopic gastrostomy in 41 patients: indications and clinical outcome. *Journal of the Royal Society of Medicine.* **85**:320–1.

78 Rabeneck L *et al.* (1997) Ethically justified, clinically comprehensive guidelines for percutaneous endoscopic gastrostomy tube placement. *Lancet.* **349**:496–8.

79 Britton J *et al.* (1997) The use of percutaneous endoscopic gastrostomy (PEG) feeding tubes in patients with neurological disease. *Journal of Neurology.* **244**:431–4.

80 McCamish M and Crocker N (1993) Enteral and parenteral nutrition support of terminally ill patients: practical and ethical perspectives. *The Hospice Journal.* **9**:107–29.

81 Bozzetti F (1996) Guidelines on artificial nutrition versus hydration in terminal cancer patients. *Nutrition.* **12**:163–7.

82 NCHSPCS (1997) Artificial hydration (AH) for people who are terminally ill. *European Journal of Palliative Care.* **4**:124–8.

83 Feins R et al. (1996) Palliation of inoperable esophageal carcinoma with the Wallstent endoprosthesis. Annals of Thoracic Surgery. 62:1603–7.

84 Cwikiel W et al. (1998) Malignant dysphagia: palliation with esophageal stents – long-term results in 100 patients. Radiology. 207:513–18.

85 Raijman I et al. (1998) Palliation of malignant dysphagia and fistulae with coated expandable metal stents: experience with 101 patients. Gastrointestinal Endoscopy. 48:172–8.

86 Twycross RG and Lack SA (1986) Control of Alimentary Symptoms in Far Advanced Cancer. Churchill Livingstone, Edinburgh.

87 Nelson K et al. (1993) Assessment of upper gastrointestinal motility in the cancer-associated dyspepsia syndrome (CADS). Journal of Palliative Care. 9:27–31.

88 Hawkey C et al. (1998) Omeprazole compared with misoprostol for ulcers associated with nonsteroidal antiinflammatory drugs. New England Journal of Medicine. 338:727–34.

89 Yeomans N et al. (1998) A comparison of omeprazole with ranitidine for ulcers associated with nonsteroidal antiinflammatory drugs. Acid suppression trial. New England Journal of Medicine. 338:719–26.

90 Lichter I (1993) Results of antiemetic management in terminal illness. Journal of Palliative Care. 9:19–21.

91 Tjeerdsma H et al. (1993) Voluntary suppression of defecation delays gastric emptying. Digestive Diseases and Sciences. 38:832–6.

92 Barkin J et al. (1986) Pancreatic carcinoma is associated with delayed gastric emptying. Digestive Diseases and Sciences. 31:265–7.

93 Schuurkes JAJ et al. (1986) Stimulation of gastroduodenal motor activity: dopaminergic and cholinergic modulation. Drug Development Research. 8:233–41.

94 De-Conno F et al. (1991) Continuous subcutaneous infusion of hyoscine butylbromide reduces secretion in patients with gastrointestinal obstruction. Journal of Pain and Symptom Management. 6:484–6.

95 Mercadante S et al. (2000) Comparison of octreotide and hyoscine butylbromide in controlling gastrointestinal symptoms due to malignant inoperable bowel obstruction. Supportive Care in Cancer. 8:188–91.

96 Barnes J and Barnes N (1991) Effective management of nausea and vomiting. Prescriber. 29–34.

97 Twycross R et al. (1997) The use of low dose levomepromazine (methotrimeprazine) in the management of nausea and vomiting. Progress in Palliative Care. 5:49–53.

98 Feuer D and Broadley K (1999) Systematic review and meta-analysis of corticosteroids for the resolution of malignant bowel obstruction in advanced gynaecological and gastrointestinal cancers. Annals of Oncology. 10:1035–41.

99 Laval G et al. (2000) The use of steroids in the management of inoperable intestinal obstruction in terminal cancer patients: do they remove the obstruction? Palliative Medicine. 14:3–10.

100 Baines M (1987) Medical management of intestinal obstruction. Baillière's Clinical Oncology. 1:357–71.

101 Krebs H and Goplerud D (1987) Mechanical intestinal obstruction in patients with gynecologic disease: a review of 368 patients. American Journal of Obstetrics and Gynecology. 157:577–83.

102 Harris A and Cantwell B (1986) Mechanisms and treatment of cytotoxic-induced nausea and vomiting. In: C Davis, G Lake-Bakaar and D Grahame-Smith (eds) *Nausea and Vomiting: Mechanisms and Treatment.* Springer-Verlag, Berlin, pp 78–93.

103 Ashby M *et al.* (1991) Percutaneous gastrostomy as a venting procedure in palliative care. *Palliative Medicine.* **5**:147–50.

104 Sykes N (1998) The relationship between opioid use and laxative use in terminally ill cancer patients. *Palliative Medicine.* **12**:375–82.

105 Muller S *et al.* (1996) Genotoxicity of the laxative drug components emodin, aloe-emodin and danthron in mammalian cells: Topoisomerase II mediated? *Mutation Research.* **371**:165–73.

106 Mueller S and Stopper H (1999) Characterization of the genotoxicity of anthraquinones in mammalian cells. *Biochimica et Biophysica Acta.* **1428**: 406–14.

107 Twycross RG and Harcourt JMV (1991) The use of laxatives at a palliative care centre. *Palliative Medicine.* **5**:27–33.

108 Fallon M and Hanks G (1999) Morphine, constipation and performance status in advanced cancer patients. *Palliative Medicine.* **13**:159–60.

109 Radbruch L *et al.* (2000) Constipation and the use of laxatives: a comparison between transdermal fentanyl and oral morphine. *Palliative Medicine.* **14**:111–19.

110 Daeninck P and Bruera E (1999) Reduction in constipation and laxative requirements following opioid rotation to methadone: a report of four cases. *Journal of Pain and Symptom Management.* **18**:303–9.

111 Wilder-Smith C and Bettiga A (1997) The analgesic tramadol has minimal effect on gastrointestinal motor function. *British Journal of Clinical Pharmacology.* **43**:71–5.

112 Yuan C *et al.* (1999) Effects of intravenous methylnaltrexone on opioid-induced motility and transit time changes in subjects receiving chronic methadone therapy: a pilot study. *Pain.* **83**:631–5.

113 Meissner W *et al.* (2000) Oral naloxone reverses opioid-associated constipation. *Pain.* **84**:105–9.

114 Ramesh P *et al.* (1998) Managing morphine-induced constipation: a controlled comparison of an Ayurvedic formulation and senna. *Journal of Pain and Symptom Management.* **16**:240–4.

115 Roth von W and Beschke von K (1988) Pharmakokinetik und laxierende wirkung von bisacodyl nach gabe verschiedener zubereitungsformen. *Arzneim-Forsch/ Drug Research.* **38**:570–4.

116 Goldman M (1993) Hazards of phosphate enemas. *Gastroenterology Today.* **3**:16–17.

117 Culbert P *et al.* (1998) Highly effective new oral therapy for faecal impaction. *British Journal of General Practice.* **48**:1599–600.

118 Culbert P *et al.* (1998) Highly effective oral therapy (polyethylene glycol/ electrolyte solution) for faecal impaction and severe constipation. *Clinical Drug Investigation.* **16**:355–60.

119 Attar A *et al.* (1999) Comparison of a low dose polyethylene glycol electrolyte solution with lactulose for treatment of chronic constipation. *Gut.* **44**:226–30.

120 Rolston K *et al.* (1989) Diarrhea in patients infected with the human immuno-deficiency virus. *The American Journal of Medicine.* **86**:137–8.

121 Dean AP and Reed WD (1991) Diarrhoea – an unrecognised hazard of coeliac plexus block. *Australian and New Zealand Journal of Medicine.* **21**:47–8.

122 Anonymous (1995) Antibiotic-induced diarrhoea. *Drug and Therapeutics Bulletin.* **33**:23–4.

123 Cascinu S *et al.* (2000) High-dose loperamide in the treatment of 5-fluorouracil-induced diarrhea in colorectal cancer patients. *Supportive Care in Cancer.* **8**:65–7.

124 Yavuz M *et al.* (2000) A randomized study of the efficacy of octreotide versus diphenoxylate on radiation-induced diarrhea. *ASCO Online.* Visited 21: Abstract 2370.

125 Govindarajan R *et al.* (2000) Effect of thalidomide on gastrointestinal toxic effects of irinotecan. *Lancet.* **356**:566–7.

126 Runyon B (1994) Care of patients with ascites. *New England Journal of Medicine.* **330**:337–42.

127 Hird V *et al.* (1989) Malignant ascites: review of the literature, and an update on monoclonal antibody-targeted therapy. *European Journal of Obstetrics, Gynaecology and Reproductive Biology.* **32**:37–45.

128 Parsons S *et al.* (1996) Malignant ascites. *British Journal of Surgery.* **83**:6–14.

129 Osterlee J (1980) peritoneovenous shunting for ascites in cancer patients. *British Journal of Surgery.* **67**:663–6.

130 Soderlund C (1986) Denver peritoneovenous shunting for malignant or cirrhotic ascites. A prospective consecutive series. *Scandinavian Journal of Gastroenterology.* **21**:1167–72.

131 Fogel M *et al.* (1981) Diuresis in the ascitic patients: a randomized controlled trial of three regimens. *Journal of Clinical Gastroenterology.* **3**:73–80.

132 Greenway B *et al.* (1982) Control of malignant ascites with spironolactone. *British Journal of Surgery.* **69**:441–2.

4 Respiratory symptoms

Breathlessness · Terminal breathlessness · Cough
Bronchorrhoea · Pleural effusion · Lymphangitis
carcinomatosa · Death rattle · Noisy tachypnoea in the
moribund · Cheyne-Stokes respiration · Hiccup

Breathlessness

Breathlessness is the subjective experience of breathing discomfort. It comprises qualitatively distinct sensations which vary in intensity. The experience derives from interactions among multiple physiological, psychological, social and environmental factors and may induce secondary physiological and behavioural responses.[1] Breathlessness on exertion is a normal (physiological) experience. It becomes pathological when it limits normal activities or is associated with disabling anxiety.

Breathlessness is present in 70% of patients with cancer in the last few weeks before death and is severe in 25% of patients in their last week of life.[2] Breathlessness is an independent predictor of survival second only to performance status.[3]

Physiology

Involuntary rhythmic respiration is generated by the central pattern generator in the brain stem and is primarily concerned with the regulation of arterial carbon dioxide (and thus acid–base balance) and maintenance of adequate arterial oxygen (Figure 4.1). It is modulated by various neurotransmitters and neuromodulators relaying information from:

- higher centres, e.g. level of arousal, emotion, motor cortex activity, temperature
- chemoreceptors, e.g. hypoxia, hypercapnia, acidosis
- airways, e.g. distortion or collapse
- respiratory muscles, e.g. weakness, fatigue (Table 4.1).

The voluntary control of respiration allows the central pattern generator to be overridden temporarily to allow activities such as talking, swallowing and coughing.

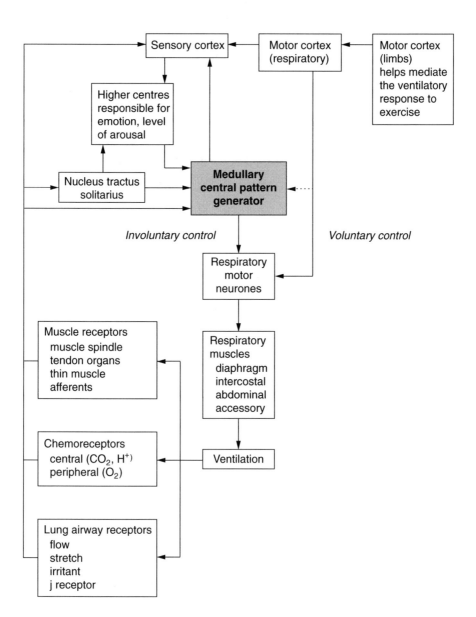

Figure 4.1   The control of breathing.

Breathlessness occurs when changes in pressure, airflow or movement of the lungs and chest wall are not appropriate for the motor command, i.e. there is a mismatch between the motor command and the mechanical response of the

Table 4.1   Neurotransmitters and neuromodulators involved in the control of breathing[4]

Substance	Effect on respiration
Neurotransmitters responsible for respiratory rhythm	
Glutamate	Stimulates central generation and transmission of respiratory rhythm
GABA	Transmission of phasic waves of inhibition
Glycine	Transmission of phasic waves of inhibition
Neuromodulators responsible for shaping respiratory pattern	
Acetylcholine	Stimulatory or inhibitory
Serotonin (5HT)	Mainly inhibitory
Noradrenaline (norepinephrine)	Mainly stimulatory
Adrenaline (epinephrine)	Mainly stimulatory
Dopamine	Mainly stimulatory (respiratory frequency)
Opioids	Inhibitory (interfere with the effect of glutamate)
Substance P	Mainly stimulatory (tidal volume)
Somatostatin	Inhibitory
Cholecystokinin	Stimulatory or inhibitory
Thyrotropin-releasing hormone	Stimulatory

respiratory system (known as neuromechanical dissociation).[1] Such a mismatch may arise in conditions associated with:

- increased ventilatory demand, e.g. diseases of the lung parenchyma and pulmonary vasculature
- abnormal ventilatory impedance, e.g. an increased resistive and/or elastic load
- respiratory muscle abnormalities, e.g. neuromuscular diseases
- blood gas abnormalities.

Causes

Breathlessness in advanced cancer is often multifactorial (Box 4.A). Most patients will have:

- parenchymal or pleural disease
- a history of smoking
- abnormal spirometry (mixed > restrictive > obstructive pattern)
- weak inspiratory muscles.

About half are hypoxic and about 20% have evidence of concurrent cardiac ischaemia or arrhythmia.[5] Anxiety, a history of smoking and a raised $PaCO_2$ all exacerbate breathlessness.

Box 4.A   Causes of breathlessness

Cancer
Pleural effusion(s)
Obstruction of a large airway
Replacement of lung by cancer
Lymphangitis carcinomatosa
Tumour cell micro-emboli
Pericardial effusion
Phrenic nerve palsy
SVC obstruction
Massive ascites
Abdominal distension
Cachexia-anorexia syndrome
    respiratory muscle weakness

Debility
Anaemia
Atelectasis
Pulmonary embolism
Pneumonia
Empyema
Muscle weakness

Treatment
Pneumonectomy
Radiation-induced fibrosis
Chemotherapy-induced
    pneumonitis
    fibrosis
    cardiomyopathy
Progestogens
    stimulate ventilation
    increase sensitivity to carbon dioxide

Concurrent
COPD
Asthma
Heart failure
Acidosis
Fever
Pneumothorax
Panic disorder, anxiety,
    depression

A patient's experience of breathlessness will be shaped by their previous experience, expectation, personality, behavioural style and emotional state. Patients with lung cancer commonly report that breathlessness:

- is intermittent, occurring in episodes lasting 5–15min precipitated by exertion, bending over, talking etc., and is associated with feelings of exhaustion

- restricts general activities of daily living and social functioning leading to a loss of independence and of role resulting in frustration, anger and depression[6]

- induces feelings of anxiety, fear, panic and impending death (Figure 4.2).[7]

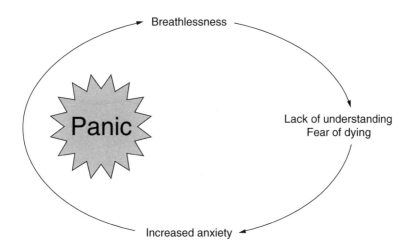

Figure 4.2   Breathlessness is a common trigger for panic.[7]

Management

Breathlessness in advanced cancer can be divided into three types:

- breathlessness on exertion (prognosis = months-to-years)
- breathlessness at rest (prognosis = weeks-to-months)[8]
- terminal breathlessness (prognosis = days-to-weeks).[9]

The relative importance of the three treatment categories (*correct the correctable, non-drug treatment, drug treatment*) changes as the patient's condition deteriorates (Figure 4.3).

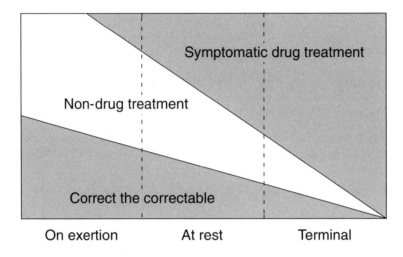

Figure 4.3   Treatment for severe breathlessness at different stages in advanced cancer.

Correct the correctable

Particularly while the patient is still ambulant, consideration should be given to the identification and correction of correctable causes (Table 4.2).

Is the breathlessness caused by the cancer?

Can the cancer be modified?

Can the impact of the cancer be modified?

The history, examination and appropriate investigation(s) will identify pulmonary, cardiac or neuromuscular abnormalities (Box 4.B). Try to determine the cause of any recent deterioration because rapid changes often present opportunities for corrective therapy, such as pleural aspiration or antibiotics.

A comprehensive evaluation will include an assessment of the patient's knowledge, beliefs and behaviours associated with their breathlessness and cancer, and the impact it has upon them.[10]

Non-drug treatment

Non-drug treatment begins by exploring the patient's experience of breathlessness (Box 4.C). Open acknowledgement of the fear and feelings of terror and panic associated with the acute exacerbations, e.g. when climbing stairs, is the key to enable the patient (and the family) to cope better. The patient must be assured that they will not die during an attack. Emphasize that 'Although you may feel you're suffocating, you've always recovered – and you always will'.

Table 4.2   Correctable causes of breathlessness

Cause	Treatment
Respiratory infection	Antibiotics Physiotherapy
COPD/asthma	Bronchodilators Corticosteroids Physiotherapy
Hypoxia	Trial of oxygen
Obstruction of bronchus, SVC	Corticosteroids Radiotherapy Stent LASER (bronchus only)
Lymphangitis carcinomatosa	Corticosteroids Diuretics Bronchodilators
Pleural effusion	Thoracocentesis Drainage and pleurodesis
Ascites	Diuretics (see p.133) Paracentesis
Pericardial effusion	Paracentesis Corticosteroids
Anaemia	Blood transfusion
Cardiac failure	Diuretics ACE inhibitors
Pulmonary embolism	Anticoagulation (see p.248)

Breathing retraining, panic management and activity pacing all ease breathlessness in patients with lung cancer.[11] Training courses for health professionals are available but the physiotherapist is often the key person in this situation.[12]

Breathing retraining

Shallow, rapid breathing is an ineffective and inefficient pattern of breathing that contributes to anxiety and panic. Breathing retraining aims to:

- promote a relaxed and gentle breathing pattern
- minimise the work of breathing
- establish a sense of control over breathing that aids confidence in coping with breathless episodes.

Box 4.B   Evaluation of the breathless patient with cancer[9]

History
Speed of onset.

Associated symptoms, e.g. pain, cough, haemoptysis, sputum, stridor, wheeze.

Exacerbating and relieving factors.

Symptoms suggestive of hyperventilation:
    poor relationship of dyspnoea to exertion
    presence of hyperventilation attacks
    breathlessness at rest
    rapid fluctuations in breathlessness within minutes
    fear of sudden death during an attack
    breathlessness varying with social situations.

Past medical history, e.g. history of cardiovascular disease.

Drug history, e.g. drugs precipitating fluid retention or bronchospasm.

Symptoms of anxiety or depression.

Social circumstances and support networks.

Level of independence:
    ability to care for themselves
    coping strategies.

What does the breathlessness mean to the patient?

How do they feel when they are breathless?

Examination
Observe the patient walking a set distance or carrying out a specific task.

Does hyperventilation reproduce symptoms?

Investigations
Common

Chest radiograph.

Haemoglobin concentration.

Less common

Ultrasound scan (useful for differentiating between pleural effusion and solid tumour).

Oxygen saturation (may be useful if assessing value of oxygen).

Peak flow/simple spirometry (assessing response to bronchodilators or corticosteroids).

Electrocardiogram.

Echocardiography.

Ventilation–perfusion scan.

Box 4.C   Non-drug treatment of breathlessness[9]

Exploring the perception of the patient and carers
What is the meaning of the breathlessness to the patient and to the carers?

Explore anxieties, particularly fear of sudden death when breathless.

Inform the patient and carers that breathlessness in itself is not life-threatening.

State what is/is not likely to happen, e.g. 'You won't choke or suffocate to death'.

Decide on realistic goals and thereby help the patient adjust to the progressive deterioration.

Help the patient to cope with and adjust to loss of role, abilities etc.

Maximizing the feeling of control over breathlessness
Breathing control advice.

Relaxation techniques.

Plan of action for acute episodes:

   simple written instructions outlining a step-by-step plan

   increase confidence in coping with acute episodes.

Use of an electric fan.

Complementary therapies benefit some patients.

Maximizing functional ability
Encourage exertion to breathlessness to increase tolerance/desensitise to breathlessness and maintain fitness.

Evaluation by district nurse, occupational therapist, physiotherapist and social worker may all be necessary to identify where additional support is required.

Reduce feelings of personal and social isolation
Meet others in a similar situation.

Attendance at a day centre.

Respite admissions.

Approaches include:

- relaxation therapies which encourage slow regular deep breathing

- diaphragmatic breathing; patients are taught to consciously expand their abdominal wall during inspiratory diaphragm descent. Outward abdominal excursion can be detected by placing one hand on the abdomen and the other on the chest. When carried out in the supine position 3 times daily for 10–20min for 6–8 weeks, improvements can be seen in breathing pattern, blood gases and expiratory muscle strength. Clear benefit from diaphragmatic breathing on function and breathlessness has not been shown.[13]

- pursed lip breathing; performed as nasal inspiration followed by expiratory blowing against partially closed lips, expiration taking twice as long as inspiration. Some patients adopt this instinctively. Encourage its use during periods of increased ventilation. Can lead to improvements in breathing pattern, respiratory muscle function and blood gases in patients with COPD, but improvement in breathlessness is variable.[13]

Positioning

Some patients with COPD find breathlessness improves in positions which:

- increase abdominal pressure, improving the efficiency of the flattened diaphragm, reducing abdominal paradoxical breathing and accessory muscle use, e.g. leaning forward with arms/elbows resting on the knees or a table, or lying prone

- maximise ventilation–perfusion matching; patients with unilateral broncho-pulmonary disease, e.g. collapse, consolidation, or pleural effusion are less likely to experience a deterioration in blood gases when lying on their side with the normal lung down (this advantage is lost with a large pleural effusion).

Desensitisation

Exposure to greater than usual levels of breathlessness in a safe environment may increase a patient's confidence to cope with the symptom. Exercise in a supervised environment enables some patients to overcome the anxiety provoked by exertional breathlessness and thereby increase their exercise tolerance.

Drug treatment

Symptomatic drug treatments for breathlessness are used after appropriate corrective and non-drug treatments have been fully exploited (Figure 4.4).

Bronchodilators

Patients with lung cancer and COPD tend to report the highest levels of breathlessness. Airflow obstruction is often underdiagnosed and undertreated. Bronchospasm is not always associated with wheeze, particularly in patients with a history of chronic asthma, chronic bronchitis or heavy smoking. Ideally, formal tests of reversibility with bronchodilators should be carried out.[14] In very ill patients an empirical trial may have to suffice.

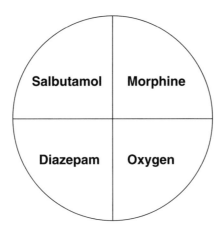

Figure 4.4 Drugs for the symptomatic relief of breathlessness.

Bronchodilator therapy, e.g. a β_2-adrenoreceptor stimulant ± an antimuscarinic, inhaled via a spacer or nebulizer, improves breathlessness in most cancer patients with COPD even without any changes in ventilatory indices.[15,16] This suggests an independent class effect of bronchodilators on breathlessness possibly by increasing muscle strength.[17]

Morphine

Opioids reduce the ventilatory response to hypercapnia, hypoxia and exercise, decreasing respiratory effort and breathlessness. Activation of μ- and δ-opioid receptors reduces tidal volume and respiratory rate respectively by interfering with the stimulatory effects of the excitatory glutamate system.[4]

Morphine reduces breathlessness by about 20% for ⩽4h.[18] Generally it is more beneficial in patients who are breathless at rest than in those who are breathless only on exertion.[18–21] In opioid-naive patients:

- start with small doses of morphine p.r.n., e.g. 2.5–5mg, and titrate the dose according to response, duration of effect and adverse effects
- if ⩾2 doses/24h are needed, prescribe morphine regularly.

In patients already taking morphine for pain and with severe breathlessness, a dose that is 100% or more of the q4h analgesic dose may be needed.[19,22] For those with less severe breathlessness, a dose equivalent to 25% of the q4h analgesic dose may suffice.[18]

In some patients diamorphine/morphine by CSCI is better tolerated and provides greater relief, possibly by avoiding the peaks (with adverse effects) and troughs (with loss of effect) of oral medication.

Nebulized morphine

Nebulized morphine is used at some centres for severe breathlessness:[23–25]

- a typical starting dose is morphine 10–20mg diluted to 5ml with 0.9% saline given q4h or p.r.n. (use a standard ampoule for injection)
- doses up to 70–100mg have been used.[23,26]

However, a randomised double-blind placebo controlled trial in patients with cancer showed no benefit.[27] Further, the use of nebulized morphine is not without risk:

- morphine can trigger the release of histamine from mast cells which may lead to bronchoconstriction
- in a patient already receiving oral morphine, 4mg caused serious respiratory depression necessitating artificial ventilation for several hours.[28]

At present, the use of nebulized morphine should be discouraged.[29]

Anxiolytics

Diazepam can be given if the patient is very anxious, e.g. 2–10mg stat, 5–20mg o.n., 2–5mg p.r.n. Reduce the dose if the patient becomes drowsy as a result of drug cumulation. Some centres use lorazepam SL b.d. and p.r.n. Patients who experience panic during acute exacerbations may also need an SSRI (*see* p.192).

Buspirone which acts predominantly via serotonin 5-HT$_{1A}$-receptors is free of sedative or respiratory depressant effects.[30] It is as effective as diazepam in the relief of generalised anxiety but *not* panic disorder.[31] Buspirone may be a useful alternative to a benzodiazepine when sedation or the risk of ventilatory depression is unacceptable but trial results in COPD are conflicting:[32–34]

- starting dose 5mg t.d.s.
- titrated to 10–20mg t.d.s.
- onset of action is 2–4 weeks.

Neuroleptics have an anxiolytic (but *not* a specific antipanic effect) and antipsychotic effect. They are helpful in patients who are anxious and delirious. Haloperidol is the neuroleptic of choice and is without marked respiratory depressant effects. When greater levels of sedation are necessary, e.g. in the terminal phase:

- levomepromazine 12.5–50mg/24h or more PO or SC
- chlorpromazine 12.5–25mg IM, IV or PR q4h–q12h.[35]

A cannabinoid, e.g. nabilone 100–250μg b.d.–q.d.s., is used at some centres in patients with severe dyspnoea at risk of developing hypercapnic respiratory failure if given opioids or benzodiazepines. With higher doses, most patients complain of drowsiness and/or dysphoria; hypotension and tachycardia may also be limiting factors.[36]

Oxygen

Oxygen therapy increases alveolar oxygen tension and decreases the work of breathing necessary to maintain a given arterial tension. The concentration given varies with the underlying condition:

- 60% in asthma, pneumonia, pulmonary embolism, fibrosing alveolitis

- 28% in COPD and other causes of hypercapnic ventilatory failure.

Inappropriate prescription can have serious or fatal effects. Patients with hypercapnic ventilatory failure who are dependent upon hypoxia for their respiratory drive should not be given a high concentration.

Domiciliary oxygen for either long-term or short-burst use can be prescribed for palliation of breathlessness in patients with cancer:[37]

- in moderately-to-severely hypoxic patients (PaO_2 <8.0kPa; oxygen saturation <90%) oxygen is generally better than air and should be available for use[37,38]

- in mildly hypoxic patients (PaO_2 8.0–9.3kPa; oxygen saturation 90–94%) the value of oxygen is more difficult to determine. Some patients obtain as much benefit from air delivered by nasal prongs.[39] This suggests that a sensation of airflow is an important determinant of benefit. Explore the benefit of a cool draught (open window or fan) before offering a trial of oxygen.

A trial of oxygen therapy can be given via nasal prongs for a fixed period of time. A pulse oximeter will help identify those patients whose oxygen saturation is objectively improved by oxygen therapy. If on review the patient has persisted in using the oxygen and has found it useful it can be continued; if the patient has any doubts to its efficacy then it should be discontinued.

Helium 80%–oxygen 20% mixture is less dense and viscous than room air.[40] Its use helps to reduce the respiratory work required to overcome upper airway obstruction. It can be used as a temporary measure pending more definitive treatment.

Terminal breathlessness

Patients often fear suffocating to death and a positive approach to the patient, their family and colleagues about the relief of terminal breathlessness is important:

- no patient should die with distressing breathlessness

- failure to relieve terminal breathlessness is a failure to utilize drug treatment correctly

- give an opioid with a sedative-anxiolytic parenterally, e.g. diamorphine/morphine and midazolam by CSCI and p.r.n.

- if the patient becomes agitated or confused (sometimes aggravated by midazolam), haloperidol or levomepromazine should be added (see p.209).

Because of distress, inability to sleep and exhaustion, patients and their carers generally accept that drowsiness may need to be the price paid for greater comfort.

Unless there is overwhelming distress, sedation is not the primary aim of treatment and some patients become mentally brighter when the breathlessness is reduced. However, because increasing drowsiness is generally a feature of the deteriorating clinical condition, it is important to stress the gravity of the situation and the aims of treatment to the relatives.

Cough

Coughing helps to clear the central airways of foreign material, secretions or pus and should generally be encouraged. It is pathological when ineffective and when it adversely affects sleep, rest, eating and social activity. It may cause embarrassment, exhaustion, muscle strain, rib or vertebral fracture, vomiting, syncope, headache, urinary incontinence or retinal haemorrhage.

Cough effectiveness is reduced by factors which:

- decrease expiratory pressure and airflow, i.e. respiratory or abdominal muscle weakness

- increase mucus tenacity, i.e. reduce the water content of secretions

- decrease mucociliary function, e.g. smoking, infection.

In patients with cancer, the prevalence of cough is 50–80%, and is highest in patients with lung cancer.[41]

Pathogenesis

Cough is caused by mechanical and/or chemical stimulation of:

- rapidly adapting myelinated stretch ('irritant') and C-fibre receptors in the airway

- other structures innervated by the vagi, trigeminal and phrenic nerves.

Afferent inputs terminate in the nucleus tractus solitarius within the brain stem (Figure 4.5). Input from higher centres allows cough to be voluntarily induced or suppressed.[9,42,43]

Acid reflux can cause cough via a vagally-mediated bronchoconstrictor reflex or by macro- or micro-aspiration into the airways. Typical symptoms of reflux are often absent and may occur predominantly during the day when upright.

In COPD, cough is caused by inflammation and/or the need to eliminate large volumes of bronchial secretions. Because ciliary clearance of mucus is slow in COPD, coughing helps to clear secretions even if it seems non-productive.

ACE inhibitors cause a dry cough in <10% of patients either immediately or after weeks/months of use. Inhibition of angiotensin-converting enzyme prevents inactivation of inflammatory mediators which cumulate and increase the sensitivity of the cough reflex. Confirmation of the diagnosis is by resolution of the cough within 4 weeks of discontinuing the ACE inhibitor. In many patients, the severity and frequency of the cough is reduced by aspirin.[44]

Evaluation

The commonest cause of acute cough is respiratory tract infection (Box 4.D). In advanced cancer chronic cough is most likely due to endobronchial tumour within the central airways.

Is the cough wet or dry?

A wet cough usually serves a physiological purpose and expectoration should be encouraged. A dry cough serves no purpose and should be suppressed. A wet cough distressing a dying patient who is too weak to expectorate should also be suppressed with antitussives (Figure 4.6).[9]

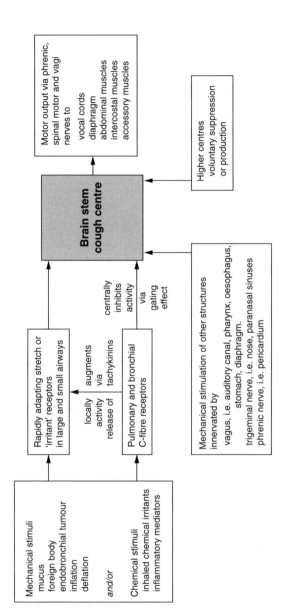

Figure 4.5 The cough reflex.

Box 4.D   Causes of cough in patients with cancer

Cardiopulmonary
Postnasal drip
Smoking
Asthma
COPD
Cardiac failure
Chest infection
Tumour
  endobronchial
    airway infiltration, distortion,
    obstruction
  lung parenchyma
    airway distortion, obstruction
    lymphangitis carcinomatosis
  mediastinum
  pleura, pericardium
  pleural effusion
Tracheo-oesophageal fistula
Vocal cord paralysis

Oesophageal
Gastro-oesophageal reflux

Aspiration
Gastro-oesophageal reflux
Bulbar muscle weakness
Neuromuscular incoordination

Treatment
Chemotherapy
  e.g. bleomycin, methotrexate,
  cyclophosphamide
Radiotherapy, dose-related
  pneumonitis in 5–15% (early onset)
  fibrosis (late onset, >6 months)
ACE inhibitors
Nitrofurantoin
β-blockers

Is the cough caused by the cancer?

It is generally obvious when the cough is caused by the cancer. Associated features such as episodic wheezing (asthma) or heartburn (gastro-oesophageal reflux) suggest an alternative cause.[45] Appropriate investigations may include:

- chest radiograph
- sputum culture
- spirometry (pre-and post-bronchodilator)
- sinus radiographs
- barium swallow.

Common causes, alone or in combination, include:

- postnasal drip syndrome
- asthma
- gastro-oesophageal reflux
- COPD.

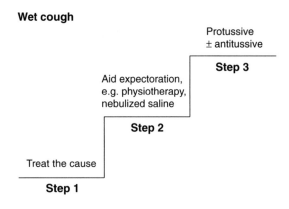

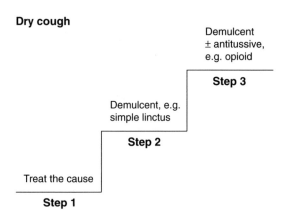

Figure 4.6   3-step therapeutic ladders for cough.

Can the cancer be modified?

Radiotherapy (teletherapy or endobronchial brachytherapy) improves cough in 50–60% of patients.[46] Other options may include chemotherapy, hormone therapy or surgery. If in doubt, seek advice from an oncologist.

Can the impact of the cancer be modified?

For example, by inserting an endobronchial stent or draining a pleural effusion.

Management

Correct the correctable

Ideally, antitussive therapy should be specific, i.e. directed at the underlying cause or the presumed mechanism responsible for cough (Table 4.3). Non-specific therapy is given when the underlying cause of the cough is not amenable to treatment or is unknown (Figure 4.6).

Wet cough

Non-drug treatment

- advise how to cough efficiently; it is impossible to cough effectively lying on your back
- physiotherapy
- steam inhalations.

A forced expiration (a huff) from a low–medium lung volume:

- is effective in clearing secretions
- is better tolerated than the assisted cough manoeuvre (involves compressing the lower thorax and abdomen with the hands)
- requires less effort for the patient
- can be augmented by postural drainage.[47]

Drug treatment

Avoid antitussives (cough suppressants) if possible, although these may be necessary to ensure sleep at night and to prevent exhaustion during the day. If used, the aim is to make expectoration more effective and less tiring.

There is a wide range of protussives (expectorants) (Box 4.E). In practice, it is best to limit choice to a few preferred drugs:

- nebulized 0.9% saline, 2.5ml q.d.s., p.r.n. and before physiotherapy
- an irritant mucolytic, which produces a greater volume but less tenacious secretions, e.g. guaifenesin, ipecacuanha or squill
- a chemical mucolytic, which reduces the viscosity of secretions, e.g. carbocisteine 750mg t.d.s.

Nebulized 0.9% saline is generally sufficient.

Table 4.3 Correctable causes of cough

Cause	Treatment
Smoking cigarettes	Stop smoking; median time to improvement = 4 weeks
Postnasal drip	
allergic rhinitis	Nasal corticosteroid ± sodium cromoglicate
	Antihistamine; second-generation antihistamines are non-sedating but are less drying than the older sedative antimuscarinic antihistamines
perennial and postinfection rhinitis	Antihistamine ± decongestant
vasomotor rhinitis	Nasal ipratropium bromide
bacterial sinusitis	Antibiotic ± decongestant ± nasal corticosteroid (acute) ± antihistamine (chronic)
Asthma	Bronchodilators ± corticosteroids
Gastro-oesophageal reflux	Avoid coffee, smoking or drugs which decrease lower oesophageal sphincter tone Prokinetic agent, increases oesophageal sphincter tone PPI to reduce gastric acid
COPD	Stop smoking Bronchodilators, e.g. ipratropium bromide Corticosteroids?

ACE inhibitor	Discontinue the ACE inhibitor; if not possible, substitute an angiotensin-II receptor antagonist, e.g. losartan
	Alternatively, consider:
	  aspirin 600mg o.m.; anti-platelet doses, e.g. 75–150mg o.m., are ineffective[44]
	  nifedipine; acts via an inhibitory effect on PG synthesis
	  theophylline
	  baclofen
	  sodium cromoglicate by inhaler

Opioid antitussives act centrally by facilitating serotonergic mechanisms which inhibit the release of glutamate, an excitatory amino acid from the afferent fibres originating in the airways. Calcium channels are also involved;

Box 4.E   Drugs for cough

Protussives	**Antitussives**
Topical mucolytics	*Peripheral*
Nebulized 0.9% saline	Simple linctus
Chemical inhalations	Benzonatate (not UK)
compound benzoin tincture (Friar's balsam)	Nebulized bupivacaine
carbol	
menthol and eucalyptus	*Central*
	Non-opioids
Irritant mucolytics	iso-aminile
Ammonium chloride	Opioid derivatives
Guaifenesin	dextromethorphan
Ipecacuanha	levopropoxyphene (not UK)
Potassium iodide	pholcodine
Squill	Opioids
Terpin hydrate	codeine
	dihydrocodeine
Chemical mucolytics	hydrocodone (not UK)
Acetylcysteine (not UK)	hydromorphone
Carbocisteine	morphine
	methadone

---

calcium-channel blockers and opioids both close calcium channels and in animals have a synergistic antitussive effect.[48]

Cough efficacy in patients with cystic fibrosis or bronchiectasis is increased by nebulized:

- hypertonic saline (commonly 6–7%, range 3–12%)

- amiloride[49]

- terbutaline after physiotherapy.[50]

Dry cough

Drug treatment

When the cause is not amenable to specific treatment or is unknown, measures should be taken to suppress the cough (Figure 4.6). If a locally soothing demulcent, e.g. simple linctus BP 5ml t.d.s.–q.d.s., is inadequate, prescribe a centrally-acting antitussive, for example:

- codeine linctus 5–10ml (15–30mg) t.d.s.–q.d.s.

- morphine solution 2.5–5mg q.d.s.–q4h.

The dose of morphine is titrated up as necessary or until unacceptable adverse effects occur. *If a patient is already receiving a strong opioid for pain relief it is nonsense to prescribe codeine or a second strong opioid for cough suppression.*

Some centres use nebulized local anaesthetics. These act by anaesthetising sensory nerves involved in the cough reflex. Their use is limited by:

- an unpleasant taste

- oropharyngeal numbness

- risk of bronchoconstriction

- a short duration of action (10–30min).[43]

The use of nebulized local anaesthetics in patients with cough caused by cancer has not been evaluated and should be used only when other measures have failed. Suggested doses are 2% lidocaine 5ml or 0.25% bupivacaine 5ml (q6h–q8h).[36]

Other possible treatments include:

- sodium cromoglicate, 10mg inhaled q.d.s. improves cough in patients with lung cancer within 36–48h[51]

- levodropropizine, 75mg PO t.d.s. is as effective as dihydrocodeine 10mg PO t.d.s. in patients with lung cancer and causes less drowsiness (not UK)[52]

- baclofen, 10mg PO t.d.s. or 20mg PO o.d. has an antitussive effect in healthy volunteers; 2–4 weeks of therapy is required to attain maximal effect[53]

- cough suppressants with local anaesthetic effects
  benzonatate 100–200mg PO t.d.s. improves cough in patients with cancer (not UK)[54]
  mexiletine 300mg PO reduces cough sensitivity but the clinical relevance is unknown.[55]

Bronchorrhoea

Bronchorrhoea is defined as the production of >100ml of sputum per day. It sometimes occurs as a late feature in bronchiolo-alveolar cell cancer. In this uncommon form of lung cancer, the tumour cells 'coat' the bronchiolar surfaces and cause mucosal inflammation. This results in the production of massive amounts of mucus in the affected areas.

Management

The inflammatory response in the bronchioles is said to be reduced by:

- oral or inhaled corticosteroids
- nebulized furosemide 20mg q.d.s.
- nebulized indometacin 25mg in 2ml q4h–q8h (pH corrected to 7.4 with sodium bicarbonate); this may work even if corticosteroids fail[56]
- macrolide antibiotics, e.g. erythromycin, clarithromycin.[57]

Anecdotal reports suggest that an antisecretory drug, e.g. hyoscine butyl-bromide or glycopyrrolate, may also be of benefit.

Pleural effusion

A small amount of fluid (20–30ml) is present in the pleural space for lubrication. It is produced by capillaries and is removed by lymphatics in the parietal inter-stitium and pleura at a rate of 100–200ml daily. These lymphatics ultimately drain into the mediastinal lymph nodes. A pleural effusion forms as a result of excess production and/or reduced resorption of fluid. The latter is most likely in malignant pleural effusion with tumour obstructing lymphatic trans-port in the pleura or regional lymph nodes. Effusions may be classified as exudates or transudates (Table 4.4). Over 95% of malignant pleural effusions are exudates.

Pleural effusions cause breathlessness as a result of:

- chest wall and diaphragm displacement, weakening respiratory muscles
- lung compression, causing ventilation–perfusion mismatch
- hypoxia.

There may also be associated cough and chest pain.

Almost 50% of patients with advanced cancer develop a pleural effusion. Most will be in patients with cancer of the lung, breast or ovary and lymphoma. Median survival for patients with malignant pleural effusion ranges from 3–12 months and is dependent upon type of cancer and the response to anticancer therapies. A low pleural fluid pH (<7.3) and/or glucose (<3.3mmol/L) is asso-ciated with more extensive pleural disease and a mean survival of 2 months.[58]

Table 4.4   Classification of pleural effusions

	Exudate	Transudate
Distinguishing features		
Protein content	>30g/L	<30g/L
Pleural fluid to serum protein ratio	>0.5	<0.5
Lactose dehydrogenase (LDH)	>200 IU	<200 IU
Pleural fluid to serum LDH ratio	>0.6	<0.6
pH	<7.3	>7.3
RBC count	>100 000mm³	<100 000mm³
WBC count	>1000mm³	<1000mm³
Glucose	Low (infection) Very low (<3.3mmol/L in cancer)	Similar to plasma glucose
Common causes		
	Cancer pleural infiltration lymphatic obstruction lymphangitis carcinomatosa venous obstruction	Cardiac failure Renal failure
	Pneumonia	
	Local pleural disease	

Evaluation

Clinical examination will detect effusions >500ml. Useful investigations include:

- chest radiographs, detect effusions >200ml

- ultrasound, helpful when there is difficulty in distinguishing pleural fluid from tumour or collapse of the lung

- cytological and biochemical examination, carried out if there is diagnostic uncertainty (Table 4.4).

Management

Treatment depends on the severity of symptoms (Table 4.5). Small asymptomatic effusions are best only monitored.

Table 4.5   Management of pleural effusion

Thoracocentesis	Drainage and pleurodesis
Preferred option when poor prognosis (<8 weeks)	Preferred option when prognosis longer (>8 weeks)
Differences	
Relatively straightforward for operator and patient	Greater operator experience required and greater inconvenience to patient
Can be carried out as an outpatient	Requires inpatient admission
Repeat treatments likely because only 1–1.5L removed short time to recurrence (50% within 4 days; 97% within 4 weeks)	Long-term control likely (>50%)[59] Tube may kink or block
May paradoxically worsen ventilation–perfusion mismatch and increase hypoxia	Rapid drainage may lead to re-expansion pulmonary oedema
Similarities	
Both may lead to pneumothorax, haemothorax, empyema fluid loculation, making further intervention difficult tumour seedling in the chest wall	

Correct the correctable

Specific anticancer treatment if available. Consider other common causes of pleural effusion, e.g. pneumonia, pulmonary embolism, cardiac failure, and treat appropriately.

Can the impact of the cancer be modified?

Large symptomatic effusions should be drained. Removal of only 500ml of fluid may provide rapid relief. In patients with a poor prognosis, e.g.

<8 weeks, or those who decline chest tube drainage, the effusion may be removed by aspiration (thoracocentesis). For all other patients, chest tube drainage and medical pleurodesis should be considered (Table 4.5). Small-bore (8–14F) catheters are increasingly being used, inserted under ultrasound scan guidance. They are as effective as the traditional large-bore intercostal tubes (24–32F), and are better tolerated.

Medical pleurodesis involves the instillation of an irritant agent into the pleural cavity to induce inflammation which in turn causes adhesion of the pleural layers, thereby obliterating the pleural space. To be successful it requires:

- removal of enough effusion to allow the lung to re-expand

- good dispersal of the irritant agent.

Suction is occasionally required to achieve complete lung re-expansion. A gradual increase in pressure up to 20cm H_2O should be applied using a high volume, low pressure system. Commonly used irritant agents in stated order of effectiveness include:

- talc slurry 5g

- bleomycin 60 IU

- doxycycline ⩾500mg (tetracycline has recently been withdrawn).

The above are added to 50ml of 0.9% saline. The tube should not be clamped and, if the lung has re-expanded, it is not necessary to rotate the patient.[60]

Adverse effects include chest pain and fever. Pain should be managed by the instillation into the pleural space of 25ml of lidocaine 1% (250mg) 10min beforehand together with systemic analgesia.[61] The tube should be removed within 72h if the lung remains fully expanded and fluid drainage is <200ml daily. *Concurrent use of corticosteroids reduces the likelihood of success.*

The drainage of loculated effusions may be helped by intrapleural streptokinase 250 000 IU b.d. or urokinase 100 000 IU o.d. in 30–100ml of 0.9% saline. These degrade fibrin and thereby disrupt adhesions. Improvement is generally seen within 3 days. Some patients become pyrexial after streptokinase but not after urokinase which is not antigenic. Haemorrhagic complications have not been reported.[59,62,63]

Patients with a reasonable prognosis with loculated or recurrent effusions despite drainage and medical pleurodesis can be considered for video-assisted thoracoscopy and talc instillation with an atomiser (poudrage). This prevents recurrence in >90% of patients and has superseded surgical pleurectomy.

Pleuroperitoneal shunts and indwelling pleural catheters may have to be considered for recurrent pleural effusions or when the lung fails to re-inflate (trapped lung) making pleurodesis impossible. Trapped lung may be caused by:

- a thick visceral peel

- pleural loculations

- proximal large airway obstruction

- a persistent pneumothorax.

Lymphangitis carcinomatosa

Lymphangitis carcinomatosa is a term used to describe the diffuse infiltration of lymphatics of the lungs by cancer cells. Clinically it is characterized by increasing breathlessness and cough ± pleuritic chest pain and central cyanosis. Prognosis is poor with a median survival of 3 months from presentation; only 10% survive longer than 10 months.[64]

Physiology

Lymphatic channels in the lungs follow the bronchi, the pulmonary arterial and venous system and form an extensive network in the pleura. These become distended with tumour cells causing lymph stasis which in turn stimulates fibrosis and smooth muscle proliferation.

Evaluation

Chest radiographs

These are generally abnormal but not always diagnostic. Abnormalities reflecting lymphatics permeated with tumour cells, fibrous tissue or oedema include:

- small nodular opacities, 1–5mm with hazy border

- a diffuse reticular pattern

- a combination of the above (reticulonodular)

- Kerley A lines <1mm thick, straight >2cm, pointing towards hilum and not touching the pleura

- Kerley B lines <1mm thick, straight <2cm, perpendicular to and touching the pleura (reflects peripheral septal thickening)

- irregular thickening of interlobular septal lines associated with tumour cells, fibrous tissue or oedema.[65]

Hilar lymphadenopathy and/or pleural effusions may also be present.

CT

High resolution CT 1.5mm in thickness increases diagnostic accuracy.[66]

Pulmonary function tests

These show a restrictive ventilatory disturbance, i.e. vital capacity, residual volume, total lung capacity, diffusing capacity for carbon monoxide and pulmonary compliance all reduced. Tidal volume is also reduced and the respiratory rate increases. Reduced compliance increases the work of breathing. Hypoxia is common because of impaired gas exchange from involvement of the alveolar capillary membrane by tumour and interstitial oedema associated with impaired lymphatic drainage.[67]

Management

Correct the correctable

Can the cancer be modified?

Chemotherapy or hormonal therapy in responsive tumours improves survival by 6–30 months.[64]

Can the impact of the cancer be modified?

Corticosteroids, e.g. dexamethasone 4–8mg PO o.d., may improve the breathlessness with an objective improvement in lung function. Give initially on a trial basis for 1 week.

Theoretically diuretics may reduce alveolar membrane congestion. Furosemide 20–40mg PO stat is used at some centres on presentation; if benefit is seen ≤4h, it is continued o.m. indefinitely.

Drug treatment

Benzodiazepines often help patients who are breathless at rest, and can be given concurrently with dexamethasone. PO morphine should be considered (*see* p.376). Oxygen is administered to correct hypoxia.

Death rattle

Death rattle is a term used to describe a rattling noise produced by secretions in the hypopharynx oscillating in time with inspiration and expiration. Generally death rattle is seen only in patients who are extremely weak and close to death. It occurs in 30–50% of patients and is distressing for relatives, carers and other patients.[68]

Management

If the patient is not distressed by the secretions the treatment is purely cosmetic, i.e. for the benefit of the relatives, other patients and staff.

Non-drug treatment

* support of those in attendance; the most effective measure for easing the family's disquiet is explanation that the semiconscious or unconscious patient is not distressed by the rattle[68,69]

* position semiprone to encourage postural drainage

* oropharyngeal suction.

Most patients dislike suctioning; generally this should be reserved for unconscious patients.

Drug treatment

An antimuscarinic antisecretory drug needs to be given promptly because it does not affect existing pharyngeal secretions (Table 4.6). Such drugs are probably most effective for rattle associated with the pooling of saliva in the pharynx and least effective for rattle caused by bronchial secretions (as a result of infection or oedema) or related to the reflux of gastric contents.

Table 4.6 Antisecretory drugs for death rattle

Drug	Stat SC dose	CSCI rate/24h
Hyoscine hydrobromide	0.4–0.6mg	1.2–2.4mg
Hyoscine butylbromide	20mg	20–40mg
Glycopyrrolate	0.2–0.4mg	0.6–1.2mg

The efficacy of hyoscine hydrobromide, hyoscine butylbromide or glyco-pyrrolate appears similar with the rattle reduced in 1/2–2/3 of patients.[68] However, the onset of action of glycopyrrolate is slower than with hyoscine hydrobromide.[70] Further, hyoscine hydrobromide crosses the blood-brain barrier and possesses anti-emetic and sedative properties; this is reflected in a reduced need for analgesic, anti-emetic and sedative medication.[70] Any potential cost savings with hyoscine butylbromide and glycopyrrolate are largely illusory.[70,71]

Noisy tachypnoea in the moribund

Noisy tachypnoea in the moribund is distressing for the family and other patients, even though the patient is not aware. It represents a desperate last attempt by a patient's body to respond to irreversible terminal respiratory failure ± airway obstruction.

Management

Drug treatment

Consider alleviating the noise by reducing the depth and rate of respiration to 10–15/min with IV diamorphine/morphine. It may be necessary to give double or treble the previously satisfactory analgesic dose. Rarely, there is associated heaving of the shoulders and chest; in this case, midazolam should be given as well, e.g. 10mg SC stat and hourly as needed.

Cheyne-Stokes respiration

Cheyne-Stokes respiration is an eponymous term use to describe recurrent apnoea alternating with a crescendo–diminuendo pattern of tidal volume. Nocturnal Cheyne-Stokes respiration is commonly associated with congestive cardiac failure (present in about 50% of patients) and may contribute to symptoms such as orthopnoea, paroxysmal nocturnal dyspnoea, insomnia and excessive daytime sleepiness.[72] Its presence during the day is associated with a poor prognosis.[73] Cheyne-Stokes respiration is also seen after strokes and in sporadic cases of brain stem degeneration or injury.[74–76] In advanced cancer, it is mostly seen in moribund patients, possibly as a result of brain stem hypoxia.

Physiology

Hypoxia induces unstable breathing primarily through the increase in the peripheral chemoreceptor gain to CO_2, with associated direct depression of the respiratory centre (known as hypoxic ventilatory depression).[77] There is a secondary increase in muscle sympathetic nerve activity.[78]

In congestive cardiac failure, increased pulmonary vagal afferent traffic and increased sympathetic activity induce hyperventilation leading to a fall in $PaCO_2$ to a level which triggers apnoea. The $PaCO_2$ subsequently increases and stimulates the peripheral chemoreceptors causing a further episode of hyperventilation.

Management

Congestive cardiac failure

- treat the underlying heart failure
- administer nocturnal oxygen[79]
- consider continuous positive airway pressure (CPAP)[80]
- if distressing during daytime, consider aminophylline.[76,81]

Moribund patients

No specific treatment is necessary.

Hiccup

Hiccup is a pathological respiratory reflex characterized by spasm of the diaphragm, resulting in sudden inspiration followed by abrupt closure of the glottis.

Causes

There are innumerable potential causes of hiccup. In advanced cancer, the following account for most cases:

- gastric distension
- gastro-oesophageal reflux

- diaphragmatic irritation
- phrenic nerve irritation
- toxicity
  uraemia and other biochemical disturbances
  fever, infection
- CNS tumour.

Of these, gastric distension probably accounts for most cases.

Acute management options

Pharyngeal stimulation

This triggers a 'gating' mechanism which inhibits hiccup. Most of 'granny's remedies' for hiccup involve pharyngeal stimulation either directly or indirectly, for example:

- rapidly ingest two heaped teaspoons of granulated sugar
- rapidly ingest two glasses of liqueur
- swallow dry bread
- swallow crushed ice
- drink from the wrong side of a cup
- a cold key dropped inside the back of one's shirt or blouse
- someone shouts 'Boo!' loudly in order to produce a startle response.[82]

Medical variations include:

- nebulized 0.9% saline (2ml over 5min)[83]
- forceful tongue traction sufficient to induce a gag reflex
- a nasogastric tube inserted as far as the oropharynx and oscillated (Figure 4.7).[84]

Massage of the junction between hard and soft palate with a cotton bob is also an effective gating mechanism.[85]

Reduce gastric distension

- peppermint water facilitates belching by relaxing the lower oesophageal sphincter (an old-fashioned remedy)

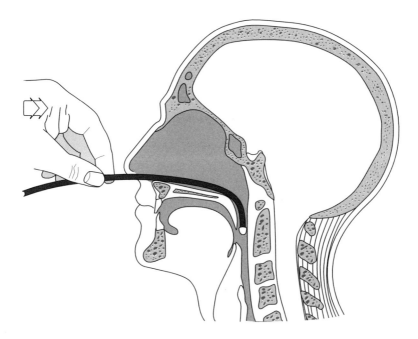

Figure 4.7 Pharyngeal stimulation to stop hiccup. A nasal catheter is inserted 8–12cm so that it is opposite the second cervical vertebrae. Jerky to-and-fro movements lead to the immediate cessation of hiccup. Afferent innervation = vagus and glossopharyngeal nerves. Reproduced with permission from Salem *et al.*, 1967.[84]

- antiflatulent, e.g. Asilone 10ml (a proprietary antacid containing dimeticone)
- metoclopramide 10mg (tightens the lower oesophageal sphincter and hastens gastric emptying).

Peppermint water and metoclopramide should not be used concurrently.

Elevation of $PaCO_2$

This inhibits processing of the hiccup reflex in the brain stem:

- rebreathing from a paper bag
- breath holding.

Muscle relaxant

- baclofen 5mg PO

- nifedipine 10mg PO/SL
- midazolam 2mg IV, followed by 1–2mg increments every 3–5min.

All of these also have central suppressant effects.

Central suppression of the hiccup reflex

Blockade of dopamine or the potentiation of GABA.

Dopamine antagonists:

- metoclopramide as above
- haloperidol 5–10mg PO or IV if no response
- chlorpromazine 10–25mg PO or IV if no response.

GABA agonists:

- baclofen as above
- sodium valproate 200–500mg PO.

Maintenance treatment

Gastric distension

- antiflatulent, e.g. Asilone 10ml q.d.s. and/or
- prokinetic, e.g. metoclopramide 10mg q.d.s.

Gastro-oesophageal reflux

- prokinetic and/or
- H_2-receptor antagonist, PPI.

Diaphragmatic irritation or other cause

- baclofen 5–20mg t.d.s., occasionally more[86,87]
- nifedipine 10–20mg t.d.s., occasionally more[88,89]
- haloperidol 1.5–3mg o.n.[90,91]
- sodium valproate, aim for 15mg/kg/24h in divided doses[92]
- midazolam 10–60mg/24h by CSCI if all else fails.[93]

References

1   American Thoracic Society (1999) Dyspnea, mechanisms, assessment and management: a consensus statement. *American Journal of Respiratory and Critical Care Medicine.* **159**:321–40.

2   Reuben DB and Mor V (1986) Dyspnoea in terminally ill cancer patients. *Chest.* **89**:234–6.

3   Reuben DB *et al.* (1988) Clinical symptoms and length of survival in patients with terminal cancer. *Archives of Internal Medicine.* **148**:1586–91.

4   Bianchi A *et al.* (1995) Central control of breathing in mammals: neuronal circuitry, membrane properties, and neurotransmitters. *Physiological Reviews.* **75**:1–45.

5   Dudgeon D and Lertzman M (1999) Dyspnea in the advanced cancer patient. *Journal of Pain and Symptom Management.* **16**:212–19.

6   O'Driscoll M *et al.* (1999) The experience of breathlessness in lung cancer. *European Journal of Cancer Care.* **8**:37–43.

7   Davis C (1997) Breathlessness, cough, and other respiratory problems. *British Medical Journal.* **315**:931–4.

8   Morita T *et al.* (1999) Survival prediction of terminally ill cancer patients by clinical symptoms: development of a simple indicator. *Japanese Journal of Clinical Oncology.* **29**:156–9.

9   Wilcock A (1998) The management of respiratory symptoms. In: C Faull, Y Carter and R Woof (eds) *The Handbook of Palliative Care.* Blackwell Scientific, London, pp 157–76.

10 Corner J and O'Driscoll M (1999) Development of a breathless assessment guide for use in palliative care. *Palliative Medicine.* **13**:375–84.

11 Bredin M *et al.* (1999) Multicentre randomized controlled trial of nursing intervention for breathlessness in patients with lung cancer. *British Medical Journal.* **318**:901–4.

12 Connolly M and O'Neill J (1999) Teaching a research-based approach to the management of breathlessness in patients with lung cancer. *European Journal of Cancer Care.* **8**:30–6.

13 Breslin E (1995) Breathing retraining in chronic obstructive pulmonary disease. *Journal of Cardiopulmonary Rehabilitation.* **15**:25–33.

14 British Thoracic Society (1997) BTS guidelines for the management of chronic obstructive pulmonary disease. *Thorax.* **52**:S1–S28.

15 Congelton J and Meurs M (1995) The incidence of airflow obstruction in bronchial carcinoma, its relation to breathlessness and response to bronchodilator therapy. *Respiratory Medicine.* **89**:291–6.

16 Janssens J-P *et al.* (2000) Management of dyspnea in severe chronic obstructive pulmonary disease. *Journal of Pain and Symptom Management.* **19**:378–92.

17 Heijden Hvd *et al.* (1996) Pharmacotherapy of respiratory muscles in chronic obstructive pulmonary disease. *Respiratory Medicine.* **90**:513–22.

18 Allard P *et al.* (1999) How effective are supplementary doses of opioids for dyspnea in terminally ill cancer patients? A randomized continuous sequential clinical trial. *Journal of Pain and Symptom Management.* **17**:256–65.

19 Bruera E *et al.* (1993) Subcutaneous morphine for dyspnoea in cancer patients. *Annals of Internal Medicine.* **119**:906–7.

20   Boyd K and Kelly M (1997) Oral morphine as symptomatic treatment of dyspnoea in patients with advanced cancer. *Palliative Medicine* **11**:277–81.

21   Mazzocato C *et al.* (1999) The effects of morphine on dyspnoea and ventilatory function in elderly patients with advanced cancer: A randomized double-blind controlled trial. *Annals of Oncology.* **10**:1511–14.

22   Bruera E *et al.* (1990) Effects of morphine on the dyspnea of terminal cancer patients. *Journal of Pain and Symptom Management.* **5**:341–4.

23   Davis C (1995) The role of nebulized drugs in palliating respiratory symptoms of malignant disease. *European Journal of Palliative Care.* **2**:9–15.

24   Quelch P *et al.* (1997) Nebulized opioids in the treatment of dyspnea. *Journal of Palliative Care.* **13**:48–52.

25   Zeppetella G (1997) Nebulized morphine in the palliation of dyspnoea. *Palliative Medicine.* **11**:267–75.

26   Ahmedzai S and Davis C (1997) Nebulised drugs in palliative care. *Thorax.* **52**:S75–S77.

27   Davis C *et al.* (1996) Single dose randomized controlled trial of nebulized morphine in patients with cancer related breathlessness. *Palliative Medicine.* **10**:64–5.

28   Lang E and Jedeikin R (1998) Acute respiratory depression as a complication of nebulised morphine. *Canadian Journal of Anaesthesia.* **45**:60–2.

29   Davis C (1999) Nebulized opioids should not be prescribed outside a clinical trial. *American Journal of Hospice and Palliative Care.* **16**:543.

30   Rapoport D *et al.* (1991) Differing effects of the anxiolytic agents buspirone and diazepam on control of breathing. *Clinical Pharmacology and Therapeutics.* **49**:394–401.

31   Smoller J *et al.* (1996) Panic anxiety, dyspnea, and respiratory disease. Theoretical and clinical considerations. *American Journal of Respiratory and Critical Care Medicine.* **54**:6–17.

32   Argyopoulou P *et al.* (1993) Buspirone effect on breathlessness and exercise performance in patients with chronic obstructive pulmonary disease. *Respiration.* **60**:216–20.

33   Singh N *et al.* (1993) Effects of buspirone on anxiety levels and exercise tolerance in patients with chronic airflow obstruction and mild anxiety. *Chest.* **103**:800–4.

34   Datta A *et al.* (1994) Palliation of breathlessness in patients with COAD and anxiety without provoking sedation or respiratory depression. *Progress in Palliative Care.* **2**:11.

35   McIver B *et al.* (1994) The use of chlorpromazine for symptom control in dying cancer patients. *Journal of Pain and Symptom Management.* **9**:341–5.

36   Ahmedzai S (1997) Palliation of respiratory symptoms. In: D Doyle, G Hanks and N MacDonald (eds) *Oxford Textbook of Palliative Medicine.* Oxford University Press, Oxford, pp 583–616.

37   Royal College of Physicians of London (1999) *Domiciliary Oxygen Therapy Services.* Royal College of Physicians. London.

38   Bruera E *et al.* (1993) Effects of oxygen on dyspnoea in hypoxaemic terminal cancer patients. *Lancet.* **342**:13–14.

39   Booth S *et al.* (1996) Does oxygen help dyspnea in patients with cancer? *American Journal of Respiratory and Critical Care Medicine.* **153**:1515–18.

40   Boorstein J *et al.* (1989) Using helium-oxygen mixtures in the emergency management of acute upper airway obstruction. *Annals of Emergency Medicine.* **18**:688–90.

41 Meurs M and Round C (1993) Palliation of symptoms in non-small cell lung cancer: a study by the Yorkshire Regional Cancer Organisation thoracic group. *Thorax*. **48**:339–43.

42 Widdicombe J (1995) Neurophysiology of the cough reflex. *European Respiratory Journal*. **8**:1193–202.

43 Fuller R and Jackson D (1990) Physiology and treatment of cough. *Thorax*. **45**:425–30.

44 Tenenbaum A *et al*. (2000) Intermediate but not low doses of aspirin can suppress angiotensin-converting enzyme inhibitor-induced cough. *American Journal of Hypertension*. **13**:776–82.

45 Mello C *et al*. (1996) Predictive values of the character, timing, and complications of chronic cough in diagnosing its cause. *Archives of Internal Medicine*. **156**: 997–1003.

46 Awan A and Weichselbaum R (1990) Palliative radiotherapy. *Haematology/ Oncology Clinics of North America*. **4**:1169–81.

47 Irwin R *et al*. (1993) Appropriate use of antitussives and protussives. A practical review. *Drugs*. **46**:80–91.

48 Kamei J (1995) Recent advances in neuropharmacology of the centrally acting antitussive drugs. *Methods and Findings: Experimental and Clinical Pharmacology*. **17**:193–205.

49 App E *et al*. (1990) Acute and long-term amiloride inhalation in cystic fibrosis lung disease: a rational approach to cystic fibrosis therapy. *American Review of Respiratory Disease*. **141**:605–12.

50 Irwin R *et al*. (1998) Managing cough as a defense mechanism and as a symptom. A consensus panel report of the American College of Chest Physicians. *Chest*. **114**:133s–181s.

51 Moroni M *et al*. (1996) Inhaled sodium cromoglycate to treat cough in advanced lung cancer patients. *British Journal of Cancer*. **74**:309–11.

52 Luporini G *et al*. (1998) Efficacy and safety of levodropropizine and dihydrocodeine on nonproductive cough in primary and metastatic lung cancer. *European Respiratory Journal*. **12**:97–101.

53 Dicpinigaitis P *et al*. (1998) Inhibition of capsaicin-induced cough by the gamma-aminobutyric acid agonist baclofen. *Journal of Clinical Pharmacology*. **38**:364–7.

54 Doona M and Walsh D (1997) Benzonatate for opioid-resistant cough in advanced cancer. *Palliative Medicine*. **16**:212–19.

55 Fujimura M *et al*. (2000) Effect of oral mexiletine on the cough response to capsaicin and tartaric acid. *Thorax*. **55**:126–8.

56 Tamaoki J *et al*. (2000) Inhaled indomethacin in bronchorrhoea in bronchiolo-alveolar carcinoma: role of cyclo-oxygenase. *Chest*. **117**:1213–14.

57 Hiratsuka T *et al*. (1998) Severe bronchorrhoea accompanying alveolar cell carcinoma: treatment with clarithromycin and inhaled beclomethasone (Japanese). *Nikon Kokyuki Gakkai Zasshi*. **36**:482–7.

58 Sanchez-Armengol A and Rodriguez-Panadero F (1993) Survival and talc pleurodesis in metastatic pleural carcinoma, revisited. Report of 125 cases. *Chest*. **104**:1482–5.

59 Stretton F *et al*. (1999) Malignant pleural effusions. *European Journal of Palliative Care*. **6**:5–9.

60 Dryzer S *et al*. (1993) A comparison of rotation and non-rotation in tetracycline pleurodesis. *Chest*. **104**:1763–6.

61   Sherman S *et al.* (1988) Optimum anaesthesia with intrapleural lidocaine during chemical pleurodesis with tetracycline. *Chest.* **93**:533–6.

62   Erasmus J and Patz E (1999) Treatment of malignant pleural effusions. *Current Opinion in Pulmonary Medicine.* **5**:250–5.

63   Davies C *et al.* (1999) Intrapleural streptokinase in the management of malignant multiloculated pleural effusions. *Chest.* **115**:729–33.

64   Bruce D *et al.* (1996) Lymphangitis carcinomatosa: a literature review. *Journal of the Royal College of Surgeons (Edinburgh).* **41**:7–13.

65   Trapnell D (1964) Radiological appearances of lymphangitis carcinomatosa. *Thorax.* **19**:251–60.

66   Stein M *et al.* (1987) Pulmonary lymphangitic spread of carcinoma: appearance on CT scans. *Radiology.* **162**:371–5.

67   Emirgil C (1964) Effect of metastatic carcinoma to the lung on pulmonary function in man. *American Journal of Medicine.* **36**:382–94.

68   Hughes A *et al.* (2000) Audit of three antimuscarinic drugs for managing retained secretions. *Palliative Medicine.* **14**:221–2.

69   Hughes A *et al.* (1997) Management of 'death rattle'. *Palliative Medicine.* **11**: 80–1.

70   Back I *et al.* (2001) An audit comparing hyoscine hydrobromide and glyco-pyrrolate in the treatment of death rattle. *Palliative Medicine.* In press.

71   Bausewein C and Twycross R (1995) Comparative cost of hyoscine. *Palliative Medicine.* **9**:256.

72   Quaranta A *et al.* (1997) Cheyne-Stokes respiration during sleep in congestive heart failure. *Chest.* **111**:467–73.

73   Andreas S *et al.* (1996) Cheyne-Stokes respiration and prognosis in congestive heart failure. *American Journal of Cardiology.* **78**:1260–4.

74   Escribano M *et al.* (1990) A case of dirhythmic breathing. *Chest.* **97**:1018–20.

75   Lalonde R and Botez M (1991) Death from bulbar involvement in Friedreich's ataxia. *Medical Hypotheses.* **36**:250–2.

76   Nachtmann A *et al.* (1995) Cheyne-Stokes respiration in ischemic stroke. *Neurology.* **45**:820–1.

77   Takahashi E and Doi K (1993) Destabilization of the respiratory control by hypoxic ventilatory depressions: a model analysis. *Japanese Journal of Physiology.* **43**: 599–612.

78   Borne van de P *et al.* (1998) Effect of Cheyne-Stokes respiration on muscle sympathetic nerve activity in severe congestive heart failure secondary to ischemic or idiopathic dilated cardiomyopathy. *American Journal of Cardiology.* **81**:432–6.

79   Andreas S *et al.* (1996) Improvement of exercise capacity with treatment of Cheyne-Stokes respiration in patients with congestive heart failure. *Journal of the American College of Cardiology.* **27**:1486–90.

80   Naughton M (1998) Pathophysiology and treatment of Cheyne-Stokes respiration. *Thorax.* **53**:514–18.

81   Tomcsanyi J and Karlocai K (1994) Effect of theophylline on periodic breathing in congestive heart failure measured by transcutaneous oxygen monitoring. *European Journal of Clinical Pharmacology.* **46**:173–4.

82   Lamphier TA (1977) Methods of management of persistent hiccup (singultus). *Maryland State Medical Journal.* **November**:80–1.

83 De-Ruysscher D *et al.* (1996) Treatment of intractable hiccup in a terminal cancer patient with nebulized saline. *Palliative Medicine.* **10**:166–7.
84 Salem MR *et al.* (1967) Treatment of hiccups by pharyngeal stimulation in anesthetized and conscious subjects. *Journal of the American Medical Association.* **202**:126–30.
85 Goldsmith A (1983) A treatment for hiccups. *Journal of the American Medical Association.* **249**:1566.
86 Ramirez FC and Graham DY (1992) Treatment of intractable hiccup with baclofen: results of a double-blind randomized, controlled, crossover study. *American Journal of Gastroenterology.* **87**:1789–91.
87 Guelaud C *et al.* (1995) Baclofen therapy for chronic hiccup. *European Respiratory Journal.* **8**:235–7.
88 Lipps DC *et al.* (1990) Nifedipine for intractable hiccups. *Neurology.* **40**:531–2.
89 Brigham B and Bolin T (1992) High dose nifedipine and fludrocortisone for intractable hiccups. *Medical Journal of Australia.* **157**:70.
90 Scarnati RA (1979) Intractable hiccup (singultus): report of case. *Journal of the American Osteopathic Association.* **79**:127–9.
91 Ives TJ *et al.* (1985) Treatment of intractable hiccups with intramuscular haloperidol. *American Journal of Psychiatry.* **142**:1368–9.
92 Jacobson P *et al.* (1981) Treatment of intractable hiccups with valproic acid. *Neurology.* **31**:1458–60.
93 Wilcock A and Twycross R (1996) Case report: midazolam for intractable hiccup. *Journal of Pain and Symptom Management.* **12**:59–61.

5   Psychological symptoms

Responses to loss · Family problems · Other problems
Anger · Anxiety · Panic disorder · Depression
The withdrawn patient · The difficult patient · Insomnia
Secondary mental disorders · Delirium

Patients with cancer experience psychological as well as physical symptoms.
The results of a survey at a major cancer centre in the USA illustrate this point
(Table 5.1). Problems are also common among patients' relatives.

Table 5.1   Common symptoms in cancer patients[1]

Physical	%	Psychological	%
Lack of energy	73	Worrying	72
Pain	63	Feeling sad	67
Drowsiness	60	Feeling nervous	62
Dry mouth	55	Difficulty sleeping	53
Nausea	45	Feeling irritable	47
Anorexia	45	Difficulty concentrating	40

Psychological problems are often overlooked by doctors and nurses. This is
partly because of selective attention to physical problems.[2] About 10% of
patients with advanced cancer have an identifiable psychiatric illness. Open
questions such as 'How are you feeling?' and 'How are you coping?' frequently
facilitates the expression of negative emotion.[3]

Some psychological problems can be prevented by:

• good staff–patient communication, giving information according to individual need. Unfortunately, staff do not always give as much information
  as patients and families want, even when asked directly

• good staff–patient relationships, with continuity of care

• allowing patients to have some control over the management of their
  illness.

Responses to loss

Many of the psychological problems seen in advanced cancer relate to actual or anticipated loss (Table 5.2). Similar psychological responses occur with major losses of any kind, e.g. redundancy, divorce, amputation, bereavement, as well as the anticipated loss of one's own life. These responses do not necessarily occur in sequence. Several may occur together and some may not occur at all. Oscillations in the patient's feelings are common. In cancer patients, more marked responses are often seen:

- at or shortly after the time of diagnosis
- at the time of the first recurrence
- as death approaches.

Table 5.2   Psychological responses to loss[4]

Phase	Symptoms	Typical duration
Disruption	Disbelief Denial Shock/numbness Despair	<1 week
Dysphoria	Anxiety Insomnia Anger Guilt Sadness Poor concentration Activities disrupted	Several weeks
Adaptation	Dysphoria diminishes Implications confronted New goals established Hope refocused and restored Activities resumed	Begins within 2–3 weeks

Denial

Denial is a common defence mechanism. It signifies an ability to obliterate or minimize threat by ignoring it. However, it may be associated with physiological and other non-verbal evidence of anxiety. Occasionally, because a patient is unable to accept that he is dying, he deludes himself into believing that there is a plot to kill him or that the treatment is the cause of his deterioration. However, such paranoid states are more likely to be caused by cerebral tumours, biochemical disturbances or corticosteroids. There is no one right way of responding and adjusting to a poor prognosis. The doctor's task is to help the patient adjust in the best way possible, given that particular patient's familial, cultural and spiritual background. Many people have a combination of inner resources and good support from the family and others which enable them to cope without prolonged and disabling distress.

Even so, most patients and relatives continue to make use of denial to a varying extent. Patients experience conflict between the wish to know the truth and the wish to avoid anxiety and denial is one way of coping with this. Professional intervention may be needed when denial persists and interferes with:

- the acceptance of treatment
- planning for the future
- interpersonal relationships.

Family problems

Cancer always changes family psychodynamics, either for better or for worse. Within families, there is a conflict between the wish to confide and to receive emotional and practical support on the one hand and the wish to protect loved ones from distress on the other, particularly children or frail parents. A conspiracy of silence (collusion) is a source of tension. It blocks discussion of the future and preparation for parting. If it is not resolved, the bereaved often experience much regret.

Other problems

Cancer-related

For example, impact on sexual function; difficulty in accepting a colostomy, paraplegia or the effects of cerebral secondaries.

Treatment-related

For example, adverse drug effects such as hair loss. Patients may want to share in decisions about when to stop treatment aimed at prolonging life. Fear of death may make some want to go on even when adverse effects are severe and the chance of improvement is minimal. Others may wish to opt for a shorter life with better quality at a time when doctors are advocating more aggressive measures.

Concurrent

For example, a bereavement or a pre-existing psychiatric illness.

Anger

> 'A person loses their temper when the emotional demands of the situation exceed their emotional resources.'

> 'Anger is an emotional response to the perception of an overwhelming threat.'

Anger is an uncomfortable dynamic emotion which ranges from a mild sense of irritation to uncontrollable rage. Anger is generally transient but may be chronic. Anger can:

- increase vigour/energy
- facilitate the expression of negative feelings
- disrupt relationships (temporarily or permanently)
- induce impulsive action
- help a person defend himself physically and psychologically
- instigate aggression.

If anger is unjustifiably displaced or projected onto the family or staff, it tends to alienate. Anger can also interfere with the acceptance of limitations, and may stop a patient from making positive adjustments to physical disability. If anger is suppressed, the patient may become withdrawn, uncooperative and possibly depressed.

Causes

Anger is a common response to the losses associated with advanced cancer and bereavement. However, there are many specific causes which need to be identified (Box 5.A).

Box 5.A   Selected causes of anger

Personality trait
Delay in diagnosis
Manner in which the patient was told the diagnosis
Part of an adjustment reaction to diagnosis and prognosis
Delay in treatment
Uncommunicative doctors
Failed treatment
Feeling of unfairness about illness
Feeling let down by God
Frustration because of the limitations imposed by progressive illness
Depression

Management

Anger is a normal response to bad news and may be directed at the doctor as the bearer of the bad news. It is important to:

- listen carefully to what is being expressed

- validate the patient's feelings, e.g. 'Given what you're having to cope with, you've every right to be angry'

- remember that a period of silence can be therapeutic

- clarify the cause(s) of anger, e.g. 'Are you able to tell me exactly what's making you so angry?

- consider whether anger is part of a clinical depression; if this seems probable, treat accordingly (see p.192)

- if anger becomes chronic, consider obtaining help from a counsellor, psychotherapist, psychiatrist or chaplain/spiritual adviser.

With time, in most patients, anger resolves to a variable extent. On the other hand, it may not; *some patients die angry.*

Anxiety

Anxiety is an unpleasant emotion with which everybody is familiar (Box 5.B). It can be acute (transient) or chronic (persistent) and varies in intensity. Many cancer patients sleep badly, have frightening dreams or are reluctant to be left alone at night, and sometimes during the day as well; these all suggest heightened anxiety.

Box 5.B   Symptoms of anxiety[5]

Persistently tense and unable to relax
Worry
Cannot distract self or be distracted
Poor concentration
Indecisiveness

Insomnia
Irritability
Sweating, tremor, nausea
Panic attacks

Severe anxiety is accompanied by physical symptoms but these vary considerably between people. They include palpitations, breathlessness, dry mouth, dysphagia, anorexia, nausea, diarrhoea, frequency of micturition, dizziness, sweating, tremor, headache, muscle tension, fatigue, weakness of the legs and chest pain.

Causes

There are many causes of anxiety in advanced cancer (Box 5.C).

Box 5.C   Causes of heightened anxiety

Situational
Adjustment reaction
Fear of hospital, chemotherapy,
   radiotherapy
Worry about family and finances

Organic
Severe pain
Insomnia
Weakness
Nausea
Breathlessness
Hypoglycaemia
Brain tumour

Psychiatric
Panic disorder
Depression
Psychosis
Delirium

Drugs
Corticosteroids
Neuroleptics (akathisia, see p.284)
Drug-induced hallucinations
   benzodiazepines
   opioids
Withdrawal from
   benzodiazepines
   antidepressants
   alcohol

Relating to a patient's inner world
Thoughts about the past, e.g wasted
   opportunities, guilt
Thoughts about the future
   fear of pain
   fear of mental impairment
   fear of loss of independence
Thoughts about after death

Evaluation

An expectation that cancer patients are bound to be anxious is a common obstacle to evaluation and treatment. A detailed assessment interview is the main method of evaluation. In addition, the family may well be able to provide useful background information.

Review medication; for example, has the patient recently started:

* a corticosteroid
* an SSRI?

Management

Correct the correctable

Management depends on the cause:

* relieve pain and other distressing symptoms
* facilitate the airing and sharing of worries and fears; 'a trouble shared is a trouble halved'
* correct misconceptions
* develop a strategy for coping with uncertainty.[6]

Non-drug treatment

There are many psychological approaches to anxiety but these are beyond the scope of this book (Box 5.D). They are also used in chronic pain management, particularly when anxiety is a concurrent feature. In practice their use depends on the availability of an appropriate therapist, e.g. psychologist, music therapist, hypnotherapist. Relaxation therapy is often provided by an occupational therapist or physiotherapist.

Box 5.D   Psychological methods for managing anxiety and/or pain

Anxiety management training	Art therapy
Cognitive-behavioural therapy	Biofeedback
Brief psychotherapy	Hypnotherapy
Music therapy	

Drug treatment

The following should be used in conjunction with psychological support:

- a benzodiazepine, e.g.
    temazepam 10–40mg o.n.
    diazepam 5–10mg o.n. and 2–5mg p.r.n.

- an antidepressant
    particularly if anxiety-depression (see p.198)
    if persistent panic attacks (see p.192)

- antipsychotics
    if the patient is psychotic, e.g. has paranoid ideas or is hallucinating
    if the anxiety is a feature of an agitated delirium
    if the situation is made worse by benzodiazepines.

Panic disorder

Panic is an episodic pathological failure of the protective 'fight or flight' response to a major threat, in which all structure and reality checks are lost. In the dying, an overwhelming sense of doom or absolute despair often supervenes. Panic is associated with various autonomic symptoms (Box 5.E). It is physiologically demanding and cannot be maintained indefinitely. Panic is therefore episodic but attacks may occur in clusters.

Box 5.E   DSM-IV criteria for a panic disorder[7]

A discrete period of intense fear or discomfort in which four or more of the following symptoms develop abruptly and reach a peak within 10 minutes:

Palpitations, pounding heart or accelerated heart rate
Sweating
Trembling or shaking
Sensations of shortness of breath or smothering
Feeling of choking
Chest pain or discomfort
Nausea or abdominal distress
Feeling dizzy, unsteady, lightheaded or faint
Derealisation (feelings of unreality) or depersonalisation (being detached from oneself)
Fear of losing control or going crazy
Fear of dying
Paraesthesias (numbness or tingling sensations)
Chills or hot flushes

Physiology

Serotonin (5HT) plays a central role in panic disorder.[8] Supporting evidence for this comes from the clinical efficacy of SSRIs.[9] Impairment of the brain's inhibitory GABA-ergic system probably also plays a part. Noradrenaline (norepinephrine) is also involved but is not the primary mediator. Various neuropeptides have also been implicated, notably corticotrophin-releasing factors.[8] Serotonin improves anxiety (and hyperventilation) by inhibiting:

- excitatory cortical inputs to the amygdala
- excitatory stimulation of the peri-aqueductal gray area, locus ceruleus and, chronically, the hypothalamo-pituitary-adrenal axis
- corticotrophin-releasing factor production and/or release
- ventilatory control abnormalities associated with low serotonergic tone.

The amygdala is instrumental in the generation of the fear response.[10] Anxiety-provoking sensory stimuli from the cardiorespiratory and gastro-intestinal systems or cognitions from the sensory cortex are relayed to the central nucleus of the amygdala (Table 5.3). This generates fear-related responses mediated by corticotrophin-releasing factor activation of:

- peri-aqueductal gray area (facilitates the panic response)
- noradrenergic cells of the locus ceruleus (further stimulating the amygdala)
- hypothalamic-pituitary-adrenal axis (increase in plasma cortisol)
- parabrachial nucleus and dorsal motor nucleus of the vagus (activating cardiorespiratory responses, i.e. hyperventilation).

Table 5.3 Afferent pathways in panic disorder[8]

Inputs	Modifiers	Output
Viscerosensory		
Respiratory panicogens	Changes in pH	Amygdaloid-
Baroreceptor stimulation	Locus ceruleus	hippocampal
Neuropeptides		activation
Visuospatial-auditory-cognitive		
Visual stimuli	Hippocampus	Amygdaloid-thalamic-
Auditory stimuli	Peri-aqueductal	cortical-amygdaloid
Catastrophic thoughts	gray area	circuit activation

Many of the areas which mediate panic are also chemosensitive to carbon dioxide and pH and thereby influence the respiratory neurones in the medulla. Depletion of serotonin increases respiratory rate, ventilation and ventilatory response to carbon dioxide which is reversed by administration of a serotonin precursor.[11] Hypersensitivity to carbon dioxide is present in many patients with panic disorder; this is reduced by treatment with a serotonergic antidepressant.[12]

Evaluation

In cancer, panic may be:

- an exacerbation of a pre-existing anxiety disorder (in which case the onset of panic attacks may well predate the diagnosis of cancer)
- a reaction to the patient's current circumstances
- secondary to uncontrolled symptoms, e.g. breathlessness
- a feature of agitated delirium
- precipitated by medication, e.g. corticosteroids.

In patients with brain tumours, the differential diagnosis includes temporal lobe epilepsy (Box 5.F). In panic disorder, the symptoms can often be reproduced by voluntary hyperventilation. Patients with breathlessness are at increased risk of panic attacks associated with exacerbations of their breathlessness. A common feature is the persistent fear about the attacks and their consequences, e.g. fear of suffocation and death during an attack.[13] Other features include:

- episodes of breathlessness occurring at rest
- poor relationship of breathlessness to exertion
- rapid fluctuations of breathlessness within minutes
- breathlessness associated with certain social situations
- previous/concurrent panic or generalised anxiety disorder.

Some patients with end-stage motor neurone disease/amyotrophic lateral sclerosis appear fearful at times but are unable to vocalize their feelings. As many such patients have incipient respiratory failure, it is probable that the non-verbally expressed fear reflects episodes of panic.

Box 5.F   Temporal lobe epilepsy

The temporal lobe is the most common site of origin for complex partial seizures.

Clinical features include:
  impaired consciousness
  hallucinations are characteristic but need not occur
    olfactory (most frequent), e.g. burning rubber
    taste
    hearing (infrequent)
    sight (infrequent)
  cognitive impairment
    jamais-vu, i.e. feelings of unreality which may provoke despair, anxiety, or panic
    déjà-vu, i.e. a feeling of excessive familiarity with events and environment
  autonomic activity
    pilo-erection ('gooseflesh')
    flushing
    sexual.

Management

Correct the correctable

If panic is really a manifestation of temporal lobe epilepsy, anti-epileptic drugs should be introduced or adjusted.

Non-drug treatment

With all breathless patients, enquire specifically about panic attacks because discussion about them is the key to successful management (Figure 5.1). Panic often responds to a calming presence and encouraging the hyper-ventilating patient to breathe more slowly and deeply. Patients should also be taught about optimal breathing techniques, respiratory control and relaxation.[13] These are most commonly provided by a physiotherapist or, in a breathless-ness clinic, by a specialist nurse.[14]

With panic attacks not associated with breathlessness, it is important to ex-plore possible reasons for the attacks. In physically healthy people, panic may relate to chronic existential anxiety. In contrast, in cancer patients there is an obvious precipitating cause, namely the fear of impending death, signifying disintegration and anihilation. Often such fears are only thinly disguised and empathic discussion can help by bringing them into the open.

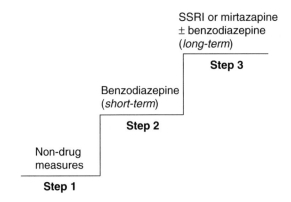

Figure 5.1   Management of panic disorder.

Drug treatment

Immediate treatment is with a benzodiazepine. Although any benzodiazepine can be used, high potency ones such as alprazolam and clonazepam seem to be better.[15] The longer halflife and high potency of clonazepam make it the benzodiazepine of choice.[16] It is best given b.d. to prevent break-through or rebound anxiety.

For some patients, propranolol 20mg PO stat is effective. An antipsychotic drug such as haloperidol or thioridazine is indicated if an organic cause is suspected and if there are concomitant psychotic symptoms such as delusions or hallucinations.

Maintenance treatment is with either a benzodiazepine, an SSRI, or both.[15,17] It is generally best to continue the benzodiazepine for a few weeks when starting an SSRI in order to prevent an initial exacerbation of anxiety. It is for this reason that a low starting dose is sometimes recommended, e.g. sertraline 25mg o.d. The dose is then titrated upwards if necessary at intervals of 1–2 weeks to sertraline 50–100mg o.d.[9] Mirtazapine with its sedative and specific serotonergic effects provides an alternative.[18,19] In breathless patients with a short prognosis, a benzodiazepine is likely to remain the treatment of choice.

Depression

A depressive illness occurs in about 5–15% of patients with advanced cancer.[20,21] Another 10–15% will have some depressive symptoms, often as part of an adjustment disorder or because of a loss of morale associated, for example, with unremitting distressing symptoms.

It is important to identify depression particularly because conventional treatment achieves a good response in >80% of cases. Untreated depression:

- intensifies other symptoms
- leads to social withdrawal
- prevents the patient from completing 'unfinished business'.

Depression may be undiagnosed because:

- low mood is ignored by doctors and nurses because it is considered 'understandable' or 'reactive'
- the patient may be feeling better when seen by the doctor compared with earlier in the day (diurnal variation)
- social skills mask the depressed mood (smiling depression)
- the depression is expressed through physical symptoms, e.g. pain (somatization)
- the depression is masked by concurrent symptoms of anxiety
- the depression manifests as a worsening of a personality trait, e.g. attention-seeking.

On the other hand, depression may be over-diagnosed if all patients who are sad and sometimes cry are said to have a depressive illness.

Clinical features

For major depression, at least five of the following symptoms must be present, including one or both of the first two. In addition, symptoms must be present most of the day, on most days, for at least two weeks:

- *depressed mood*
- *markedly diminished interest or pleasure in almost all activities*
- significant weight loss or gain
- insomnia or hypersomnia
- psychomotor agitation or retardation
- impaired concentration (indecisiveness)
- fatigue (lack of energy)

- feelings of worthlessness (or guilt)
- suicidal ideas.[22]

Causes

Many psychosocial and physiological factors predispose to depression (Box 5.G). There is a relationship between the site and nature of an organic brain disorder and the subsequent development of depression (Box 5.H).

Box 5.G   Risk factors for depression

Psychosocial
Past history of depression
Obsessional personality
Inability to express emotions
Conspiracy of silence
Lack of supportive/confiding relationship
Mutilation
Threat of death
Loss of independence (greater risk in men)
Recent bereavement(s)

Physiological
Unrelieved pain
Drugs
  corticosteroids
  chemotherapy
  phenothiazines, e.g. chlorpromazine
  antihypertensives, e.g. methyldopa
Paraneoplastic[a]
Biochemical
  hypokalaemia
  hypercalcaemia
Endocrine
  hyperparathyroidism
  hypoparathyroidism
  hypercortisolism
    (Cushing's syndrome)[b]
  hyperprolactinaemia
Vitamin deficiency
  folate
  nicotinic acid (Pellagra)
  thiamine (B_1)
Cerebral
  stroke
  head injury
  cerebral tumour
  epilepsy
  parkinsonism
  multiple sclerosis

---

a   incidence higher in cancer of pancreas[23,24]

b   nearly 50% become depressed; more likely when caused by pituitary dysfunction.

Box 5.H   Organic brain disorders and depression

Epilepsy
Higher suicide rate, particularly with temporal lobe epilepsy.

Brain tumours
Depression more common with supratemporal tumours and with frontal and temporal lobe tumours.[25]

Cerebrovascular accident (CVA) and head injury
Location of lesion relevant for the first 6 months; psychosocial factors more relevant later. Greater risk with *left*-sided lesion, particularly *left anterior* brain.[26]

Positive emission tomography shows that the brain serotonin concentration is lower after a left-sided CVA than after a right-sided CVA.[27]

Parkinson's disease
Left-sided Parkinson's disease (i.e. right brain) is associated with more depression (*the opposite of poststroke depression*).[28] Responds well to antidepressants.

Multiple sclerosis
Up to 1/3 become depressed and cognitively impaired; a similar proportion are relatively euphoric.[29] There is a higher than expected incidence of depression in *the year before diagnosis*,[30] and a greater likelihood of a past history of bipolar depression.

Motor neurone disease
Less depression than in multiple sclerosis.[31]

Evaluation

Diagnosing depression is difficult in the presence of a debilitating physical illness.[32]

Some patients are seemingly depressed but in reality are simply close to death with no residual energy and a corresponding loss of pleasure in life. In more robust patients, in the absence of confounding factors such as severe pain, it is necessary to differentiate between a severe adjustment reaction, i.e. sadness provoked by the change in personal circumstances, and depression (Figure 5.2 and Table 5.4).

Evaluation is made more difficult by the fact that the somatic symptoms of depression overlap with the symptoms of cancer:

- anorexia
- weight loss

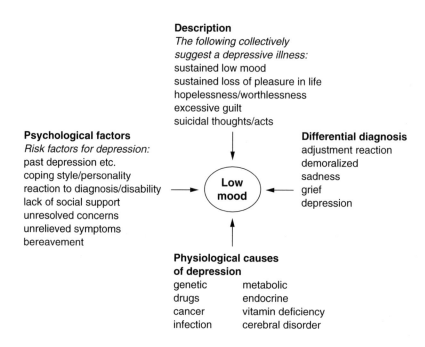

Figure 5.2   The four dimensions of the evaluation of low mood.

Table 5.4   Distinguishing a depressive illness from sadness[33]

Features of both	Features more typical of depression
Loss of interest	Loss of all emotion and pleasure in life
Decreased concentration	Social withdrawal
Tearfulness	Not distractable (but with diurnal variation)
Anxiety	Irritability
Decreased sleep	Physical anxiety (sweating, tremor, panic attacks)
Tiredness	Hopelessness and worthlessness
Anorexia	(particularly with regard to family and friends)
Suicidal ideas	Excessive guilt
	Intractable pain
	Requests for euthanasia
	Suicide attempts

- constipation
- sleep disturbance
- loss of libido.

Proxies, including close relatives, cannot reliably be used to determine a person's emotional state. Although some centres recommend the use of the HAD scale as a screening tool,[3,20,34] its validity in patients with advanced disease is questionable.[35,36] The Edinburgh depression scale, developed for use in postnatal (physically fit) women is said to be more reliable.[37,38] The International Neuropsychiatric Interview has also been recommended.[39] However, asking the patient directly about their mood, i.e. 'Are you depressed?', has been shown to be a reliable and sensitive screening question.[40,41] If a patient denies being depressed, the use of a validated diagnostic tool only rarely shows the presence of depression.

Explanation

The nature of the explanation will vary according to the patient's physical and psychological state. Patients are often helped by being told that depression is not shameful. For example:

> 'It seems to me that you've developed a depressive illness … Being physically ill is hard work and emotionally exhausting. Ongoing stress reduces certain chemicals in the brain and this results in depression … Antidepressants are tablets which help the brain replenish these chemicals.'

Management

Guidelines 5.1: Depression (p.389).

In patients who have had depression in the past, ask them what helped before and consider together whether such measures might help again.

Non-drug treatment

Attendance at a palliative care day centre is helpful for patients who are isolated at home because of weakness and/or other debilitating symptoms. A day centre provides:

- social interaction

- psychological support
- medical supervision.

Drug treatment

The range of antidepressants has increased considerably in recent years (Box 5.1). The choice of antidepressant is dictated partly by cost, availability and fashion but also by a desire to keep adverse effects to a minimum. For example, amitriptyline is a cheap and widely available tricyclic antidepressant but it causes more adverse effects than, say, imipramine and dosulepin (dothiepin). Sometimes the choice of antidepressant will be influenced by the type of depression, e.g. retarded rather than agitated. However, increasingly, newer antidepressants are being used, e.g. SSRIs, venlafaxine and mirtazapine. Adverse effects can still be troublesome particularly with SSRIs. Nausea and anxiety are common reasons for discontinuing an SSRI.[42] Each palliative care service needs to agree on its own preferred antidepressants and become familiar with their use (see p.390).

Box 5.1   Classification of antidepressants according to principal actions

Enzyme inhibitors (mono-amine oxidase inhibitors, MAOIs)
Phenelzine, moclobemide (reversible inhibitor of mono-oxidase, RIMA)

Re-uptake inhibitors (mono-amine *re-uptake* inhibitors, MARIs)
Serotonin and noradrenaline (norepinephrine)
Amitriptyline, imipramine, dosulepin (dothiepin), venlafaxine

Serotonin (selective serotonin re-uptake inhibitors, SSRIs)
Fluoxetine, paroxetine, sertraline, citalopram

Noradrenaline (norepinephrine)
Desipramine[a], lofepramine[a], maprotiline, reboxetine

Receptor antagonists[b]
Trazodone (α_1, $5HT_2$)
Nefazodone ($5HT_2$); also a MARI
Mirtazapine (central α_2, $5HT_2$, $5HT_3$)[c]

---

a also has a clinically unimportant effect on serotonin re-uptake

b antagonism of $5HT_2$- and $5HT_3$-receptors facilitates increased $5HT_{1A}$ binding; this enhances the antidepressant effect

c mirtazapine is described as a noradrenaline (norepinephrine) and specific serotonin antagonist (NaSSA).

Antidepressants take time to work. A latency of 1–2 weeks for SSRIs and 2–3 weeks for tricyclics are misleadingly optimistic for many patients, particularly when slow dose escalation is preferable. The *median* response time is 2–3 months in older patients.[43]

St. John's wort

St. John's wort (hypericum extract) is a popular over-the-counter (OTC) antidepressant. It is as effective as imipramine and amitriptyline in treating mild–moderate depression and causes fewer adverse effects.[44–47] However, if OTC hypericum is combined with prescription antidepressants, there is a risk of developing a central serotonergic syndrome, i.e. agitated delirium, tachycardia, myoclonus, hyperreflexia and possibly hyperthermia (>40°C).[48]

Hypericum induces several cytochrome P450 iso-enzymes in the liver and gastro-intestinal tract, particularly CYP 3A4 but also 1A2 and 2C9, thereby reducing the blood levels of some drugs and potentially impairing their effectiveness.[49] In palliative care the most important interactions occur with HIV protease inhibitors and HIV non-nucleoside reverse transcriptase inhibitors. With these drugs, hypericum may reduce plasma concentrations by >50%, and possibly lead to treatment failure.[50]

Psychostimulants

The place of psychostimulants in depression is controversial, although a consensus panel in the USA has recommended their use.[32] They seem to be of greater benefit in medically ill patients than in the physically healthy.[51] Because of a rapid onset of action (days rather than weeks), psychostimulants have a place in a severely retarded patient with a prognosis of less than 2–3 months.[52–54]

Methylphenidate is the current preferred psychostimulant:

- start with 5mg b.d. (*0800, 1200h*)
- increase if necessary after 3–4 days to 10mg b.d. → 15mg b.d.
- response is variable.[54,55]

Psychostimulants are used at some centres for other purposes:

- troublesome opioid-induced drowsiness
- restoring a normal day and night rhythm of waking and sleeping.[56]

Psychostimulants are rarely used by the authors.

The withdrawn patient

Some patients seem to be psychologically inaccessible. Although this may not be detrimental to the patient, there are times when the patient's facial expression and behaviour suggests considerable underlying psychological distress.

Causes

These fall into several categories (Box 5.J). Sometimes there may be several concurrent causal factors.

Box 5.J   Differential diagnosis of the withdrawn patient[57]

Personality

Pathological
Brain tumour(s)
Cerebrovascular disease
Secondary mental disorders (see p.204)
Concurrent illness, e.g. hypothyroidism

Pharmacological
Oversedation
Tardive dyskinesia (see p.285)

Psychological

Anger, Collusion, Distrust	'no point in talking about my feelings'
Fear	'too painful'
Guilt, Shame	'too embarrassed'

Psychiatric

| Depression | 'no point in talking about my feelings' |
| Paranoia | 'too dangerous' |

Management

Management depends on the cause. If a psychological cause seems likely, try to find a 'window' in the patient's protective shell in order to help him acknowledge the problem and to begin to move forward to a healthier/more comfortable frame of mind. Good communication skills are essential to achieve this:

- acknowledge *your* difficulty, 'We seem to be finding it difficult to get into conversation'

- offer the patient an invitation which he can accept or reject, e.g. 'Are you able to tell me why you find it difficult to talk to me about things?'

- if the patient then gives a clue as to the reason for the reticence, this should be gently but firmly followed up, e.g. 'Can you tell me exactly what's troubling you?'

- it is important to establish the frequency and intensity of any mood disturbance in case the patient is psychiatrically ill rather than just psychologically disturbed

- ask for specialist help if you feel you are getting nowhere.

The difficult patient

It is not possible to be equally positive towards all patients. Some patients we find difficult. It is important to remember that the problem is primarily *ours* and not the patient's, although it could be a joint problem. Thus it is better to say, 'I find Mrs Brown difficult to look after' and not, 'Mrs Brown is difficult'.

Causes

There are many reasons why a patient may be difficult to care for (Box 5.K). The difficulties elicit feelings of impotence and inadequacy in us; we feel we have failed and we have come to the end of our therapeutic resources.

Management

Acknowledge your difficulty with the rest of the team.

Explore possible reasons why the patient seems difficult.

Box 5.K   Reasons why patients can be difficult to care for

Patients or relatives perceived as
Unpleasant
Seductive
Ungrateful
Critical
Antagonistic
Demanding
Manipulative
Overdependent

Patient's behaviour
Withdrawn
Psychologically volatile, angry
Depressed

Patient's symptoms
Gross disfigurement
Malodour
Poor response to symptom management
Somatization

Transference and countertransference

Consider transference and countertransference reactions, i.e. negative feelings evoked by behaviour or personality traits in the patient because of your past experiences (transference), or your personality evoking negative feelings in the patient (countertransference). Both parties sense the negative 'vibes' and react to them.

Agree on a management plan with the rest of the team and record it in the notes, including short-term goals and time to be spent with the patient and family. Accept that some problems cannot be solved.

Insomnia

Some patients catnap during the day so much that they do not sleep well at night. If this is the case it is important to determine whether being awake during the night is a problem for the patient. Or is the concern about wakeful nights a problem only for the family or carers?

Causes

If the patient is not sleeping well at night, the situation needs to be evaluated; there may be an easily correctable cause (Box 5.L).

Box 5.L   Causes of wakeful nights

Physiological
Wakeful stimuli
  light
  noise
  urinary frequency
Sleep during day
  long siesta
  catnaps
  sedative drugs
Normal old age

Psychological
Anxiety (see p.185)
Depression (see p.192)
Fear of dying in the night

Unrelieved symptoms
Pain
Breathlessness
Vomiting
Incontinence
Diarrhoea
Pruritus
Restless legs

Drugs
Diuretics
Corticosteroids
Caffeine
Sympathomimetics
Night sedative withdrawal
Alcohol (can cause rebound wakefulness)

Management

Correct the correctable

- relieve disturbing symptoms

- if night pain, consider increasing the bedtime dose of morphine from double to *treble* the daytime q4h dose or supplement bedtime m/r morphine with ordinary morphine tablets or solution; in practice this is rarely necessary.

Non-drug treatment

- change mattress/bed if not comfortable

- facilitate expression of anxieties and fears

- increase daytime activity

- reduce light and noise at night

- hot drink at bedtime

- soothing music

- relaxation therapy/tape

- massage, e.g. of hands or feet

- brief psychotherapy.[58,59]

Drug treatment

Modify the drug regimen:

- corticosteroids, give as a single morning dose
- anxiolytics, if receiving diazepam in the daytime, convert to a single dose at 2200h
- diuretics, give as a single morning dose.

Prescribe one or more of the following:

- a night sedative, e.g. temazepam 10–40mg o.n.
- an antidepressant if the patient is depressed or wakes early (see p.390)
- haloperidol 3–5 mg o.n., particularly if sleep is disturbed by unpleasant dreams
- levomepromazine or chlorpromazine 50–200 mg if haloperidol fails.

Secondary mental disorders

These are mental disorders which are secondary to organic disease or related to chemical substances (drugs, alcohol) or both (synonym: organic mental disorders). All types of secondary mental disorders are seen in patients with advanced cancer (Box 5.M).

Box 5.M   Secondary mental disorders

Delirium	Personality disorder
Dementia	Intoxication
Amnestic disorder	Withdrawal state
Anxiety disorder	Psychosis
Mood disorder	

Delirium (synonyms: acute brain syndrome, acute confusion), dementia (synonym: chronic brain syndrome) and amnestic disorder are all characterized by cognitive impairment. The word confusion is often used of all three conditions. Note that:

- sometimes dementia is compounded by delirium

- dementia is not generally associated with drowsiness

- some patients with cancer appear to develop dementia rapidly and this may cause difficulty in diagnosis (Box 5.N).

Box 5.N   Comparison of global cognitive impairment disorders

Delirium		**Dementia**
Acute		Chronic
Often remitting and reversible		Usually progressive and irreversible
Mental clouding (*information not taken in*)		Brain damage (*information not retained*)

Delirium		Dementia
+	Poor concentration	+
+	Impaired short-term memory	+
+	Disorientation	+
+	Living in the past	+
+	Misinterpretations	+
++	Hallucinations	+
+	Delusions	+

Speech rambling and incoherent	Speech stereotyped and limited
Often diurnal variation	Constant (in later stages)
Often aware and anxious	Unaware and unconcerned (in later stages)

Patients with cognitive impairment disorders (confusion) have identifiable cognitive defects if tested formally using, for example, the Mini-Mental State Examination. Patients manifesting the following are sometimes misdiagnosed as confused:

- not taking in what is said
    - deaf
    - anxious
    - too ill to concentrate

- muddled speech
    - poor concentration
    - nominal dysphasia.

It is also important to identify hypnagogic (going to sleep) and hypnopompic (waking up) hallucinations as these are normal phenomena, although more common in ill patients receiving sedative drugs.

Causes

Dementia is usually caused by Alzheimer's disease, Lewy body disease or cerebral atherosclerosis.[60] Other causes of other secondary mental disorders are:

- drugs
- biochemical derangement
- organ failure
- brain tumours
- paraneoplastic.

Delirium

Delirium (acute confusion) is the result of mental clouding. This leads to a disturbance of comprehension and bewilderment.

Clinical features

The clinical features of delirium are numerous (Box 5.O). The disordered level of arousal and cognition is typically of acute onset (hours to days) and is generally accompanied by evidence of the underlying causal condition.[61] Delirium can be classified as:

- hyperactive (agitated), characterized by hallucinations and delusions
- hypo-active (lethargic), characterized by confusion and sedation
- mixed, alternating features of both agitation and lethargy.

Hyperactive delirium may be associated with overactivity of the autonomic nervous system, e.g. facial flushing, dilated pupils, injected conjunctivae, tachycardia, sweating.

Identifying early signs of delirium in patients at risk allows appropriate treatment to be started sooner rather than later, thereby preventing a crisis. Inability to write one's name and address correctly may be as sensitive an indicator of early delirium as some of the more lengthy and intrusive tests.[62]

Box 5.O   Clinical features of delirium

Prodromal symptoms (restlessness, anxiety, sleep disturbance and irritability)
Fluctuating course
Disorientation for time, place or person
Memory impairment (cannot register new material)
Disorganised thinking and incoherent speech
Reduced attention (easily distractible)
Altered arousal
Increased or decreased psychomotor activity
Disturbance of the sleep–wake cycle
Affective symptoms (emotional lability, sadness, anger, euphoria)
Agitation ± noisy aggressive behaviour
Altered perceptions
  misinterpretations
  hallucinations (predominantly visual and tactile rather than auditory)
  illusions
  delusions (poorly formed)
Cortical abnormalities (dysgraphia, constructional apraxia, dysnomic aphasia)
Motor abnormalities (tremor, asterixis, myoclonus, altered tone and reflexes)
Electro-encephalogram abnormalities (global slowing of activity)

Evaluation

Delirium is precipitated or exacerbated by many factors (Box 5.P). In most instances in palliative care, delirium is probably multifactorial. Delirium is present in most moribund patients.[61]

Management

Correct the correctable

Delirium is generally a reversible condition and an underlying cause should be sought and appropriately treated (Box 5.P).[63,64] Common causes are infection and medication, e.g. psychotropics, opioids, corticosteroids. In more than 1/2 of patients with advanced cancer and delirium the cause may not be identified.[65]

If nicotine withdrawal is suspected, encourage smoking or administer a medicinal nicotine product:

- Nicorette nasal spray, containing nicotine 500µg/metered spray
- TD nicotine patches, 11mg and 22mg in 24h.

The cost of TD patches is not covered by the NHS in the UK.

Box 5.P   Precipitating factors for delirium

Change of environment
Unfamiliar excessive stumuli
   too hot
   too cold
   wet bed
   crumbs in bed
   creases in sheets
General deterioration
Fatigue
Anxiety
Depression
Pain
Faecal impaction
Urinary retention
Infection
Dehydration
Brain tumour(s)

Biochemical disturbances
   hypercalcaemia
   hyponatraemia
Drug-induced
   opioids
   antimuscarinics
   corticosteroids
   chemotherapy agents, e.g. cisplatin, 5-FU,
      ifosfamide, methotrexate
   immunomodulators, e.g. interferon,
      interleukin
Withdrawal state
   alcohol
   nicotine
   psychotropics
Thiamine deficiency

Non-drug treatment

An attempt should be made to help the patient to express their distress. Hallucinations, nightmares and misinterpretations often reflect the patient's fears and anxieties. Their content should be explored with the patient. In addition:

- keep calm and avoid confrontation

- respond to the patient's comments

- clarify perceptions, and validate those which are accurate

- explain what is happening and why

- state what can be done to help

- repeat important and helpful information

- when indicated, recommend some tablets or an injection 'to help settle things down so that you can relax and rest for a few hours'

- stress to both the patient and the family that delirium is not madness, and that they can expect lucid intervals

- continue to treat the patient with courtesy and respect

- restraints should never be used

- bed rails should be avoided, they can be dangerous

- patient should be allowed to walk about accompanied

- allay fear and suspicion, and reduce misinterpretations by
  use of night light
  not changing the position of the patient's bed
  explaining every procedure and event in detail
  the presence of a family member or close friend.

In severe delirium, the doctor should acknowledge and accept the patient's distress, e.g. 'I can see that you are very upset', and invite the patient to return to his room and/or bed so that they can discuss things further. The presence of a close relative or friend, continuity of professional carers and a single room to minimize external visual and auditory stimulation may all help to provide a safe environment.[66]

Drug treatment

Treat sooner rather than later, before symptoms are marked, persistent and cause distress to the patient and/or family. Consider:

- reduction in medication

- oxygen if cyanosed

- dexamethasone 8–16mg o.m. if cerebral tumour.

Benzodiazepines should not be used alone as they may worsen delirium.[67] The exception to this rule is delirium associated with alcohol withdrawal for which benzodiazepines are the drug of choice.[68,69] However, generally, haloperidol is the drug of choice for delirium.[61] It is as effective as phenothiazines, e.g. chlorpromazine, but is safer to use. It can be given PO, PR, SC, IM and IV.[66] Adverse effects are uncommon; extrapyramidal reactions occur occasionally, e.g. akathisia.

The initial dose of haloperidol depends on previous medication, weight, age and severity of symptoms. Subsequent doses depend on the initial response. Daily or b.d. maintenance doses are generally adequate; sometimes more frequent administration is necessary. Curiously, the effective dose in patients with AIDS is generally lower than in other patients, e.g. 1–6mg for initial treatment with a similar dose for maintenance given either o.n. or divided and given b.d.[67]

Haloperidol, e.g. 5mg, *combined* with benzodiazepines, e.g. diazepam or midazolam 10mg, can be useful when a period of sedation is required in an agitated delirious patient. If the patient is already receiving regular psychotropic medication, a higher dose may be indicated. For example, lorazepam 1mg = diazepam 5mg. Thus, if already receiving lorazepam 1mg t.d.s., a stat dose of diazepam 20mg would be indicated.

Rarely, it may be necessary to give an agitated patient who is a danger to themselves an injection against their wishes. Although dependent on the circumstances and previous medication haloperidol 5–10mg *and* midazolam 10mg would generally be a good choice, given either SC or IM. Forcing the patient to have an injection is an assault which can be justified only on the grounds of necessity (*see* p.2). This should be seen as the last resort and taken only after discussing the situation with other team members.

The doctor should stay until the patient begins to settle down. It may be necessary for a nurse to stay longer to discourage the patient from getting up and wandering about. A doctor should remain easily contactable in case further measures are necessary. In any case, the ward should be contacted after 1–2h to review the situation and to prescribe ongoing medication.

Occasionally, a dying patient becomes severely agitated despite the above measures. It is occasionally necessary to heavily sedate a patient as the only way to contain the situation, i.e. give sedation sufficient to diminish the level of consciousness (*see* p.369).[70]

References

1   Portenoy R *et al.* (1994) The memorial symptom assessment scale: an instrument for the evaluation of symptom prevalence, characteristics and distress. *European Journal of Cancer.* **30A**:1326–36.

2   Heaven C and Maguire P (1997) Disclosure of concerns by hospice patients and their identification by nurses. *Palliative Medicine.* **11**:283–90.

3   LeFevre P *et al.* (1999) Screening for psychiatric illness in the palliative care inpatient setting: a comparison between the Hospital Anxiety and Depression Scale and the General Health Questionnaire-12. *Palliative Medicine.* **13**:399–407.

4   Massie M and Holland J (1989) Overview of normal reactions and prevalence of psychiatric disorders. In: J Holland and J Rowland (eds) *Handbook of Psycho-oncology.* Oxford University Press, Oxford, pp 273–82.

5   Faulkner A and Maguire P (1994) *Talking to Cancer Patients and Their Relatives.* Oxford Medical Publications, Oxford.

6   Twycross R (1999) *Introducing Palliative Care.* Radcliffe Medical Press, Oxford, pp 28–30.

7   American Psychiatric Association (1994) Panic attacks. In: *Diagnostic and Statistical Manual of Mental Disorders, 4th edition (DSM-IV).* APA, New York.

8   Hood S and Nutt D (2000) Panic disorder. *Central Nervous System.* **2**:7–10.

9   Boyer W (1995) Serotonin uptake inhibitors are superior to imipramine and alprazolam in alleviating panic attacks: A meta-analysis. *International Clinics of Psychopharmacology.* **10**:45–9.

10 Kent J *et al.* (1998) Clinical utility of the selective serotonin reuptake inhibitors in the spectrum of anxiety. *Biological Psychiatry.* **44**:812–24.

11 Bianchi A *et al.* (1995) Central control of breathing in mammals: neuronal circuitry, membrane properties, and neurotransmitters. *Physiological Reviews.* **75**:1–45.

12 Bertani A (1997) Pharmacological effect of paroxetine, sertraline and imipramine on reactivity to the 35% carbon dioxide challenge: a double blind, random, placebo controlled study. *Journal of Clinical Psychopharmacology.* **117**:97–101.

13 Smoller J *et al.* (1996) Panic anxiety, dyspnea, and respiratory disease. Theoretical and clinical considerations. *American Journal of Respiratory and Critical Care Medicine.* **54**:6–17.

14 Bredin M *et al.* (1999) Multicentre randomized controlled trial of nursing intervention for breathlessness in patients with lung cancer. *British Medical Journal.* **318**:901–4.

15 Marshall J (1997) Panic disorder: a treatment update. *Journal of Clinical Psychiatry.* **58**:36–42.

16 Herman J *et al.* (1987) The alprazolam to clonazepam switch for the treatment of panic disorder. *Journal of Clinical Psychopharmacology.* **7**:175–8.

17 Tyrer P (1989) Treating panic. *British Medical Journal.* **298**:201.

18 Carpenter L *et al.* (1999) Clinical experience with mirtazapine in the treatment of panic disorder. *Annals of Clinical Psychiatry.* **11**:81–6.

19 Berigan T and Harazin J (1999) Mirtazapine in the treatment of panic disorder. *Primary Psychiatry.* **6**:36.

20 Hopwood P and Stephens R (2000) Depression in patients with lung cancer: prevalence and risk factors derived from quality-of-life data. *Journal of Clinical Oncology.* **18**:893–903.

21 Wilson K *et al.* (2000) Diagnosis and management of depression in palliative care. In: H Chochinov and W Breitbart (eds) *Handbook of Psychiatry in Palliative Medicine.* Oxford University Press, Oxford, pp 25–49.

22 American Psychiatric Association (1994) *Diagnostic and Statistical Manual of Mental Disorders.* APA, New York.

23 Green A and Austin C (1993) Psychopathology of pancreatic cancer: a psychobiologic probe. *Psychosomatics.* **34**:208–21.

24 Passik S and Breitbart W (1996) Depression in patients with pancreatic carcinoma. *Cancer.* **78**:615–26.

25 Hecaen H and deAjuriaguerra J (1956) *Troubles Mentaux au cours des Tumeurs Intracraniennes.* Masson, Paris.

26 Lishman W (1998) *Organic Psychiatry.* Blackwells Scientific Publication, Oxford, p.386.

27 Mayberg H *et al.* (1988) PET imaging of cortical S2 serotonin receptors after stroke: lateralized changes and relationship to depression. *American Journal of Psychiatry.* **145**:937–43.

28 Fleminger S (1991) Left-sided Parkinson's disease is associated with greater anxiety and depression. *Psychological Medicine.* **21**:629–38.

29 Surridge D (1969) An investigation into some psychiatric aspects of multiple sclerosis. *British Journal of Psychiatry.* **115**:749–64.

30 Whitlock F and Siskind M (1980) Depression as a major symptom of multiple sclerosis. *Journal of Neurology, Neurosurgery and Psychiatry.* **43**:861–5.

31 Schiffer R and Babigian H (1984) Behavioral disorders in multiple sclerosis, temporal lobe epilepsy, and amyotrophic lateral sclerosis. An epidemiological study. *Archives of Neurology.* **41**:1067–9.

32 Block S (2000) Assessing and managing depression in the terminally ill patient. *Annals of Internal Medicine.* **132**:209–18.

33 Casey P (1994) Depression in the dying – disorder or distress? *Progress in Palliative Care.* **2**:1–3.

34 Kramer J (1999) Use of the Hospital Anxiety and Depression Scale (HADS) in the assessment of depression in patients with inoperable lung cancer. *Palliative Medicine.* **13**:353–4.

35 Faull C *et al.* (1993) *The hospital anxiety and depression (HAD) scale: its validity in patients with terminal malignant disease.* Paper presented at the Palliative Care Research Forum, London.

36 Urch C *et al.* (1998) The drawback of the Hospital Anxiety and Depression Scale in the assessment of depression in hospice inpatients. *Palliative Medicine.* **12**:395–6.

37 Cox J *et al.* (1987) Edinburgh postnatal depression scale (EPDS). *British Journal of Psychiatry.* **150**:782–6.

38 Lloyd-Williams M *et al.* (2000) Criterion validation of the Edinburgh Postnatal Depression Scale as a screening tool for patients with advanced metastatic cancer. *Journal of Pain and Symptom Management.* **20**:259–65.

39 Passik S *et al.* (2000) Oncology staff recognition of depressive symptoms on videotaped interviews of depressed cancer patients: implications for designing a training program. *Journal of Pain and Symptom Management.* **19**:329–38.

40 Mahoney J *et al.* (1994) Screening for depression: single question versus GDS. *Journal of the American Geriatric Society.* **42**:1006–8.

41 Chochinov H *et al.* (1997) 'Are you depressed?' screening for depression in the terminally ill. *American Journal of Psychiatry.* **154**:674–6.

42 Trindade E *et al.* (1998) Adverse effects associated with selective reuptake inhibitors and tricyclic antidepressants: a meta-analysis. *Canadian Medical Association Journal.* **17**:1245–52.

43 Reynolds C *et al.* (1998) Effects of age at onset of first lifetime episode of recurrent major depression on treatment response and illness course in elderly patients. *American Journal of Psychiatry.* **155**:795–9.

44 Vorbach E *et al.* (1997) Efficacy and tolerability of St John's wort extract LI160 versus imipramine in patients with severe depressive episodes according to ICD10. *Pharmacopsychiatry.* **30**:81–5.

45 Wheatley D (1997) LI160, an extract of St John's wort versus amitriptyline in mildly to moderately depressed outpatients – a controlled 6-week clinical trial. *Pharmacopsychiatry.* **30**:77–80.

46 Gaster B and Holroyd J (2000) St John's wort for depression: a systematic review. *Archives of Internal Medicine.* **160**:152–6.

47 Woelk H (2000) Comparison of St John's wort and imipramine for treating depression: randomised controlled trial. *British Medical Journal.* **321**:536–9.

48 Lantz M *et al.* (1999) St John's wort and antidepressant drug interactions in the elderly. *Journal of Geriatric Psychiatry and Neurology.* **12**:7–10.

49 Roby C *et al.* (2000) St John's wort: effect on CYP3A4 activity. *Clinical Pharmacology and Therapeutics.* **67**:451–7.
50 Piscitelli S *et al.* (2000) Indinavir concentrations and St John's wort. *Lancet.* **355**:547–8.
51 Satel S and Nelson J (1989) Stimulants in the treatment of depression: A critical overview. *Journal of Clinical Psychiatry.* **50**:241–9.
52 Breitbart W and Mermelstein H (1992) An alternative psychostimulant for the management of depressive disorders in cancer patients. *Psychosomatics.* **33**:352–6.
53 Emptage R and Semla T (1996) Depression in the medically ill elderly: a focus on methylphenidate. *Annals of Pharmacotherapy.* **30**:151–7.
54 Homsi J *et al.* (2000) Methylphenidate (MP) in the management of depression in advanced cancer. *Supportive Care in Cancer.* **8**:40–1.
55 Kaufmann M *et al.* (1984) Use of psychostimulants in medically ill patients with neurological disease and major depression. *Canadian Journal of Psychiatry.* **29**:46–9.
56 Dalal S and Melzack R (1998) Potentiation of opioid analgesia by psychostimulant drugs: a review. *Journal of Pain and Symptom Management.* **16**:245–53.
57 Maguire P and Faulkner A (1993) Handling the withdrawn patient – a flow diagram. *Palliative Medicine.* **7**:333–8.
58 Moorey S *et al.* (1994) Adjuvant psychosocial therapy for patients with cancer: outcome at 1 year. *Psychooncology.* **3**:39–46.
59 Moorey S *et al.* (1998) A comparison of adjuvant psychological therapy and supportive counselling in patients with cancer. *Psychooncology.* **7**:218–28.
60 American Psychiatric Association (1994) Dementia. In: *Diagnostic and Statistical Manual of Mental Disorders, 4th edition (DSM-IV).* APA, New York.
61 Breitbart W and Strout D (2000) Delirium in the terminally ill. *Clinics in Geriatric Medicine.* **16**:357–72.
62 Macleod A and Whitehead L (1997) Dysgraphia and terminal delirium. *Palliative Medicine.* **11**:127–32.
63 American Psychiatric Association (1999) Practice guideline for the treatment of patients with delirium. *American Journal of Psychiatry.* **156**:1–18.
64 Cole M (1999) Delirium: effectiveness of systematic interventions. *Dementia and Geriatric Cognitive Disorders.* **10**:406–11.
65 Bruera E *et al.* (1992) Cognitive failure in patients with terminal cancer: A prospective study. *Journal of Pain and Symptom Management.* **7**:192–5.
66 Macleod A (1997) The management of delirium in hospice practice. *European Journal of Palliative Care.* **4**:116–20.
67 Breitbart W *et al.* (1996) A double-blind trial of haloperidol, chlorpromazine, and lorazepam in the treatment of delirium in hospitalized AIDS patients. *American Journal of Psychiatry.* **153**:231–7.
68 Lundberg J and Passik S (1997) Alcohol and cancer: a review for psychooncologists. *Psychooncology.* **6**:253–66.
69 Chick J (1998) Review: benzodiazepines are more effective than neuroleptics in reducing delirium and seizures in alcohol withdrawal. *Evidence-Based Medicine.* **3**:11.
70 Fainsinger R *et al.* (2000) Sedation for delirium and other symptoms in terminally ill patients in Edmonton. *Journal of Palliative Care.* **16**:5–10.

6　Biochemical syndromes

Hypercalcaemia
Syndrome of inappropriate ADH secretion (SIADH)

Hypercalcaemia

Hypercalcaemia is an *ionized* plasma calcium concentration above the upper limit of normal. In most centres, the total plasma calcium concentration is measured. This includes both protein-bound and ionized calcium. If a patient is hypo-albuminaemic, the total plasma concentration may give a false impression of normality. Hence, it is necessary to 'correct' for hypo-albuminaemia using a formula based on the *mean normal plasma albumin concentration* for that particular biochemical laboratory (Box 6.A).

Box 6.A　Correcting plasma calcium concentrations (Oxford Radcliffe Hospitals Trust)

Corrected calcium (mmol/L) = measured calcium + 0.022 × (42 − albumin (g/L))

　　e.g. measured calcium = 2.45; albumin = 32

　　　　corrected calcium = 2.45 + 0.022 × 10 = 2.67mmol/L

Incidence

All malignant disease 10–20%. Up to 50% in breast cancer and myeloma.

Common in cancer of the lung (squamous cell), head and neck, kidney and cervix uteri.

Uncommon in cancer of the prostate, lung (small cell), gastric and large bowel.

Cancer-related hypercalcaemia is generally associated with disseminated disease and, despite treatment, survival is often <3 months. Only 20% will be alive after 12 months.[1]

Pathogenesis

Any type of cancer with or without skeletal metastases may be associated with hypercalcaemia. However, more than 80% of patients with cancer-related hypercalcaemia have skeletal metastases.[2] The extent of bony disease does not correlate with the level of hypercalcaemia.[3]

Biochemical evidence of humoral mechanisms is detectable in almost all cases of hypercalcaemia in cancer (Box 6.B). In solid tumours, the most common mediator of hypercalcaemia is tumour-secreted parathyroid hormone-related protein (PTHrP). This is not detected by radio-immuno-assay for parathyroid hormone (PTH); in hypercalcaemia in cancer, plasma PTH concentrations are low or undetectable.

In myeloma, hypercalcaemia is caused by osteoclast-activating factors (Box 6.B). In lymphoma, similar factors to myeloma are responsible in some cases; in others, PTHrP is present. Some lymphomas also produce an enzyme which converts 25-hydroxyvitamin D into biologically active 1, 25-dihydroxyvitamin D (1,25 DHCC). This leads to increased intestinal absorption of vitamin D and an increased production of vitamin D during exposure to sunlight.

PTHrP impairs calcium excretion by the distal renal tubule, and vomiting leads to sodium loss and to sodium-linked calcium resorption by the proximal renal tubule. Renal impairment in myeloma is exacerbated by nephrotoxic immuno-globulin light chains.

Clinical features

The severity of the symptoms is not always related to the severity of the hypercalcaemia. Sometimes a small elevation causes definite symptoms, and vice versa (Box 6.C). Polyuria and polydipsia are not constant features. Severe symptoms may develop rapidly without a clearly defined prodrome.

If untreated, severe hypercalcaemia >4mmol/L is generally fatal because of renal failure and cardiac arrhythmias. Neurological symptoms and signs are seen occasionally, e.g. upper motor neurone deficits, scotomata, ataxia, fits. These can mimic cerebral secondaries. Severe dysphagia for food and fluid occasionally occurs.[4] *Pain may be precipitated or exacerbated by hypercalcaemia.*[5–7]

Evaluation

Hypercalcaemia is seldom associated with an occult cancer. Diagnosis is based on a high level of clinical suspicion and confirmed by appropriate blood tests. Alternative causes should be considered, e.g. hyperparathyroidism.

Box 6.B   Humoral factors and hypercalcaemia of malignancy

Parathyroid hormone-related protein (PTHrP)
Most common mediator of cancer-related hypercalcaemia.

Produced by many solid tumours, notably lung, breast and kidney.

Acts by activating PTH receptors in tissue.

Stimulates osteoclastic bone resorption; enhances renal tubular calcium resorption.

Transforming growth factors (TGF)
Produced by many solid tumours, including cancers of the lung (squamous cell), head and neck, breast, kidney.

Epidermal growth factor is secreted by tumour cells and is a potent bone resorber.

TGF-α is secreted by many tumours; it is structurally and functionally similar to epidermal growth factors and is a potent bone resorber.

TGF-β is produced by normal and malignant cells and enhances the production of PTHrP in breast cancer cells.

Osteoclast-activating factors
Tumour necrosis factor-alpha (TNF-α) is a potent osteoclast-activating factor.

Lymphotoxin (TNF-β) is a cytokine produced by activated T lymphocytes and myeloma cells.

Interleukin-6 (IL-6) is a cytokine produced by T lymphocytes, myeloma cells and uterine endometrial cells.

IL-1 is a cytokine produced by monocytes and inhibits osteoblastic bone formation.

1,25-dihydroxyvitamin D (vitamin D)
Generally plays a minor role in cancer-related hypercalcaemia.

However, in certain lymphomas tumour cells metabolize vitamin D, thereby increasing gastro-intestinal absorption of calcium.

Also has a direct bone-resorbing action.

In malignant hypercalcaemia there is *hypochloraemic alkalosis* whereas primary hyperparathyroidism is associated with *hyperchloraemic acidosis* because of impaired renal bicarbonate resorption. Thus, plasma chloride concentration is:

- generally <98mmol/L in malignant disease
- generally >103mmol/L in hyperparathyroidism.

Plasma PTH concentration is low or undetectable in malignant disease but is raised in primary hyperparathyroidism.

Box 6.C   Symptoms of hypercalcaemia

Mild	Severe
Patient ambulatory	*Patient increasingly incapacitated*
Fatigue	Nausea ⎫ → dehydration and
Lethargy	Vomiting ⎬ cardiovascular collapse
Mental dullness	Ileus
Weakness	Delirium
Anorexia	Drowsiness
Constipation	Coma

Management

Stop and think! Are you justified in correcting a potentially fatal complication in a moribund patient?

The following together comprise a set of indications for the correction of hypercalcaemia:

- corrected plasma calcium concentration of >2.8mmol/L

- symptoms attributable to hypercalcaemia

- first episode or long interval since previous one

- previous good quality of life (in the patient's opinion)

- medical expectation that treatment will achieve a durable effect (based on the results of previous treatment)

- patient willing to have IV therapy and requisite blood tests.

Not all symptoms respond equally to treatment (Box 6.D). This may be because some are caused by other factors, principally the underlying disseminated disease.

Fluid replacement

Some centres give IV fluid replacement routinely. Others do so only when there are severe symptoms or renal impairment, e.g. 0.9% saline 2–3L/24h, with potassium supplements, until oral fluid intake is adequate.

Saline improves hypercalcaemia by improving the glomerular filtration rate and by promoting a sodium-linked calcium diuresis. Saline alone will reduce plasma calcium concentrations by 0.2–0.4 mmol/L.

Box 6.D   Impact of correcting hypercalcaemia[8]

Consistent response	**Variable response**
Thirst	General malaise
Polyuria	Fatigue
Delirium	Anorexia
Mental dullness	
Constipation	

Bisphosphonates

Bisphosphonates inhibit osteoclast activity and thereby inhibit bone resorption, but have no impact on the effect of PTHrP on renal tubular resorption of calcium. Bisphosphonates are generally given IV, at least initially, because of poor alimentary absorption. Bisphosphonates are adsorbed onto the bone surface where they remain bound to hydroxyapatite for weeks or months. A single infusion therefore has a prolonged duration of action on osteoclasts. The two most widely used bisphosphonates are clodronate and pamidronate.

Before using any bisphosphonate, it is important to check the manufacturer's recommendations. With pamidronate, the dose depends on the corrected plasma calcium concentration (Table 6.1):

- the maximum recommended dose is 90mg IV/treatment

- the infusion rate should not exceed *60mg/h* (*20mg/h* in patients with renal impairment)

- the concentration should not exceed *60mg/250ml*

- repeat after 1 week if the initial response is inadequate

- repeat every 3–4 weeks according to plasma calcium concentration (Table 6.2).

Table 6.1   IV pamidronate for hypercalcaemia

Corrected plasma calcium concentration (mmol/L)	Dose (mg)
<3	30
3–3.5	30–60
3.5–4	60–90
>4	90

Table 6.2   Bisphosphonates and the treatment of hypercalcaemia[9,10]

	Clodronate	Pamidronate
Initial IV dose	(a) 1500mg (b) 300–600mg daily for 5 days	30–90mg
Onset of effect	<2 days	<3 days
Maximum effect	3–5 days	5–7 days
Median duration of effect	(a) 2 weeks (b) 3 weeks	4 weeks
Restores normocalcaemia	40–80%	70–90%

Mechanism of action
  inhibits osteoclasts
  stimulates osteoblasts
	
	+
	–
		
		+
		+

Initial PO treatment	Effective	Effective but gastro-intestinal intolerance common
Maintenance	Tablets generally prevent relapse	IV infusion every 3–4 weeks

With clodronate:

- the maximum recommended dose is 1500mg IV/treatment
- the infusion rate should not exceed *400mg/h* (slower in patients with renal impairment, e.g. *200mg/h*)
- the concentration should not exceed *3mg/ml* (1500mg/500ml)
- repeat after 5 days if the initial response is inadequate
- maintain normocalcaemia by prescribing anhydrous sodium clodronate capsules 1600mg (400mg × 4) PO o.d. or 800mg (400mg × 2) PO b.d.
- in patients with renal impairment the PO dose should be halved to 800mg/24h
- if necessary the PO dose may be increased to 3200mg/24h.

Clodronate can also be given SC over 6–12h (*see* p.28).[11] Swelling, erythema or bruising occurs in about 25%. SC pamidronate is possibly more irritant; it commonly causes pain, erythema and pruritus.[12]

Calcitonin

Calcitonin (salmon) has a rapid calcium-lowering effect which is evident within 2h. It inhibits both osteoclast activity and renal tubular resorption of calcium. It is generally given SC or IM but PR is also effective. Maximum effect is seen with 100 IU/24h and the effect lasts 2–3 days.

More calcitonin is less effective because of down-regulation of calcitonin receptors in osteoclasts. Relapse is delayed to 6–9 days by the concurrent use of a corticosteroid.[13] The combination of calcitonin and corticosteroids long-term is not as effective as bisphosphonates. The main use of calcitonin is in combination with a bisphosphonate in order to obtain a rapid early response.

Corticosteroids

No longer recommended for cancer-related hypercalcaemia because of the poor response rate.[13] However, they are beneficial when used as an adjunct to SC calcitonin.[14]

If more effective treatments are not available, the use of prednisolone 60mg o.d. or dexamethasone 8mg o.d. should be considered in patients with breast and renal cancer or with myeloma and lymphoma.[15] Smaller doses are unlikely to be effective.

Octreotide

Octreotide is a somatostatin analogue. It has been used successfully in the treatment of hypercalcaemia associated with neuro-endocrine tumours resistant to other meausres.[16]

Syndrome of inappropriate ADH secretion (SIADH)

Inappropriate secretion of antidiuretic hormone (ADH) occurs in 2% of patients with malignant disease. The most common association is small cell lung cancer with an incidence of about 10%,[17] accounting for 75% of cancer-related cases of SIADH.[18] In head and neck cancer, the incidence is 3%.[19]

Pathogenesis

There are many causes of SIADH (Box 6.E). In cancer-related SIADH there is ectopic secretion of arginine vasopressin (ADH) or vasopressin-like peptides by the cancer.[20,21] In small cell lung cancer an elevated arginine vasopressin can be detected in about 40% of patients but in the majority it is asymptomatic.

Box 6.E   Causes of SIADH

Cancer
Small cell lung
Head and neck
Pancreas
Prostate
Carcinoid
Lymphoma
Acute myeloid leukaemia

Treatment
After neurosurgery
Chemotherapy, e.g.
  cyclophosphamide
  vincristine
Drugs
  tricyclic antidepressants
  SSRIs
  carbamazepine
  phenothiazines
  lorazepam
  barbiturates

Miscellaneous
Pulmonary
  pneumonia
  tuberculosis
  lung abscess
  positive pressure ventilation
Central nervous system
  meningitis
  encephalitis
  subarachnoid haemorrhage
  cerebral thrombosis
  head injury
Psychiatric
  schizophrenia
  psychosis
Recreational drugs
  ethanol
  nicotine

Hyponatraemia, possibly caused by SIADH, should be considered in all patients who develop drowsiness, confusion or convulsions while taking a tricyclic antidepressant or SSRI. Most cases associated with SSRIs involve elderly people, particularly women.[22,23]

Clinical features

Clinical features depend on both the level and the rate of decline of the plasma sodium concentration (Box 6.F). Given time, brain cells can compensate against cerebral oedema by secreting potassium and other solutes; asymptomatic hyponatraemia therefore indicates chronic rather than acute SIADH.

Box 6.F Clinical features of SIADH

Plasma sodium 110–120mmol/L	**Plasma sodium <110mmol/L**
Anorexia	Multifocal myoclonus
Nausea and vomiting	Drowsiness
Lassitude	Seizures
Confusion	Coma
Oedema	

Evaluation

The diagnosis of SIADH is based on the following criteria:

*   hyponatraemia (<125mmol/L)

*   low plasma osmolality (<270mosmol/L)

*   raised urine osmolality (>100mosmol/L)

*   urine sodium concentration
     always >20mmol/L
     often >50mmol/L

*   normal plasma volume.[24]

In practice, a plasma sodium concentration of <120mmol/L is sufficient to make a clinical diagnosis of SIADH in the absence of:

*   severe vomiting

*   diuretic therapy

*   hypo-adrenalism

*   hypothyroidism

*   severe renal failure.

Management

Treat the patient and not the biochemical results.

Correct the correctable

Successful anticancer treatment will lead to a remission of SIADH.

Non-drug treatment

Restrict fluid intake to 700–1000ml/day or daily urine output to <500ml. Although standard treatment for SIADH, fluid restriction to this extent is an added burden for most patients struggling to cope with end-stage cancer.

Drug treatment

Demeclocycline, a tetracycline derivative, is the drug treatment of choice, and is given in a dose of 300mg PO b.d.–q.d.s. In patients unable to take demeclocycline reliably PO, it can be given PR dispersed in 5ml of a methylcellulose carrier.[25] It acts by inducing nephrogenic diabetes insipidus, i.e. inhibits the action of ADH on renal tubules.

The effect of demeclocycline is apparent after 3–5 days, and persists for several days after stopping treatment. There is no need to restrict fluid during treatment. Adverse effects include uraemia, particularly with higher doses. Nausea and photosensitivity also occur.

Vasopressin V2-receptor antagonists which selectively block the action of ADH on renal tubules are being developed for PO and IV use.

References

1   Bower M *et al.* (1997) Endocrine and metabolic complications of advanced cancer. In: D Doyle, G Hanks and N MacDonald (eds) *Oxford Textbook of Palliative Medicine.* Oxford University Press, Oxford, pp 709–25.

2   Glick J and Glover D (1998) Metabolic emergencies. In: G Murphy, W Lawrence and R Lenhard (eds) *Clinical Oncology.* American Cancer Society, Atlanta, Georgia, pp 609–10.

3   Mundy G (1997) Malignancy and the skeleton. *Hormone and Metabolic Research.* **29**:120–6.

4   Grieve R and Dixon P (1983) Dysphagia: a further symptom of hypercalcaemia. *British Medical Journal.* **286**:1935–6.

5   Parsons V *et al.* (1974) The effects of calcitonin on the metabolic disturbances surrounding widespread bony metastases. *Acta Endocrinologica.* **76**:286–301.

6   Davies J *et al.* (1979) Effect of mithramycin on widespread painful bone metastases in cancer of the breast. *Cancer Treatment Reports.* **63**:1835–8.

7   Coombes R *et al.* (1979) Agents affecting osteolysis in patients with breast cancer. *Cancer Chemotherapy and Pharmacology.* **3**:41–4.

8   Ralston S *et al.* (1990) Cancer-associated hypercalcaemia: morbidity and mortality. *Annals of Internal Medicine.* **112**:449–504.

9   Ralston S (1994) Pathogenesis and management of cancer associated hypercalcaemia. In: G Hanks (ed) *Cancer Surveys: Palliative Medicine: Problem areas in pain and symptom management.* Cold Spring Harbor Laboratory Press, pp 179–96.

10 Purohit O *et al.* (1995) A randomised, double-blind comparison of intravenous pamidronate and clodronate in hypercalcaemia of malignancy. *British Journal of Cancer.* **72**:1289–93.

11 Walker P *et al.* (1997) Subcutaneous clodronate: a study evaluating efficacy in hypercalcaemia of malignancy and local toxicity. *Annals of Oncology.* **8**: 915–16.

12 Constans T *et al.* (1991) hypodermoclysis in dehydrated elderly patients: local effects with and without hyaluronidase. *Journal of Palliative Care.* **7**:10–12.

13 Percival R *et al.* (1984) Role of glucocorticoids in management of malignant hypercalcaemia. *British Medical Journal.* **289**:287.

14 Ralston S *et al.* (1985) Comparison of aminohydroxypropylidene diphosphonate, mithramycin, and corticosteroids/calcitonin in treatment of cancer-associated hypercalcaemia. *Lancet.* **ii**:907–10.

15 Mannheimer I (1965) Hypercalcaemia of breast cancer. Management with corticosteroids. *Cancer.* **18**:679–91.

16 Harrison M *et al.* (1990) Somatostatin analogue treatment for malignant hypercalcaemia. *British Medical Journal.* **300**:1313–4.

17 van Oosterhout A *et al.* (1996) Neurologic disorders in 203 consecutive patients with small cell lung cancer. *Cancer.* **77**:1434–41.

18 List A *et al.* (1986) The syndrome of inappropriate secretion of antidiuretic hormone (SIADH) in small-cell lung cancer. *Journal of Clinical Oncology.* **4**: 1191–8.

19 Ferlito A *et al.* (1997) Syndrome of inappropriate antidiuretic hormone secretion associated with head and neck cancers. Review of the literature. *Annals of Otology, Rhinology and Laryngology.* **106**:878–83.

20 Meinders A (1993) Hyponatraemia: SIADH or SIAD? *Netherlands Journal of Medicine.* **43**:1–4.

21 Sorensen J *et al.* (1995) Syndrome of inappropriate secretion of antidiuretic hormone (SIADH) in malignant disease. *Journal of Internal Medicine.* **238**: 97–110.

22 ADRAC (Adverse Drug Reactions Advisory Committee) (1996) Selective serotonin reuptake inhibitors and SIADH. *Medical Journal of Australia.* **164**:562.

23 Liu B *et al.* (1996) Hyponatremia and the syndrome of inappropriate secretion of antidiuretic hormone associated with the use of selective serotonin reuptake inhibitors: a review of spontaneous reports. *Canadian Medical Association Journal.* **155**:519–27.

24 Saito T (1996) SIADH and other hyponatremic disorders: diagnosis and therapeutic problems. *Nippon Jinzo Gakkai Shi.* **38**:429–34.

25 Hussain I *et al.* (1998) Rectal administration of demeclocycline in a patient with syndrome of inappropriate ADH secretion. *International Journal of Clinical Practice.* **52**:59.

7 Haematological symptoms

Haematological changes in cancer · Anaemia of chronic disease · Bleeding · Surface bleeding · Nosebleeds Haemoptysis · Haematemesis and melaena · Rectal and vaginal haemorrhage · Haematuria · Severe haemorrhage Venous thrombosis · Pulmonary embolism · Disseminated intravascular coagulation

Haematological changes in cancer

Haematological changes are common in cancer, and sometimes are the presenting feature (Table 7.1). Anaemia is the most common abnormality.

Anaemia of chronic disease

Anaemia is defined in adults as a haemoglobin concentration of <13.5g/dL in men and <11.5g/dL in women. It occurs in up to 50% of patients with solid tumours and in most patients with myeloma and lymphoma. Symptoms vary but can have a major impact on a patient's lifestyle (Box 7.A). In some patients there may be more than one cause, e.g. iron deficiency as well as anaemia of chronic disease (ACD).

ACD is caused by a cytokine-mediated (interleukin-1) suppression of erythropoietin production and erythropoiesis. ACD is associated with:

- reduced response to erythropoietin (Figure 7.1)[1]

- impaired transferrin production, resulting in reduced availability of stored iron

- shortened red blood cell (RBC) survival.

Table 7.1   Haematological changes in malignant disorders[2,3]

Haematological changes	Common association
RBC	
Anaemia of chronic disease	All
Iron deficiency anaemia	Gastro-intestinal, cervix, uterus
Megaloblastic anaemia	Myeloma
Sideroblastic anaemia	Myeloproliferative disorders
Leuco-erythroblastic anaemia	Breast, bronchus, kidney, prostate, stomach, thyroid
Micro-angiopathic haemolytic anaemia	Mucin-secreting tumours, stomach
Selective red cell aplasia	Thymus, lymphoma, bronchus
Immune haemolytic anaemia	Ovary, lymphoma
Polycythaemia	Kidney, liver, posterior fossa, uterus
Secondary myelosclerosis	As for leuco-erythroblastic anaemia, also reticuloses
WBC	
Leucocytosis	All
Leukaemoid reactions	As for leuco-erythroblastic anaemia
Eosinophilia	Many
Monocytosis	All
Basophilia	Myeloproliferative disease, mastocytosis
Lymphopenia	Cancer, reticulosis
Platelets	
Thrombocytosis	Gastro-intestinal with bleeding Bronchus and others without bleeding
Thrombocytopenia	As for micro-angiopathies
Acquired thrombocytopathy	Macroglobulinaemia, other paraproteinaemias
Coagulation	
Thrombophlebitis	All
Disseminated intravascular coagulation	Many (*see* p.252)
Primary activation of fibrinolysis	Prostate
Miscellaneous	
Abnormal proteins, e.g. cryofibrinogens	Prostate, others
Foetal proteins	
α-fetoprotein	Liver and others
carcino-embryonic	Gastro-intestinal neoplasms
foetal haemoglobin	Leukaemia, other tumours

Box 7.A   Anaemia and cancer

Main causes	**Symptoms**
Anaemia of chronic disease (ACD)	Tiredness (fatigue)
Iron and folate deficiency	Lack of energy (lethargy)
Malignant infiltration of the marrow	Shortness of breath
Haemolytic anaemia	Angina
Renal failure	Loss of appetite
	Loss of libido
	Low mood

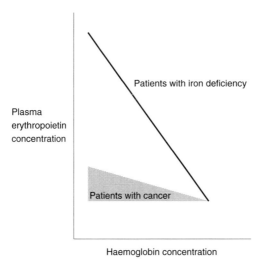

Figure 7.1   Relationship between haemoglobin and erythropoietin concentrations in patients with iron deficiency and cancer-associated anaemia. Reproduced with permission from Miller et al., 1990.[1]

Evaluation

It is important to differentiate between ACD and iron deficiency (Table 7.2). Diagnostic features of ACD are:

- normochromic–normocytic anaemia
- reticulocytopenia
- low/low-normal plasma transferrin (TIBC) concentration

- low plasma iron
- high/high-normal plasma ferritin concentration
- hypoplastic bone marrow appearances
- increased marrow iron stores
- reduced iron within maturing erythroblasts.

Table 7.2   Iron deficiency anaemia compared with anaemia of chronic disease[4]

Test	Normal[a]	Iron deficiency	ACD
Blood film	Normochromic– normocytic	Hypochromic– microcytic	Normochromic or hypochromic– normocytic; rarely microcytic
TIBC (μmol/L)	45–75	High/high-normal	Low/low-normal
Plasma iron (μmol/L)	14–31	Low/very low	Low
Plasma ferritin (μg/L)	17–230	Low	High/high-normal

a   reference values, Oxford Radcliffe Hospitals.

Management

Treat the patient and not the laboratory results. Although tiredness and weakness can be caused by the cancer itself, if associated with anaemia they are strong indicators for a trial blood transfusion (Box 7.B). Alternatively, epoetin (recombinant human erythropoietin) can be used; this is generally given SC three times a week. Maintenance treatment with a weekly injection may be adequate for some patients.

Erythropoietin stimulates the production of RBC. Its plasma concentration is often low in patients with cancer particularly those receiving chemotherapy. Epoetin 150–300 IU/kg SC three times a week leads to:

- an increase in haemoglobin of >2g/dL in 50–60% of patients
- improved quality of life with each increment in haemoglobin up to a level of around 12g/dL.[7,8]

Patients most likely to benefit from its use are those with:

- a low plasma erythropoietin concentration (<100mg/ml)

Box 7.B   Non-emergency blood transfusion in palliative care

Indications
Generally the following criteria should all be met:
* symptoms attributable to anaemia, e.g. fatigue, weakness and breathlessness on exertion, which
     are troublesome to the patient
     limit routine activity
     are likely to be corrected by transfusion
* expectation that a blood transfusion will achieve a durable effect, e.g. at least 2 weeks
* patient willing to have a transfusion and requisite blood tests.

Contra-indications for blood transfusion
* no benefit from previous transfusion
* patient is moribund, i.e. the patient's condition is terminal
* if the transfusion can best be described as simply prolonging a patient's death
* if the main reason is a demand by the family that 'something must be done'.

Blood transfusion helps about 75% of patients in terms of wellbeing, strength and breathlessness.[5] Benefit occurs equally in patients with haemoglobin <8g/dL and in those with haemoglobin 8–11g/dL.[5,6]

---

* adequate bone marrow reserve (neutrophils >1.5 × 10⁹/L, platelets >100 × 10⁹/L)

* an increase in haemoglobin of >1g/dL within 4 weeks of commencing treatment with epoetin.

It is expensive. An excessive increase in red cell mass is avoided by:

* reducing the dose by 25% when haemoglobin rises by >2g/dL/month

* aiming to maintain a haemoglobin of 11g/dL in women and 12g/dL in men

* discontinuing treatment if the haemoglobin rises >15g/dL (Table 7.3).

Table 7.3   Comparison of epoetin and blood transfusion

	Epoetin	*Transfusion*
Rise in haemoglobin	Long-lasting	Transient (2–4 weeks)
Speed of effect	4–6 weeks	Immediate
Safety	Adverse effects rare and generally minor	Risk of transfusion reactions and infections
Inconvenience to patient	SC injection	IV infusion
Cost	£100–£250/week	£500–£750/transfusion

Bleeding

Bleeding occurs in about 20% of patients with advanced cancer. It contributes significantly to the patient's death in about 5%. External catastrophic bleeding is less common than internal occult bleeding. *Stop and think! Are you justified in treating a potentially fatal complication in a moribund patient?*

Excessive bruising and bleeding from the gums and nose or the gastrointestinal tract suggests a platelet abnormality whereas bleeding into joints or muscles suggests a deficiency of at least one coagulation factor.

Check the prothrombin time and the activated partial thromboplastin time (aPTT), and obtain a full blood count. In patients with cancer, an elevated prothrombin time and an elevated aPTT are seen with:

• severe hepatic impairment

• phytomenadione (vitamin K_1) deficiency

• disseminated intravascular coagulation (DIC) (*see* p.252).

Thrombocytopenia

Thrombocytopenia is defined as a platelet count of $<150 \times 10^9$/L. With platelet counts of $10–20 \times 10^9$/L the risk of a major bleed is small (0.1% per day). Below 10×10^9/L the risk rises (2% per day) with severe bleeds occurring mostly with counts below 5×10^9/L. Risk of intracranial haemorrhage is present only below 1×10^9/L. Treatment varies with the cause (Box 7.C). Platelet function may also be impaired without thrombocytopenia by most NSAIDs (*see* p.36), and also in myeloma and renal failure.[9]

Box 7.C   Causes of thrombocytopenia

Decreased production of platelets
Marrow replacement with tumour
Chemotherapy
Carbamazepine
Thiazide diuretics
Excessive alcohol (recovers within 3–5 days of cessation)

Platelet sequestration by the spleen
Increased venous pressure resulting from liver disease
Cardiac failure
Respiratory failure

Increased platelet destruction (immune)
Sepsis
Heparin
After transfusion of blood products

Increased platelet destruction (non-immune)
Disseminated intravascular coagulation (DIC)

Correct the correctable

- modify or stop chemotherapy

- prescribe antibiotics if caused by sepsis

- review drug Data Sheets and stop any drug which is potentially causal.

Heparin-induced thrombocytopenia (HIT)

Heparin causes thrombocytopenia. An early (<4 days) mild fall in platelet count is often seen after starting heparin therapy, particularly after surgery. This corrects spontaneously despite the continued use of heparin and is asymptomatic.[10] However, occasionally, an immune thrombocytopenia develops associated with heparin-dependent IgG antibodies. The antibodies form a complex with platelet factor 4 and bind to the platelet surface, *causing disruption of the platelets and a release of procoagulant material.* It can occur up to 4 weeks after starting heparin and manifests as venous or arterial thromboembolism which may be fatal (Box 7.D). Heparin should be stopped immediately if there is a dramatic fall in the platelet count (Box 7.D). If continued anticoagulation is desirable, a heparinoid or hirudin should be used, e.g. danaparoid. Cross-reactivity is rare.

HIT is less common with prophylactic regimens (low doses) than with therapeutic ones (higher doses). The risk is further reduced by using low molecular

---

Box 7.D   Clinical events associated with HIT[11]

Platelet count
Thrombocytopenia.

Falling platelet count that does not reach thrombocytopenic levels, i.e. a fall in the platelet count of ⩾50% beginning on or after day 5 of heparin use.

Venous thrombosis
Deep vein thrombosis (mostly proximal vein); if gross swelling, arterial supply may be compromised → limb gangrene.

Pulmonary embolism.

Adrenal haemorrhagic infarction (probably secondary to adrenal vein thrombosis).

Cerebral vein or cerebral dural sinus thrombosis.

Arterial thrombosis or thrombo-embolism
Arterial thrombosis, e.g. cerebral, coronary, aorta (may cause spinal cord infarction), mesenteric, renal, limb.

Vascular graft occlusion.

Reactions at heparin injection sites
Erythematous plaques.

Skin necrosis.

Sequelae after IV heparin bolus in patients with HIT-IgG
Acute systemic reaction (inflammatory or respiratory).

Transient global amnesia.

---

weight heparin (LMWH) rather than unfractionated heparin. HIT typically develops 5–8 days after starting heparin and, for this reason, some centres check the platelet count at this time (Box 7.E). HIT is more common in the USA (where more bovine heparin is used) than in the UK (where more porcine heparin is used). The risk in the USA has been put at 3% for unfractionated heparin.[11]

Non-drug treatment

In a relatively well patient with a platelet count $<5 \times 10^9$/L, platelet transfusions should be considered as an emergency measure. They are not indicated if the platelet count is above 10×10^9/L and there is no bleeding. Each transfusion is generally of 6 units (each unit raises the platelet count by $5–7 \times 10^9$/L).[12] Patients for whom both life-supporting treatment is appropriate and who are

---

Box 7.E   Diagnosis and management of HIT[11]

High clinical suspicion for HIT

Platelet count fall generally of 50% or more, or to below $100 \times 10^9/L$, beginning after 5 days of heparin use.

New thrombotic or thrombo-embolic event.

Laboratory confirmation

Do one of the following tests but if negative or borderline, do both.

Functional assay for antibodies using washed platelets or citrated platelet-rich plasmas.

Antigen assay (platelet factor 4/heparin ELISA).

Therapeutic approach

Stop heparin.

Start treatment with danaparoid or hirudin.

Unless already fully anticoagulated with warfarin, do not start warfarin until the thrombocytopenia has resolved and the patient is satisfactorily anticoagulated with danaparoid or hirudin.

---

bleeding, have sepsis or DIC should be given platelets sufficient to maintain a count of $>50 \times 10^9/L$. In reversible renal and hepatic failure, emergency treatment with cryoprecipitate infusions 10 units q12h should be considered.

Drug treatment

In relatively well patients, consider the following:

- corticosteroids, e.g. prednisolone 1mg/kg, or immunoglobulin infusions 1g/kg if there is auto-immune destruction of platelets

- desmopressin 0.3µg/kg IV over 30min or 150µg in each nostril (effect lasts 4–8h); this augments platelet function. *Regular use will lead to water retention and a risk of thrombosis*

- blood transfusions to raise the haematocrit above 30%.

Phytomenadione deficiency

Phytomenadione (vitamin K_1) is required for the synthesis of several coagulation factors (II, VII, IX, X). It is present in green vegetables and is synthesized by bacteria in the bowel; body stores are low. Patients who are malnourished, have fat malabsorption or are receiving prolonged courses of antibiotics which sterilize the bowel are at risk of deficiency and a rapid rise in prothrombin time. Treat with:

- phytomenadione 10mg PO o.d.

- menadiol sodium phosphate 10mg PO o.d. (if fat malabsorption present).

When a more rapid response is required for serious bleeding:

- phytomenadione (e.g. Konakion MM) 10mg by slow IV injection over 15min *or*

- 4 units of fresh frozen plasma.

Hepatic impairment

Severe liver disease leads to multiple coagulation defects:

- reduced synthesis and increased consumption of nearly all of the major coagulation factors

- hypersplenism causing thrombocytopenia

- increase in fibrin degradation products and plasmin leading to platelet dysfunction

- enhanced fibrinolysis, suggested by diffuse oozing from sites of minor trauma (Box 7.D).

Despite the risk of coagulation abnormalities, paradoxically the risk of venous thrombosis is often increased in patients with hepatic failure.

Renal impairment

Patients with renal disease may have either a bleeding or a thrombotic tendency. There is a loss of natural anticoagulants in nephrotic syndrome. Patients on dialysis have a high incidence of gastro-intestinal and genito-urinary bleeding and subdural haematomas. In end-stage renal disease, gastro-intestinal bleeding due to angiodysplasia or gastritis can occur. Treatment includes:

- epoetin or blood transfusion to raise the haematocrit over 30%

- oestrogen 0.6mg/kg IV for 5 days; this reduces the risk of bleeding for up to 2 weeks.

In more acute situations, consider:

• dialysis in severe impairment
• desmopressin ⎫
                 ⎬ as for thrombocytopenia (see p.235).
• cryoprecipitate infusions ⎭

The reason for a hypercoaguable state in certain renal diseases is not understood.

Surface bleeding

Surface bleeding may be exacerbated by the effect of a NSAID on platelet function (see p.36). When this is the case, change to a non-acetylated salicylate, a preferential or selective COX-2 inhibitor or paracetamol. Other options comprise:

• physical measures
• haemostatic drugs, e.g. tranexamic acid
• radiotherapy (Box 7.F).

The maximum dose of tranexamic acid is 1.5g q.d.s., although a smaller dose is often satisfactory (Box 7.F). Improvement occurs in 2–4 days. Discontinue or reduce to 500mg t.d.s. 1 week after bleeding has stopped. Restart if bleeding recurs.

Nosebleeds

Most nosebleeds are venous. When from the anterior nasal septum (Little's area), they can often be stopped by direct pressure, i.e. by pinching the nostrils for 10–15min. If this does not work, a silver nitrate caustic pencil applied to the bleeding point is often effective. Alternatively, the nostril can be packed for 2 days with calcium alginate rope (e.g. Kaltostat) or with ribbon gauze soaked in adrenaline (epinephrine) (1 in 1000) 1mg in 1ml.

If bleeding continues into the nasopharynx, the source is more posterior and may require referral to an ENT department for:

• the insertion of a Merocel tampon for 36h with antibiotic cover *or*
• packing with gauze impregnated with bismuth iodoform paraffin paste (BIPP) for 3 days *or*
• balloon catheter *or*
• cauterization under local anaesthetic.

Box 7.F   Management of surface bleeding

Physical

Gauze applied with pressure for 10min soaked in:

- adrenaline (epinephrine) (1 in 1000) 1mg in 1ml *or*

- tranexamic acid 500mg in 5ml

} use standard ampoules.

Silver nitrate sticks applied to bleeding points in the nose and mouth, and on skin nodules and fungating tumours.

Haemostatic dressings, i.e. alginate (e.g. Kaltostat, Sorbsan).

Diathermy.

Specialist therapy:
    cryotherapy
    LASER
    embolization.[13,14]

Drugs

Topical

Sucralfate paste 2g (two 1g tablets crushed in 5ml KY jelly).[15]

Sucralfate suspension 2g in 10ml b.d. for the mouth and rectum.[16]

Tranexamic acid 5g in 50ml warm water b.d. for rectal bleeding.[17]

1% alum solution (*see* p.245).

Systemic

Antifibrinolytic drug, e.g. tranexamic acid 1.5g stat and 0.5–1g b.d.–t.d.s., reduces capillary oozing by inhibiting fibrinolysis.[18] *Do not use if DIC suspected.*

Haemostatic drug, e.g. etamsylate 500mg q.d.s., restores platelet adhesiveness.

Desmopressin, augments platelet function.[19]

Radiotherapy

Teletherapy and brachytherapy are both used to control haemorrhage from:

skin	bladder	rectum.
lungs	uterus	
oesophagus	vagina	

Chronic recurrent mild epistaxis is often related to nasal vestibulitis which can be treated with chlorhexidine and neomycin cream (e.g. Naseptin) applied b.d. for 2 weeks followed by petroleum jelly (Vaseline). If bleeding is heavy, consider checking the prothrombin time and the aPTT, and obtain a full blood count to check platelet count and haemoglobin concentration.

Haemoptysis

One third of patients with lung cancer experience haemoptysis. The incidence of acute fatal bleeds is 3%, of which some occur without warning. Haemoptysis need not be massive to cause respiratory embarassment. When death results, it is generally caused by suffocation and not exsanguination. Haemoptysis of 400ml within 3h or 600ml within 24h has a mortality of about 75%.[20]

Physiology

The lungs have two blood supplies:

- low-pressure pulmonary circulation which supplies blood for gas exchange

- high-pressure bronchial circulation which supplies blood to the structures of the respiratory tract; *this is the more important in haemoptysis.*

Causes

In cancer, haemoptysis may be caused by the cancer itself or by other factors:

- lung cancer; massive haemoptysis is most likely with squamous cell cancer lying centrally or causing cavitation. Generally there is necrosis of vessels within the tumour bed rather than direct tumour invasion into the pulmonary vasculature

- metastatic lung disease; particularly cancers of the breast, colorectum and kidney, and melanoma

- chest infection (acute and chronic); in haematological malignancies, pulmonary haemorrhage ± haemoptysis is associated with fungal infection

- pulmonary embolus.

Pattern recognition generally helps to identify non-cancerous causes, e.g. infection is associated with purulent sputum and a pulmonary embolus with pleuritic pain. These should be treated as appropriate.

Note: coughed up blood may not originate from the lungs. Particularly in patients with a bleeding tendency or thrombocytopenia, fresh blood can be from the nose, pharynx or lungs. Dark blood is more likely from the lungs.

Management

Validate the patient's concern, i.e. never say, 'Don't worry about it' but 'I'm glad you mentioned it, I imagine you must be very concerned about it'. Assure the patient that, although it is a nuisance and unpleasant, life-threatening haemoptysis is rare.

Correct the correctable

Can the cancer be modified?

Radiotherapy leads to prolonged relief in 85% of patients.[18] A palliative dose of teletherapy is generally given as 1–2 treatments, which permits retreatment if necessary. For patients with unrelieved or recurrent haemoptysis in whom further external beam radiation is not possible, other options will vary according to local availability:

- brachytherapy (endobronchial radiation). A fine catheter is placed at bronchoscopy which is afterloaded for a short time with a radio-active source by remote control. Can be carried out as a day case procedure and is effective in >80% of patients[21]

- cryotherapy, in which the tumour is cooled by a liquid nitrogen probe to −70°C. Multiple treatments may be required; it requires rigid bronchoscopy and a general anaesthetic

- LASER therapy, requires rigid bronchoscopy and a general anaesthetic.

Can other factors be modified?

Consider discontinuing drugs with an antiplatelet effect. In relation to the commonly used NSAIDs, substitute one of the following:

- a non-acetylated salicylate (e.g. diflunisal) which does not interfere with platelet function

- a preferential COX-2 inhibitor (e.g. meloxicam, nimesulide) or selective COX-2 inhibitor (e.g. celecoxib, rofecoxib)

- paracetamol.

Consider checking the prothrombin time, aPTT and the full blood count.

Non-drug treatment

Massive haemoptysis is an emergency, but conventional life-saving interventions, i.e. bronchoscopy, intubation and bronchial artery embolization, are generally not appropriate in palliative care. Often there will have been several warning haemorrhages which will have prompted team discussion and a decision that the patient is 'not to be resuscitated' will have been taken. The family and patient should be brought into the discussions in an appropriate way.

Adequate maintenance of the airway is essential. Lying on the bleeding side, if known, reduces the impact on the other lung. When the site of bleeding is unknown, the patient may benefit by being placed in a head down position with oxygen and suctioning as needed. Some patients feel safer sitting upright in a comfortable highbacked chair with the head supported, tilted forward with chin down.[22] Others feel safer reclining in bed with the head and neck well-supported.

Tilting the head backwards because of boredom or exasperation may restart the bleeding. On the other hand, standing up after 1–2h, bending forward and taking deep breaths helps to dislodge clots by coughing and reduces wheezing.

If life-threatening haemoptysis seems likely, it may be sensible to have a syringe containing diamorphine/morphine and one containing midazolam 10mg drawn up and kept in a convenient safe place, or to have ampoules readily available. The dose of the opioid will depend on whether the patient is already receiving diamorphine/morphine regularly. If not, 10mg will be appropriate; otherwise use the equivalent of a q4h dose. The aim is to reduce fear, not necessarily to render the patient unconscious. If the patient is shocked and peripherally vasoconstricted, medication can be given IV or IM.

A fall in blood pressure helps bleeding to stop but a subsequent rise could lead to renewed bleeding. It is important that the patient is not left alone until the situation has resolved one way or the other.

Drug treatment

Drug treatment is often helpful for persistent mild–moderate haemoptysis. Options include:

- nebulized adrenaline (epinephrine) (1 in 1000) 1mg in 1ml diluted to 5ml in 0.9% saline used up to q.d.s. as a short-term measure; not used by authors

- a corticosteroid, e.g. dexamethasone 2–4mg or prednisolone 15–30mg/24h, may stop or reduce mild persistent haemoptysis, i.e. blood-streaked sputum

- an antifibrinolytic drug, e.g. tranexamic acid 1.5g stat and 1g t.d.s.; maximum dose 1.5g q.d.s., with improvement in 2–4 days[18]

- a haemostatic drug, e.g. etamsylate 500mg q.d.s.

Haematemesis and melaena

Bleeding from the gastroduodenum, manifesting as haematemesis and/or melaena, is uncommon in advanced cancer, with an incidence of about 2%.[23] Melaena occurs more frequently than haematemesis and they often occur together. Patients with liver cancer or hepatic metastases have a much increased risk of haemorrhage, some 200 times greater than other cancer patients.[23] NSAIDs are an added risk factor.

For some, the haematemesis and/or melaena is a preterminal event, with death ensuing within days. With those who survive, a decision may need to be taken about a blood transfusion (see Box 7.B). In patients taking a NSAID, consider modifying the patient's medication, for example:

- stop the NSAID and prescribe paracetamol instead

- change to a less gastrotoxic NSAID, preferably one that does not impair platelet function, e.g. meloxicam, celecoxib, rofecoxib

- prescribe a PPI or H_2-receptor antagonist to reduce gastric acid

- prescribe a gastroprotective agent, e.g. sucralfate (Box 7.G).

Box 7.G   Strategies to prevent NSAID-associated gastropathy

Prescribe paracetamol instead of a NSAID.

Use smallest dose of NSAID necessary.

Use enteric-coated aspirin.

Use a NSAID which is less likely to cause gastric injury, e.g. ibuprofen, available without prescription because of this, or diclofenac.

Use a NSAID which is only poorly absorbed in the stomach, e.g. diclofenac, diflunisal, ibuprofen.

Use a preferential COX-2 inhibitor (e.g. meloxicam, nimesulide) or a selective COX-2 inhibitor (e.g. celecoxib, rofecoxib) which do not impair platelet function.

Administer acid-reducing or gastroprotective drugs concurrently, i.e. H_2-receptor antagonist, PPI, sucralfate, misoprostol.[24,25]

Rectal and vaginal haemorrhage

Haemorrhage from the rectum or vagina in advanced cancer is generally associated with local tumour or radiotherapy. Bloody diarrhoea is a complication of intrapelvic radiotherapy, e.g. in cancers of the cervix uteri and prostate. It is caused by acute inflammatory damage to the mucosa of the rectum and sigmoid colon and is self-limiting. If particularly troublesome, it can be treated with retention enemas of:

* prednisolone 20mg in 100ml (Predsol retention enema) o.d.–b.d. *or*

* prednisolone 5mg and sucralfate 3g in 15ml b.d. (made up by local pharmacy).

Bleeding associated with chronic ischaemic radiation proctocolitis does *not* benefit from prednisolone but generally responds to:

* PO or PR tranexamic acid

* PO etamsylate

* PR sucralfate suspension (*see* Box 7.F).

With these treatments, bleeding generally stops in 1–2 weeks. Treatment should be continued for 1 more week after which it can be stopped.

With bleeding from a rectal or vaginal tumour, palliative radiotherapy should be considered unless the patient is thought to be within 2–3 weeks of death.

Haematuria

Haematuria in advanced cancer is generally associated with urinary tract cancer, notably bladder cancer, but may be caused by chronic radiation cystitis (Box 7.H). In many cases it is mild and nothing need be done. If the haematuria is more marked, tranexamic acid (even though there is a risk of clot retention until the bleeding has completely stopped) and/or etamsylate generally stops it (*see* Box 7.F).

Other options include bladder instillations and irrigations (Table 7.4). Alum may also be given as an instillation, e.g. 50ml of 1% alum instilled through a catheter and retained for 1h, repeated b.d.–q.d.s. according to response. Rarely, it may be necessary to consider:

* cauterization

* arterial embolization.[26,27]

Box 7.H   Causes of haemorrhagic cystitis[28]

Drugs	**Viruses**, e.g.
Tiaprofenic acid	Cytomegalovirus
Methenamine	Herpes simplex
Anabolic steroids	Influenza A
Chemotherapy	
busulfan	**Toxins**
cyclophosphamide	Dyes
ifosfamide	Insecticides
thiotepa	Turpentine
Immune agents	
	Radiotherapy
Diseases	Bladder
Cancer	Pelvis
Amyloidosis	Prostate
Rheumatoid arthritis	Rectum

Daily bladder instillations of carboprost tromethamine, a PGE_1 analogue, are occasionally used. Although no anaesthesia is required, such treatment is expensive and requires close monitoring.[28]

Severe haemorrhage

In a patient who is close to death, it is often appropriate to regard severe haemorrhage as a terminal event, and not to intervene with resuscitative measures. However, sometimes there is uncertainty and, if the patient's condition stabilizes, a blood transfusion after 24–48h may be indicated.

Acute haematemesis, fresh melaena, vaginal bleeding

While accepting the possibility of death and therefore adopting a conservative approach, the possibility that the patient may survive must be borne in mind. This prognostic uncertainty is reflected in an ambiguous approach to management:

- a nurse or doctor should stay with the patient if death seems imminent or until things have settled down

- if the patient is distressed, give midazolam 10mg buccal/SC or diazepam 10mg PR (if haematemesis) or PO (if melaena or vaginal bleeding)

Table 7.4   Bladder instillations and irrigations for hemorrhagic cystitis[28]

Therapy	Administration	Duration	Comment
Preferred options			
Saline 0.9%	Continuous irrigation	Until urine is clear	No adverse effects but not effective in severe cases
Alum 1%	Continuous irrigation (2L costs about £10)	Until urine is clear	Mild adverse effects, no anaesthesia required. Recurrence common, aluminium toxicity rare
Silver nitrate 0.5–1.0%	Instillation, retain for 10–20min	Repeat if no response	*Anaesthesia required.* Often successful; short duration of response
If the above fail			
Formalin 3%	Instillation, retain 20–30min	Repeat if no response	*Anaesthesia required.* Often successful; risk of ureteric stenosis and obstruction if formalin refluxes into the ureters
Phenol 100%	Instillation, retain for 1min	Single application	Use in refractory cases. Limited published data; risk of ureteric stenosis and obstruction if phenol refluxes into the ureters

- note the pulse every 30min to monitor the patient's condition; if it is steady or decreases, this suggests that bleeding has stopped; *measurement of blood pressure is intrusive and unnecessary*
- possibly take blood for grouping and cross-matching
- review the need for continuing a NSAID and/or corticosteroid
- consider prescription of a PPI, an H_2-receptor antagonist or sucralfate
- if patient survives 24h, consider a blood transfusion (*see* Box 7.A).

As always, prevention is better than cure (*see* Box 7.F).

Erosion of an artery by a malignant ulcer (e.g. neck, axilla, groin)

If one or more warning haemorrhages have occurred, consider prescribing an anxiolytic prophylactically, e.g. diazepam 5–10mg PO o.n.

Local pressure should be applied with packing. The more superficial material can be changed if it becomes saturated with blood. A green surgical towel may make extent of blood loss less obvious and less disturbing to the patient and family. Consider midazolam 10mg buccal/SC or diazepam 10mg PR (rectal solution/suppository). A nurse or doctor should stay with the patient until the bleeding is under control.

Massive haemorrhage from the *carotid artery* in recurrent neck cancer is more likely after surgery and radiotherapy and results in death in minutes; the only sensible response is to stay with the patient.

Venous thrombosis

Older patients with venous thrombosis may have a previously undiagnosed underlying cancer (10–20%) or a cancer manifests within the next 2 years (25%).[29,30] This is most likely with cancers of the:

- lung
- breast
- gastro-intestinal tract, particularly pancreas
- brain.

The propensity to thrombosis is related to an increase in tissue factor which triggers the extrinsic coagulation cascade. Excessive tissue factor is produced either directly by the cancer or indirectly by induction of WBC (Figure 7.2). Central venous catheters can also cause an increase in tissue factor, which is the reason why prophylactic low-dose warfarin or low-dose LMWH is prescribed by some centres for patients with an indwelling catheter.[31]

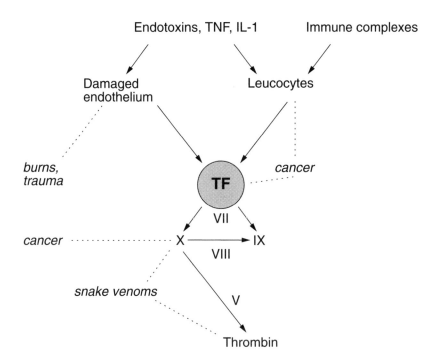

Figure 7.2 Cancer causes excessive tissue factor (TF) formation and leads to a hypercoagulable state.

Evaluation

Evaluation and management of acute deep vein thrombosis (DVT) or pulmonary embolism (PE) depends on the patient's general condition and the overall aims of care. For some patients, it is appropriate to confirm the diagnosis and to treat with anticoagulants. *If the patient is close to death, no investigations are indicated and anticoagulants are contra-indicated.*

Making a clinical diagnosis of DVT on the basis of a warm, swollen and tender limb is unreliable. DVT can be relatively asymptomatic or mimicked by lymphatic obstruction or external compression of the large veins by tumour or nodes in the pelvis/axilla. If the patient is well enough, investigations should be considered:

- venography, diagnostic gold standard but there is a small risk of exacerbating the thrombosis

- B-mode ultrasound[32]

- impedence plethysmography   } screening tests.

- light reflection rheography

If a screening test is negative, DVT is excluded; if positive, venography is indicated to confirm or refute the diagnosis.

Ultrasound is good for detecting proximal DVT but not distal ones. However, the risk of a pulmonary embolus from a distal DVT is low, and only about 20% of calf vein thromboses progress to a proximal thrombosis. It is reasonable, therefore, not to treat if ultrasound for a proximal DVT is negative, but to repeat the test after 1 week. If there is now evidence of thrombosis, anticoagulation treatment can be started.

Management

Symptom relief only

A NSAID should be prescribed ± compression (TED stockings or Tubigrip) ± elevation. Compression stockings ease the symptoms of venous hypertension; they also reduce the incidence of post-thrombotic syndrome.

Anticoagulation

Treat with LMWH, e.g. dalteparin 200 IU/kg SC o.d. Warfarin should also be started. When a therapeutic INR level is achieved with warfarin, continue LMWH for a further 2 days to ensure that the warfarin is fully effective.

Paracetamol can interfere with the metabolism of warfarin leading to a dose-dependent increase in INR within 18–48h.[33,34] Doses as little as 2.5–4g taken over a week can lead to a three-fold increase in the risk of anticoagulation. There may well be genetic polymorphism, i.e. the risk is dependent on what are the main metabolic pathways for warfarin and paracetamol in each individual (Figure 7.3). In patients on warfarin, it has been recommended that the intake of paracetamol is kept to <1.3g/day for no longer than 2 weeks.[34] Alternatively, the INR should be checked more often and the dose of warfarin adjusted until a new steady-state is achieved.

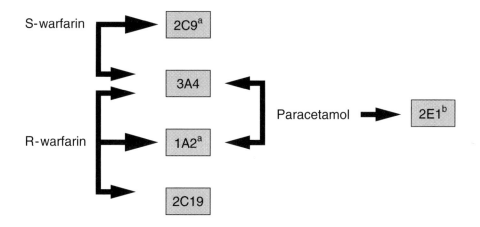

Figure 7.3 Major cytochrome P450 metabolic pathways for warfarin and paracetamol. Reproduced with permission from Shek *et al.*, 1999.[34]

a   predominant metabolizing enzymes for warfarin
b   predominant metabolizing enzyme for paracetamol.

Following the first episode of DVT, anticoagulant therapy is commonly given for 2–3 months and as long-term therapy if there is a recurrence. However, because of the hypercoagulable state associated with many cancers and leukaemia, long-term therapy is theoretically advisable even after one episode.

The risks of an unstable INR and bleeding with long-term warfarin treatment are higher in patients with advanced cancer.[35] The use of LMWH o.d. provides a more stable and hence safer method of anticoagulation. In high-risk patients, safety is further increased by dividing the o.d. dose and giving it b.d. In patients with highly vascular brain metastases, i.e. renal cell and melanoma, the risk of bleeding is even higher and is a relative contra-indication for anti-coagulation.

Thrombosis in uncommon sites

Upper limb

Treat as for lower limb DVT but, if associated with a venous catheter, remove the catheter. Extensive thrombosis may require angiography-guided thrombolytic therapy.

Cerebral vein

Dehydrated patients are particularly at risk. Cerebral vein thrombosis presents with:

- non-specific symptoms or signs
- symptoms and signs of raised intracranial pressure; if CT normal then suspect thrombosis
- focal neurological signs ± altered level of consciousness.

Visceral vein

The mesenteric vein is the third commonest site of thrombosis in hyper-coagulable states in cancer after DVT and cerebral vein thrombosis. It presents with:

- severe abdominal pain
- extensive bowel infarction.

Priapism

This is caused by blockage of the venous drainage of the cavernosa and can occur as a result of direct tumour infiltration or DIC.

Non-bacterial endocarditis

This manifests as systemic embolization.

Hepatic vein thrombosis (Budd-Chiari syndrome)

This manifests as a painful swollen liver and ascites and can lead to hepatic failure.

Pulmonary embolism

Most pulmonary emboli (PE) occur as a complication of DVT in the legs. The risk of PE from untreated DVT is estimated to be 50% and the mortality rate of untreated PE 30–40%. Most deaths from PE occur within the first hour.

Clinical features

- breathlessness and cough (generally first)
- tachypnoea (70–90%)
- hypoxia (85%)
- tachycardia (50%)
- haemoptysis (33%)
- syncope (10–20%)
- chest pain hours or days later with the development of lung infarction.

Evaluation

Investigations include:

- D-dimer levels (often raised in malignant disease and therefore of limited diagnostic value)
- chest radiograph, shows non-specific infiltrate or effusion (70%)
- V/Q scan, not specific for pulmonary embolism and less helpful in patients with a previous PE or cardiorespiratory disease. 40–50% of patients with PE have high probability scans but up to 25% have low probability scans which can neither confirm nor exclude a PE. Thus, unless either a high probability or normal scan, other investigations may be necessary
- bilateral leg venography
- pulmonary angiography, the traditional gold standard but invasive
- spiral CT detects some 60–80% of PE in the main pulmonary, lobar or segmental vessels[36]
- MRI angiogram, the emerging gold standard.

Management

Symptom relief only

- oxygen
- SC/IV diamorphine/morphine
- anxiolytic, e.g. diazepam, midazolam.

Antithrombotic treatment

Thrombolytics, e.g. streptokinase, should be limited to patients to be resuscitated but who are not candidates for embolectomy. In other situations thrombolytics provide no advantage over heparin and their use is not without risk. Generally, therefore, immediate treatment comprises:

- LMWH, e.g. dalteparin, tinzaparin
- warfarin (see p.248).

Non-drug treatment

IVC filters are used at some centres in selected cancer patients for whom anticoagulation is contra-indicated (about 20%) or ineffective (about 20%).[37] However, limb- or life-threatening thrombo-embolic complications develop in about 20% of those so treated. Generally patients with advanced cancer do not survive long enough to justify the expense.

Disseminated intravascular coagulation

Disseminated intravascular coagulation (DIC) is a consequence of the hyper-coagulable state detectable in many cancer patients, particularly with adenocarcinoma and leukaemia. Clinical manifestations vary from asymptomatic to a fulminant haemorrhagic thrombotic state. DIC results from inappropriate thrombin formation. Thrombin catalyses the activation and consumption of fibrinogen and other coagulant proteins, and the resulting fibrin thrombi consume platelets. Fibrinolysis is also activated and leads to depletion of fibrinogen.

Causes

As well as being a paraneoplastic phenomenon, DIC occurs in other circumstances, for example:

- parturition
- intra-uterine death
- after surgery
- infection.

The common factor is an increased expression of tissue factor (TF) which forms a complex with coagulation factor VII, and triggers the extrinsic coagulation pathway (see Figure 7.2).

Clinical features

Acute DIC

Acute DIC is uncommon in cancer. The clinical features of acute DIC are a mixture of the manifestations of abnormal thrombosis and abnormal bleeding, and depend on the extent and site of thrombus formation and secondary thrombocytopenia.[38] In practice it is generally the haemorrhagic features which alert the doctor to the possibility of DIC. In the skin, microvascular thrombosis of endarterioles and associated haemorrhage result in:

- petechiae
- purpura
- haematomas
- haemorrhagic bullae
- cyanosis of the extremities
- gangrene in areas of end circulation, i.e. digits, nose and ear lobes.

Areas of trauma tend to bleed because even small wounds cannot display normal haemostasis if there are profound deficiencies of coagulation factors and secondary concurrent activation of fibrinolytic pathways. The following are all common:

- oozing from venepuncture sites
- surgical wound bleeding
- haematuria in catheterized patients
- gastro-intestinal blood loss
- blood-stained secretions from endotracheal tubes.

Hypotension may also occur as a result of bradykinin release secondary to activation of the kallikrein–kinin system. This is seen in about 1/2 of patients with acute DIC. Poor tissue perfusion and acidosis prolongs the hypotension.

Chronic DIC

Although many patients with disseminated cancer have laboratory findings consistent with DIC, most remain asymptomatic. Clinical manifestations are usually thrombotic. However, a significant haemostatic stress such as surgery or an invasive procedure may result in abnormal bleeding. Thrombotic manifestations include:

- DVT
- PE
- migratory thrombophlebitis (Trousseau's syndrome), mostly in lung (adeno-carcinoma), pancreas, stomach and colorectal cancers
- microvascular thrombi with micro-angiopathic haemolytic anaemia
- venous catheter thrombosis.

In DIC the most commonly clinically affected organs are:

- lungs
- kidneys
- CNS
- skin.

DIC can lead to adult respiratory distress syndrome, a common terminal event. At autopsy, microthrombi are found in most organs including the heart, pancreas, adrenals and testes.

Evaluation

Particularly in the early phase of DIC, coagulation tests may be normal or only mildly abnormal. Treatment may have to be based on clinical suspicion. Repeating coagulation tests after several hours may demonstrate significant changes. DIC is highly probable when the following features co-exist:

- thrombocytopenia, platelet count $<150 \times 10^9$/L in 95% of cases
- decreased plasma fibrinogen concentration
- elevated plasma D-dimer concentration in 85% of cases (Figure 7.4)
- prolonged prothrombin time and/or aPTT.[39]

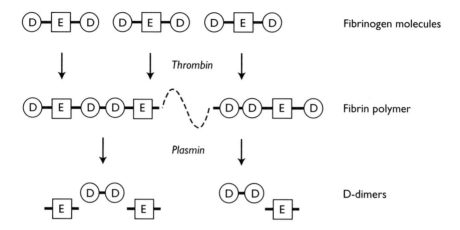

Fibrinogen molecules

Thrombin

Fibrin polymer

Plasmin

D-dimers

Figure 7.4 D-dimers are created by enzymatic degradation of 'cross-linked' fibrin polymers. D-dimer concentrations cannot be elevated unless fibrin polymers are being formed. D and E are the designated nomenclature for the main domains of the fibrinogen molecule.

A normal plasma fibrinogen concentration (200–250mg/100ml) is also suspicious because fibrinogen levels are usually raised in cancer (e.g. 450–500mg/100ml) unless there is extensive hepatic disease. Infection and cancer both may be associated with an increased platelet count which may also mask an evolving thrombocytopenia.

Management

DIC results from a triggering mechanism activating the coagulation pathways. Treatment of the underlying disorder, e.g. infection, is curative but this is not possible if caused by advanced cancer.

Acute DIC

When haemorrhagic manifestations predominate, consider:

- phytomenadione (vitamin K_1) and folic acid
- IV fluids
- oxygen
- blood products
     fresh frozen plasma (to keep the prothrombin time <2)
     cryoprecipitate (if fibrinogen <800mg/L despite fresh frozen plasma)
     platelet transfusions (to keep count at 50–75 × 10^9/L)
- the cautious use of heparin if there is concurrent thrombosis.

Tranexamic acid, an antifibrinolytic drug, should *not* be used as it increases the risk of clot formation.

Chronic DIC

Chronic DIC most commonly presents as recurrent thrombosis in both superficial and deep venous systems. It does not always respond to warfarin.[40,41] Treatment is with low molecular weight heparin (LMWH) indefinitely, e.g. dalteparin 200 IU/kg SC o.d. up to a maximum of 18 000 IU. This is as effective as standard heparin and safer in patients with cancer.[42,43] It does not require routine monitoring and a long duration of action allows o.d. administration.[44] Alternatively, standard heparin 10 000 IU SC b.d.

References

1   Miller C *et al.* (1990) Decreased erythropoietin response in patients with the anemia of cancer. *New England Journal of Medicine.* **322**:1689–92.
2   Staszewski H (1997) Haematological paraneoplastic syndromes. *Seminars in Oncology.* **24**:329–33.
3   Bunch C (1999) The blood in systemic disease. *Medicine.* 86–8.
4   Callender S (1987) Normochromic, normocytic anaemias. In: J Ledingham and D Warrell (eds) *Oxford Textbook of Medicine.* Oxford Medical Publications, Oxford, pp 19.91–19.93.
5   Gleeson C and Spencer D (1995) Blood transfusion and its benefits in palliative care. *Palliative Medicine.* **9**:307–13.
6   Monti M *et al.* (1996) Use of red blood cell transfusions in terminally ill cancer patients admitted to a palliative care unit. *Journal of Pain and Symptom Management.* **12**:18–22.
7   Glaspy J *et al.* (1997) Impact of therapy with epoietin alfa on clinical outcomes in patients with non-myeloid malignancies during cancer chemotherapy in community oncology practice. *Journal of Clinical Oncology.* **15**:1218–34.
8   Littlewood T *et al.* (1999) Efficacy and quality of life outcomes of epoietin alfa in a double blind, placeo-controlled multicentre study of cancer patients receiving non-platinum containing chemotherapy. *ASCO.* **Abstract**: 2217.
9   Weigert A and Schafer A (1998) Uraemic bleeding: Pathogenesis and therapy. *The American Journal of the Medical Sciences.* **316**:94–104.
10   Warkentin T *et al.* (1998) Heparin-induced thrombocytopenia: towards consensus. *Thrombosis and Haemostasis.* **79**:1–7.
11   Warkentin T *et al.* (1995) Heparin-induced thrombocytopenia in patients treated with low molecular weight heparin or unfractionated heparin. *New England Journal of Medicine.* **332**:1330–5.
12   Royal College of Physicians of Edinburgh (1998) Consensus statement on platelet transfusion. Final statement. *British Journal of Cancer.* **78**:290–1.
13   Broadley K *et al.* (1995) The role of embolization in palliative care. *Palliative Medicine.* **9**:331–5.

14   Rankin E *et al.* (1988) Transcatheter embolisation to control severe bleeding in fungating breast cancer. *European Journal of Surgical Oncology.* **14**:27–32.

15   Regnard C and Makin W (1992) Management of bleeding in advanced cancer: a flow diagram. *Palliative Medicine.* **6**:74–8.

16   Kochhar R *et al.* (1988) Rectal sucralfate in radiation proctitis. *Lancet.* **332**:400.

17   McElligott E *et al.* (1991) Tranexamic acid and rectal bleeding. *Lancet.* **337**:431.

18   Dean A and Tuffin P (1997) Fibrinolytic inhibitors for cancer-associated bleeding problems. *Journal of Pain and Symptom Management.* **13**:20–4.

19   Mannucci P (1997) Desmopressin (DDAVP) in the treatment of bleeding disorders: the first 20 years. *Blood.* **90**:2515–21.

20   Lyons H (1976) Differential diagnosis of haemoptysis and its treatment. *Basics of RD.* **5**:1.

21   Jones D and Davies R (1990) Massive haemoptysis. *British Medical Journal.* **300**: 889–90.

22   Paton W (1990) Massive haemoptysis. *British Medical Journal.* **300**:1270.

23   Mercadante S *et al.* (2000) Gastrointestinal bleeding in advanced cancer patients. *Journal of Pain and Symptom Management.* **19**:160–2.

24   Hawkey C *et al.* (1998) Omeprazole compared with misoprostol for ulcers associated with nonsteroidal antiinflammatory drugs. *New England Journal of Medicine.* **338**:727 34.

25   Yeomans N *et al.* (1998) A comparison of omeprazole with ranitidine for ulcers associated with nonsteroidal antiinflammatory drugs. Acid suppression trial. *New England Journal of Medicine.* **338**:719–26.

26   Lang E *et al.* (1979) Transcatheter embolization of hypogastric branch arteries in the management of intractable bladder haemorrhage. *Journal of Urology.* **121**:30–6.

27   Appleton D *et al.* (1988) Internal iliac artery embolisation for the control of severe bladder and prostate haemorrhage. *British Journal of Urology.* **61**:45–7.

28   West N (1997) Prevention and treatment of hemorrhagic cystitis. *Pharmacotherapy.* **17**:696–706.

29   Levine M and Hirsh J (1990) The diagnosis and treatment of thrombosis in the cancer patient. *Seminars in Oncology.* **17**:160–71.

30   Piccioli A *et al.* (1996) Cancer and venous thromboembolism. *American Heart Journal.* **132**:850–5.

31   Monreal M *et al.* (1996) Upper extremity deep venous thrombosis in cancer patients with venous access devices – prophylaxis with a low molecular weight heparin (Fragmin). *Thrombosis and Haemostasis.* **75**:251–3.

32   Wells P *et al.* (1997) Value of assessment of pretest probability of deep-vein thrombosis in clinical management. *Lancet.* **350**:1795–8.

33   Hylek E *et al.* (1998) Acetaminophen and other risk factors for excessive warfarin in anticoagulation. *Journal of the American Medical Association.* **279**:657–62.

34   Shek K *et al.* (1999) Warfarin-acetaminophen drug interaction revisited. *Pharmacotherapy.* **19**:1153–8.

35   Johnson M (1997) Problems of anticoagulation within a palliative care setting: an audit of hospice patients taking warfarin. *Palliative Medicine.* **11**:306–12.

36   Bates S and Ginsberg J (2000) Helical computed tomography and the diagnosis of pulmonary embolism. *Annals of Internal Medicine.* **132**:240–2.

37 Ihnat D *et al.* (1998) Treatment of patients with venous thromboembolism and malignant disease: should vena cava filter placement be routine? *Journal of Vascular Surgery.* **28**:800–7.

38 Colman R and Rubin R (1990) Disseminated intravascular coagulation due to malignancy. *Seminars in Oncology.* **17**:172–86.

39 Spero J *et al.* (1980) Disseminated intravascular coagulation: findings in 346 patients. *Thrombosis and Haemostasis.* **43**:28–33.

40 Naschitz J *et al.* (1993) Thromboembolism in cancer. *Cancer.* **71**:1384–90.

41 Bona R *et al.* (1995) The efficacy and safety of oral anticoagulation in patients with cancer. *Thrombosis and Haemostasis.* **74**:1055–8.

42 Pineo G (1997) Decreased mortality in cancer patients treated for deep vein thrombosis with low molecular weight heparin as compared with unfractionated heparin (Abstract). *Thrombosis and Haemostasis.* **Supplement**: 384.

43 Anonymous (1998) Low molecular weight heparins for venous thromboembolism. *Drug and Therapeutics Bulletin.* **36**:25–9.

44 Boneu B (1994) Low molecular weight heparin therapy: is monitoring needed? *Thrombosis and Haemostasis.* **72**:330–4.

8 Neurological symptoms

Weakness · Corticosteroid myopathy · Paraneoplastic
neurological disorders · Lambert-Eaton myasthenic
syndrome (LEMS) · Spinal cord compression · Cramp
Spasticity · Myoclonus · Grand mal convulsions
Patulous Eustachian tube · Stopping dexamethasone
in patients with intracranial malignancy · Drug-induced
movement disorders

Weakness

Localized

Localized weakness may be caused by:

- cerebral neoplasm, e.g. monoparesis, hemiparesis

- spinal cord compression, generally bilateral (*see* p.267)

- peripheral nerve lesions, e.g.
    brachial plexus lesion
    Pancoast's tumour
    axillary recurrence
    lumbosacral plexus lesion
    lateral popliteal nerve palsy

- proximal limb muscle weakness, e.g.
    corticosteroid myopathy (*see* p.261)
    paraneoplastic myopathy and/or neuropathy
    paraneoplastic polymyositis
    LEMS (*see* p.264).

Peripheral neuropathy secondary to diabetes mellitus or vitamin B_{12} deficiency
is occasionally seen in advanced cancer. Correction of hyperglycaemia or
vitamin deficiency prevents further deterioration but improvement takes time.
Corrective measures are unnecessary in patients close to death.

Generalized

Generalized progressive weakness may mean that the patient is close to death. Other possibilities should be considered (Table 8.1).

Table 8.1   Causes of generalized weakness in advanced cancer

Causes	Treatment possibilities
Cancer	
Progression of disease	Modify pattern of life
Anaemia	Haematinics, blood transfusion, erythropoietin
Hypercalcaemia	Bisphosphonates (*see* p.219)
Hypo-adrenalism	
Neuropathy	Corticosteroid
Myopathy	
Treatment	
Surgery	
Chemotherapy	Supervised rehabilitation
Radiotherapy	
Hypokalaemia	Potassium supplements
Debility	
Insomnia	Night sedative
Prolonged bed rest	
pain	Relieve symptom
breathlessness	Physiotherapy
Infection	Antibiotic
Dehydration	Hydration
Malnutrition	Dietary advice

Management

When weakness relates to an easily correctable cause, specific measures should be considered (Table 8.1). For example, if associated with iron-deficiency anaemia, it may respond to iron supplements. On the other hand, anaemia of chronic disease does not respond to haematinics but is often corrected by erythropoietin injections (*see* p.231).

If weakness relates mainly to disease progression and is troubling the patient, consider a 1 week trial of corticosteroids, e.g. dexamethasone 4mg o.d. or prednisolone 20–30mg o.d. There is about a 50% chance of benefit lasting several weeks, sometimes longer.[1] However, often the best course is to help the patient adjust their goals, i.e. living within the constraints debility imposes and not hankering after the increasingly impossible. IV hyperalimentation is not indicated for weakness in advanced cancer; it only occasionally leads to weight gain but weakness persists.[2]

Corticosteroid myopathy

The onset of corticosteroid myopathy generally occurs in the third month of treatment with dexamethasone $\geqslant$4mg o.d. or prednisolone $\geqslant$40mg o.d.[3,4] It can occur earlier and with lower doses. An appropriate level of suspicion is the main prerequisite for diagnosis (Box 8.A). For example, a patient may walk into the consultation room with no difficulty but subsequently have difficulty getting up from the sitting position. If the chronological sequence fits with corticosteroid myopathy, a presumptive diagnosis should be made and the following steps taken:

• explanation to patient and family

• discuss the need to compromise between maximizing therapeutic benefit and minimizing adverse effects

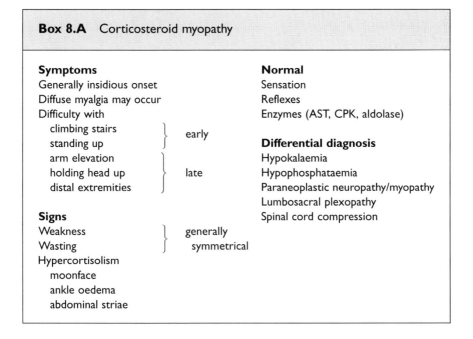

Box 8.A   Corticosteroid myopathy

Symptoms
Generally insidious onset
Diffuse myalgia may occur
Difficulty with
   climbing stairs ⎫
   standing up   ⎬ early
   arm elevation ⎫
   holding head up ⎬ late
   distal extremities ⎭

Signs
Weakness ⎫ generally
Wasting   ⎬ symmetrical
Hypercortisolism
   moonface
   ankle oedema
   abdominal striae

Normal
Sensation
Reflexes
Enzymes (AST, CPK, aldolase)

Differential diagnosis
Hypokalaemia
Hypophosphataemia
Paraneoplastic neuropathy/myopathy
Lumbosacral plexopathy
Spinal cord compression

- halve the corticosteroid dose (generally possible as as a single step)
- arrange for physiotherapy (disuse exacerbates myopathy)
- emphasize that weakness should improve after 3–4 weeks
- review after 2–3 weeks to ensure that there is no further deterioration
- consider changing from dexamethasone to prednisolone (non-fluorinated corticosteroids cause less myopathy).

Paraneoplastic neurological disorders

A paraneoplastic neurological disorder is a disorder in which a particular neoplasm is associated with a specific non-metastatic effect on the nervous system more frequently than expected by chance.[5] Only a limited number of tumours can provoke these disorders. The commonest is small cell lung cancer (SCLC), in which the incidence is about 3%.[5] This means about 250 new cases a year in the UK but in practice the diagnosis is probably often not made. Other neoplasms commonly implicated in paraneoplastic disorders are:

- breast cancer
- ovarian cancer
- neuroblastoma
- thymoma
- lymphoma.

Sometimes the onset of the neurological syndrome precedes the cancer by as much as five years.

Pathogenesis

The relationship between a neurological syndrome and the associated tumour is complex. A particular syndrome can occur with several different tumours, and several syndromes have been associated with a single tumour, notably small cell lung cancer. The basic mechanism is the production by the tumour of a specific auto-antibody (Table 8.2). Antibodies are not detectable in all patients with paraneoplastic neurological syndromes; their absence does not therefore exclude the diagnosis.

Table 8.2   Paraneoplastic neurological disorders and associated auto-antibodies[5]

Disorder	Neoplasm	Antibody
Cerebellar degeneration	Ovary Breast Other gynaecological	} Anti-Yo
	SCLC	Anti-Hu, anti-VGCC
	Hodgkin's lymphoma	Anti-Tr
Encephalomyelitis	SCLC	Anti-Hu
	Thymoma	Anti-CV2
LEMS	SCLC	Anti-VGCC
Myasthenia gravis	Thymoma	Anti-AChR
Neuromyotonia	Thymoma SCLC	} Anti-VGKC
Opsoclonus-myoclonus	Neuroblastoma	Anti-Hu
	Breast	Anti-Ri
Sensory neuropathy	SCLC	Anti-Hu

SCLC = small cell lung cancer; VGCC = voltage-gated calcium channel; VGKC = voltage-gated potassium channel; AChR = acetylcholine receptor.

Clinical features

Symptoms are determined by the underlying pathological condition (Box 8.B). They are typically subacute in onset. More than one syndrome may be present in the same patient.[6–8]

Management

The humorally-mediated disorders may respond to:

- plasma exchange
- IV immunoglobulin
- treatment of the tumour in LEMS
- immunosuppressive treatment with prednisolone in some cases.

By contrast, neither tumour treatment nor immunosuppression is effective in the other disorders.

Box 8.B   Paraneoplastic neurological disorders

Cerebellar degeneration
Trunk and limb ataxia
Vertigo
Nausea
Diplopia (sometimes)

Encephalomyelitis
Confusion ⎫
Memory loss ⎬ limb form
Hallucinations ⎭
Paresis ⎫
Deafness ⎪
Diplopia ⎬ brain stem form
Vertigo ⎪
Central respiratory failure ⎭

LEMS (see below)

Myasthenia gravis
Fatigue
Muscle weakness
   ocular
   limb
   bulbar
   respiratory

Neuromyotonia
Myoclonus (see p.276)
Myokymia
Muscle hypertrophy
Cramps
Sweating
Mood change, occasional
Hallucinations, occasional

Opsoclonus-myoclonus
Oscillopsia (chaotic eye movements)
Vertigo
Ataxia
Limb myoclonus

Inflammatory dorsal root ganglionopathy
Painful
Asymmetrical, sometimes

Lambert-Eaton myasthenic syndrome (LEMS)

LEMS is a paraneoplastic disorder of neuromuscular transmission which occurs in 3% of patients with SCLC and occasionally with other cancers, e.g. non-small cell lung, breast and lymphoma.[9] LEMS is distinct from the myopathy which is common in lung cancer patients who have lost ⩾15% of their body weight because of cachexia–anorexia (see p.86).

Pathogenesis

In LEMS there is a presynaptic deficit in neuromuscular transmission caused by a reduction in the amount of acetylcholine released on arrival of nerve impulses at the motor nerve terminal. Neurological paraneoplastic syndromes in SCLC often occur concurrently.[9] Thus, LEMS may occur with one or more of the following:

- sensory neuropathy
- cerebellar degeneration
- limbic encephalopathy
- myelopathy
- visual failure.

LEMS is associated with auto-immunity. Antibodies against SCLC are sometimes cross-reactive against the voltage-gated calcium channel, an important component of the neuromuscular junction. SCLC is thought by some to be derived from neural crest tissue, and this is thought to explain the cross-reactivity with other neural tissues and the association with other paraneoplastic neurological syndromes.

Clinical features

The common symptoms are:

- proximal muscle weakness
     always present in the legs (and the presenting symptom in over 50%)
     seen in the arms in about 25% of cases
     onset generally insidious but can be abrupt
     often worse after exercise
- diplopia (usually transient)
- dry mouth (75%)
- erectile impotence
- constipation.

Signs include:

- a rolling or waddling gait associated with truncal and proximal weakness
- transient augmentation of strength during first few seconds of muscular contractions
- diminished or absent tendon reflexes at rest but which re-appear or increase after sustained (15 second) muscular contraction; *this is pathognomonic of a presynaptic neuromuscular transmission deficit*

- ptosis
- strabismus (uncommon, in contrast to myasthenia gravis).

Evaluation

LEMS generally manifests in otherwise asymptomatic patients with SCLC. Patients with LEMS must therefore be investigated for lung cancer. The diagnosis of LEMS is confirmed by electrophysiological tests.[10] In 90% of patients there is a positive assay for antibodies against the voltage-gated calcium channel.[11]

Patients with LEMS generally feel stronger if given edrophonium 10mg IM/IV. Edrophonium is an anticholinesterase with a duration of action of about 5min. A negative result does not exclude the diagnosis and a positive result is also seen in myasthenia gravis.

Management

Successful anticancer treatment is often accompanied by improvement of the neurological symptoms. Unlike other neurological paraneoplastic syndromes, LEMS generally responds to:

- immunosuppression
- enhanced neuromuscular transmission.[12]

Immunosupression

- prednisolone 60mg o.d. or more
- azathioprine 100–150mg o.d.
- IV immunoglobulin 400mg/kg for 5 days[13] } improvement within 2 weeks which lasts for up to 6 weeks.
- plasma exchange

It is possible that some cachectic patients who benefit from corticosteroids may have an immune-mediated paraneoplastic syndrome.

Enhanced neuromuscular transmission

- an anticholinesterase will enhance neuromuscular transmission, e.g. pyridostigmine 60–120mg q4h

- 3,4-diaminopyridine (DAP) inhibits potassium flux out of neurones and thereby prolongs acetylcholine release which enhances neuromuscular transmission. DAP 10mg q.d.s. is prescribed in the UK on a named patient basis, increasing up to 20mg q.d.s.[9] Most patients experience dose-related paraesthesiae in association with periods of increased strength. The effects of an anticholinesterase and DAP are additive.

Spinal cord compression

Spinal cord compression occurs in 3–5% of patients with advanced cancer.[14] Cancers of the breast, bronchus and prostate account for 40%. Most occur in the thorax. There is compression at more than one level in 20%. Below the level of L2 vertebra, compression is of the cauda equina (i.e. peripheral nerves) and not the spinal cord.

Pathogenesis

Spinal cord compression is caused by:

- a vertebral metastasis ± vertebral collapse (85%)

- an extravertebral tumour extending through the intervertebral foramina into the epidural space, e.g. lymphoma (10%)

- an intramedullary tumour (originates from within the spinal cord), e.g. ependymoma

- an intradural tumour, i.e. arising from the meninges or nerve roots

- an epidural blood-borne metastasis (Figure 8.1).

Clinical features

- pain   >90%
- weakness   >75%
- sensory level   >50%
- sphincter dysfunction   >40%.

The patient may be unaware of sensory loss until examined, particularly if this is confined to the sacrum or perineum. Pain generally predates other

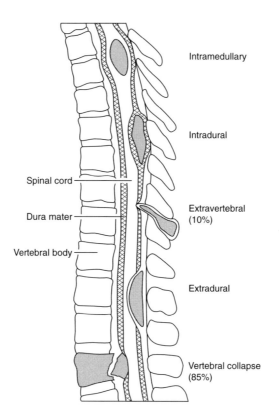

Figure 8.1   Mechanisms of spinal cord compression.

symptoms and signs of cord compression by several weeks or months. Pain may be caused by:

- vertebral metastasis
- root compression
- compression of the long tracts of the spinal cord (funicular pain).

Radicular and funicular pains are often exacerbated by neck flexion or straight leg raising, and by coughing, sneezing or straining. Funicular pain is generally less sharp than radicular pain, has a more diffuse distribution (like a cuff or garter around thighs, knees or calves) and is sometimes described as a cold unpleasant sensation.

Evaluation

- history and clinical findings
- a plain radiograph shows vertebral metastasis and/or collapse at the appropriate level in 80%
- a bone scan does not often yield additional information
- MRI is the investigation of choice
- CT with myelography may be helpful if MRI is not available.

Management

Spinal cord compression must be treated as an emergency.[15,16] Patients with paraparesis do better than those who are totally paraplegic.[17] Recovery is more likely with lesions of the cauda equina (= peripheral nerves). Loss of sphincter function is a bad prognostic sign.

Rapid onset complete paraplegia (over 24 36h) has a poor prognosis; it is almost always caused by infarction of the spinal cord secondary to tumour compression and thrombosis of a spinal artery.

The main therapeutic options are:

- corticosteroids
- radiotherapy.

These act in different ways and can be given concurrently. Corticosteroids may bring about early improvement in physical signs and pain relief by reducing peritumour inflammation. Radiotherapy brings about improvement more slowly by reducing tumour size. Dexamethasone is given in high doses initially. Regimens vary, for example:

- 12mg PO stat and 24mg PO o.d. for 3 days
- 100mg IV stat and 24mg PO q.d.s. for 3 days.[18,19]

Dexamethasone is rapidly reduced to 12–16mg o.d., after which reductions are made according to the rate and completeness of response. If there is a good result, it may be possible to completely stop dexamethasone. Surgery is occasionally indicated; it should be considered if:

- neurological symptoms and signs progress despite radiotherapy and dexamethasone

- there is a solitary vertebral metastasis
- the diagnosis is in doubt.

Laminectomy (posterior decompression) may well lead to further deterioration because cord compression is often anterior. Laminectomy is therefore likely to exacerbate spinal instability and cord injury. Vertebral body resection with anterior spinal stabilization is the operation of choice.[20]

Cramp

Cramp is a painful muscle spasm lasting from a few seconds to many hours or days. However, some authorities refer to pain lasting longer than 10min as *painful muscle stiffness*.[21]

Physiology

Ordinary muscle cramp is poorly understood. The fact that cramp can be induced by nerve stimulation distal to a nerve block suggests that a functional disturbance of the neuromuscular junctions is the final common pathway.[22]

The neuromuscular junctions are excitable when a muscle is maximally shortened. They are also excited in exercise by metabolites in the extra-cellular muscle space. These two circumstances are both triggers for cramp. Cramp is also associated with:

- acute fluid loss, e.g. diuresis, sweating, diarrhoea, renal dialysis (the mechanical effect of a contracted extracellular space)
- neural dysfunction and injury (neural hyperexcitability).[23]

Causes

Cramp is a universal experience. It occurs most commonly in a single muscle in the calf or foot. Cramp is also common in muscles close to a painful bone metastasis, particularly when movement precipitates or exacerbates pain.

In a series of 50 cancer patients with severe cramp referred to a neurological clinic, an underlying pathological condition was identified in all but nine.[23] Causes included:

- meningeal metastases
- nerve compression

- peripheral neuropathy
- polymyositis
- concurrent spinal degeneration.

In some patients, the peripheral neuropathy was secondary to diabetes mellitus. Cramp occurred in:

- arms only (about 10%)
- legs only (40%)
- arms and legs (40%)
- arms, legs and trunk (10%).

Most patients suffered frequent attacks, generally of brief duration (seconds → minutes). In patients with advanced cancer, cramp in the arm(s) in particular should alert the doctor to the possibility of an underlying neurological cause.

Cramp may be caused by drugs (Box 8.C). In the case of diuretics, cramp is triggered by electrolyte imbalance, i.e. loss of sodium and magnesium. Cramp associated with cisplatin possibly relates to the combined impact of hypo-magnesaemia and peripheral neuropathy. In many cases, the mechanism is not clear.

Box 8.C   Drug-induced cramps[23–25]

Diuretics	β_2-adrenergic agonists
Chemotherapy	salbutamol
vincristine	terbutaline
cisplatin	Amitriptyline
Medroxyprogesterone acetate	Amphotericin B
Prednisolone	Cimetidine
Beclometasone (by inhaler)	Clofibrate
	Lithium

Management

Correct the correctable

If associated with a neurological condition, treatment should be directed to the underlying cause. If feasible, causal drugs should be reduced in dose or stopped at least temporarily.

Non-drug treatment

Cramp cannot be induced or sustained in a stretched muscle.[22] Stretching movements (both active and passive) are an important non-drug measure. Daily stretching of the calf and foot muscles is a time-honoured way of reducing the frequency and severity of nocturnal calf and foot cramps. In debilitated patients, this is best done by a physiotherapist, nurse or relative.

Forced dorsiflexion of the foot for 5–10 seconds repeated for up to 5min stretches both calf and foot muscles. It is an uncomfortable procedure but the nocturnal benefit generally outweighs the short-term discomfort.

Some patients may be fit enough to stretch their own muscles by leaning with both hands against a wall and with one leg bent to provide stability and the other stretched back with the dorsiflexed foot firmly on the floor. Stretching is aided by 'rocking' on the dorsiflexed foot. After stretching the muscles of one leg, the positions of the two legs are reversed and the procedure repeated.

Massage and relaxation therapy are particularly important for cramp associated with myofascial trigger points (see p.23).

Drug treatment

Trigger points are often made less sensitive by injection with a local anaesthetic, e.g. lidocaine 1% or bupivacaine 0.5%. If the trigger point is secondary to muscle trauma, injection of a depot preparation of a corticosteroid (methylprednisolone or triamcinolone) may help to disrupt the trigger.

Drugs used to prevent cramp include:

* quinine
* diazepam
* baclofen
* dantrolene.

For nocturnal calf or foot cramp, quinine sulphate 200mg (or quinine bisulphate 300mg) o.n. is a time-honoured remedy.[26,27] Alternatively, quinine sulphate 200mg may be taken with the evening meal and a further 100mg o.n.[28] Quinine reduces the frequency of cramps and sleep disturbance but does not always reduce cramp severity.[29] The maximum benefit of quinine may not be obtained for about 4 weeks. Smoking can block the effect of quinine.[29] Quinine is an antimalarial drug and is toxic in overdose; accidental fatalities have occurred in children.

In patients with advanced disease and recurrent or persistent cramp, diazepam 5–10mg o.n. is probably the drug of choice. Alternatively, baclofen

10–20mg b.d.–t.d.s. can be tried. Both drugs work via a central inhibitory GABA mechanism, thereby reducing muscle tone. In anxious patients, diazepam is of double benefit; it relaxes both muscles and mind.

Dantrolene acts directly on skeletal muscle and is less sedating. It is a further option and if necessary can be used in conjunction with diazepam or baclofen. The recommended starting dose is 25mg o.d., increasing by 25mg weekly to 100mg q.d.s. The modal dose is 75mg t.d.s. In palliative care it may be necessary to titrate the dose at a faster rate because of the need for rapid relief.

Spasticity

Spasticity is a condition in which muscles are continuously contracted. This causes stiffness or tightness of the muscles and can interfere with gait, movement and speech.

Causes

Spasticity is generally caused by damage to the spinal cord or to the area of the brain which controls voluntary movement. Causes include:

- spinal cord injury
- multiple sclerosis
- motor neurone disease (amyotrophic lateral sclerosis)
- brain injury, e.g. anoxic brain damage, cerebral palsy.

Clinical features

Clinical features include:

- hypertonicity (increased muscle tone)
- clonus (a series of rapid contractions provoked by forcibly stretching the affected muscle)
- exaggerated deep tendon reflexes
- muscle spasms
- scissoring (involuntary crossing of the legs)
- fixed joints.

The degree of spasticity varies from mild muscle stiffness to severe painful uncontrollable muscle spasms which greatly interfere with daily activities.

Management

Non-drug treatment

As with cramp, physiotherapy is important in the management of spasticity. In patients with chronic disease, surgery is sometimes of benefit, e.g. muscle and tendon lengthening, release of contractures, tendon transfers.[30,31]

Drug treatment

The drug treatment of spasticity is similar to that for cramp.[32] However, quinine sulphate is of no value. Baclofen, diazepam, dantrolene and tizanidine are all currently approved for use in patients with spasticity (Table 8.3). Dose escalation to the maximum recommended dose may take 4–8 weeks.

More invasive treatments include IT phenol. This is neurotoxic and can cause urinary and faecal incontinence. Indwelling devices to deliver IT baclofen has largely replaced the use of IT phenol.[32]

Tizanidine

Tizanidine is a central α_2-receptor agonist, like clonidine, and is licensed for use in spasticity.[33,34] It is comparable in efficacy to diazepam and baclofen. Tizanidine reduces the sympathetic outflow which in turn reduces muscle tone. Tizanidine causes sedation, weakness and dry mouth in more than 2/3 of those taking it,[35] although sedation and weakness may be less than with diazepam and baclofen.[36]

Botulinum toxin (BTX)

The BTX-type A light chain acts as a zinc endopeptidase and interferes with acetylcholine release.[37] The toxin is injected into the spastic muscles and reduces spasticity in a dose-dependent manner. Its use is rarely relevant in palliative care.

Table 8.3   Oral drugs used to treat spasticity

Agent	Starting dose	Maximum dose	Adverse effects	Monitoring	Precautions
Diazepam	2mg b.d. or 5mg o.n.	60mg/day	Weakness, sedation, cognitive impairment, depression	Cumulation, prolongation of plasma halflife with cimetidine	Withdrawal syndrome
Baclofen	5mg o.d.–t.d.s.	20mg q.d.s.	Weakness, sedation, fatigue, dizziness, nausea, hepatotoxicity	Periodic LFT	Abrupt cessation is associated with seizures
Tizanidine	2–4mg o.n.	12mg t.d.s.	Drowsiness, dry mouth, dizziness, hepatotoxicity	Periodic LFT	Do not use with antihypertensives or clonidine
Dantrolene	25mg o.d.	100mg q.d.s.	Weakness, sedation, diarrhoea, hepatotoxicity	Periodic LFT	

Myoclonus

Myoclonus is sudden, brief, shock-like involuntary movements caused by either primary muscle contractions or secondary to CNS stimulation. Myoclonus may be:

- focal (a single muscle or group of muscles), regional or multifocal (generalized)
- unilateral or bilateral (either asymmetrical or symmetrical)
- mild (twitching) or severe (jerking).

Secondary multifocal myoclonus is a central pre-epileptiform phenomenon and should not be ignored. It occurs mainly in moribund patients.

Causes

Myoclonus may be:

- physiological
- primary ('essential')
- secondary to
    neurological disorders
    biochemical disorders, e.g. hypoglycaemia, renal failure
    drug toxicity, e.g. antimuscarinics, opioids (see p.43).[38]

Management

If of recent onset, review medication and, if possible, reduce or stop causal drugs. In moribund patients, consider:

- diazepam 5mg PR stat and 5–10mg PR o.n. *or*
- midazolam 5mg buccal/SC p.r.n, and 10mg/24h by CSCI.

Adjust the dose upwards if several p.r.n. doses are needed.

Even if longstanding, it is worth trying clonazepam 0.5mg o.n. for troublesome primary myoclonus.

Grand mal seizures

Common causes of grand mal seizures in patients receiving palliative care include:

- longstanding epilepsy
- previous cerebrovascular accident
- brain tumour, primary or secondary
- biochemial disturbance, e.g. renal failure, severe hyponatraemia.

In relatively fit patients, the cause of the seizure(s) needs to be investigated, and an appropriate oral anti-epileptic regimen started and monitored according to standard practice.

Occasionally a patient may develop status epilepticus. This has been defined as a continuous seizure which lasts more than 30min, or two or more discrete seizures between which the patient does not recover consciousness.[39] Because isolated tonic-clonic seizures rarely last more than a few minutes, a working definition of continuous seizures lasting more than 5min has been suggested.[40]

Management

If a patient has a grand mal seizure, give:

- diazepam 10mg PR/IV and repeat after 15 and 30min if not settled *or*
- midazolam 10mg buccal/SC/IV and repeat after 15–20min if not settled
- if the above fail, phenobarbital 100mg SC *or*
- phenobarbital 100mg in 100ml of 0.9% saline IV over 30min.

Status epilepticus

One approach to the management of status epilepticus is provided in Figure 8.2.[40,41] As with all IV regimens, there is need for close monitoring. After the seizures have been controlled, treatment should be continued with an appropriate maintenance regimen. However, in palliative care it is generally a matter of managing a single discrete seizure.

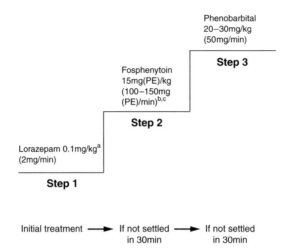

Figure 8.2 IV treatment for status epilepticus. Some centres reverse step 2 and step 3. If all else fails, proceed to general anaesthesia with thiopental, propofol etc.

a   BNF recommendation; clonazepam, diazepam or midazolam can be used instead

b   fosphenytoin is a pro-drug of phenytoin and can be given more rapidly; fosphenytoin sodium
    1.5mg ≡ phenytoin sodium 1mg. Dose is expressed as *phenytoin sodium equivalent (PE)*

c   IV phenytoin 20–30mg/kg (50mg/min) can be used instead with ECG monitoring.

Moribund patients

When patients are no longer able to swallow, convert to PR diazepam or midazolam by CSCI. Although, higher doses may be necessary, maintenance treatment in moribund patients typically comprises:

- diazepam 10–30mg PR o.n. or b.d. *or*
- midazolam 30–60mg/24h by CSCI *or*
- phenobarbital 200–600mg/24h by CSCI.

If some hours have elapsed since the last oral dose, it may be wise to give a stat dose of diazepam 10mg PR or midazolam 10mg SC. Remember:

- phenytoin and sodium valproate have long plasma halflives and will be present in the patient for some time after stopping oral therapy. The continuing but diminishing effects of phenytoin and sodium valproate supplement the benzodiazepine
- phenobarbital sodium for injection is made up in 90% propylene (200mg/1ml). If given by CSCI, it should be diluted with water. Of drugs commonly given by CSCI, phenobarbital is miscible only with diamorphine and hyoscine.

Patulous Eustachian tube

The Eustachian tube is normally closed and opens only temporarily during swallowing. The tube is patulous (i.e. remains open), free passage of air and sound occurs between the nasopharynx and the middle ear. The air causes flapping of the tympanic membrane and this is responsible for the annoying auditory discomfort linked to breathing.

The Eustachian tube becomes patulous particularly in pregnant women and in association with a rapid marked loss of weight. The incidence in advanced cancer is not known; possibly 2–3% of patients. It is often misdiagnosed as serious otitis media.

Clinical features

Symptoms are either continuous or intermittent, and vary from a minor annoyance to a major cause of distress:

- a feeling of aural fullness/pressure, generally interpreted as a blocked ear which is not relieved by swallowing
- blowing sound in ear(s) synchronous with breathing
- crackling sound when chewing
- voice sounds excessively loud and hollow, resembling an echo (autophony)
- postural variation: symptoms often diminish or disappear when patient is supine.

Auroscopy generally shows movement of the tympanic membrane synchronous with nasal inspiration and expiration.

Management

Symptoms are not often severe and explanation alone is generally adequate. Patients benefit by discovering that in certain positions the symptoms remit, e.g. when supine. A sharp forceful sniff may also bring temporary relief. Other options include:

- nasal drops containing hydrochloric acid, chlorbutanol, benzyl alcohol and propylene glycol[42]

- intratubal injection of
   atropine
   liquid paraffin
   gelatine sponge
   Teflon

- insertion of a grommet (ventilating tube) in the tympanic membrane under local anaesthetic by an ENT specialist.

Stopping dexamethasone in patients with intracranial malignancy

Most patients stop taking dexamethasone automatically when they become moribund and can no longer swallow. They may need diamorphine/morphine by CSCI to prevent distressing headaches and PR diazepam/SC midazolam to prevent seizures.

Occasionally the patient requests that the dexamethasone is stopped because of deterioration, despite the continued use of dexamethasone, and an unacceptable quality of life. This is a situation which tends to cause considerable staff distress.

It is probably best to reduce the dexamethasone step by step on a daily basis, because this gives the patient time to reconsider. At the same time prescribe extra analgesics in case headache recurs:

- if on paracetamol, prescribe co-proxamol p.r.n.

- if on co-proxamol, prescribe morphine 10–20mg PO or diamorphine/ morphine 5–10mg SC p.r.n.

- increase the dose of the regular analgesic(s) if ≥2 p.r.n. doses have been given in the previous 24h.

If the patient becomes drowsy or swallowing becomes difficult, consider changing PO anti-epileptics to SC midazolam and possibly give both diamorphine and midazolam by CSCI.

If diamorphine/morphine depresses ventilation, the increased $PaCO_2$ will result in intracranial vasodilation and a rise in intracranial pressure which exacerbate headache. If headache is suspected because of grimacing or general restlessness, p.r.n. medication should be given and the dose of the regular opioid increased until the patient appears comfortable. *It is important first to exclude the more common reasons for agitation in moribund patients, e.g. full bladder or rectum, pain and stiffness related to immobility.*

Drug-induced movement disorders

Drug-induced movement disorders encompass:

- extrapyramidal reactions
    parkinsonism
    acute dystonia
    acute akathisia
    tardive dyskinesia

- malignant neuroleptic syndrome.

The features of the various syndromes are listed in Box 8.D. Extrapyramidal reactions are caused mostly by drugs which block dopamine receptors in the CNS; these include all neuroleptics and metoclopramide.[43] Other drugs have also been implicated (Box 8.E), including antidepressants and ondansetron.[44-46]

High potency neuroleptics possess a greater affinity for dopamine receptors and a lower affinity for cholinergic receptors than low potency neuroleptics. They therefore cause a greater imbalance between dopamine and acetylcholine, and are more likely to cause extrapyramidal reactions. Thus haloperidol is high risk but, for example, levomepromazine is low risk. More extrapyramidal reactions occur at higher doses of any potentially causal drug. There is probably also a genetic factor.

To explain the mechanism by which antidepressants and ondansetron cause extrapyramidal reactions, a 'four neurone model' has been proposed which includes 5HT- and GABA-receptors.[47]

Parkinsonism

Parkinsonism develops in up to 40% of patients treated long-term with neuroleptics. It develops at any stage but not generally before the second week. It is most common in the over 60s. Although generally symmetrical, there may be asymmetry in the early stages.

The tremor of drug-induced parkinsonism is typically:

- of frequency <8 cycles per second

- worse at rest

- suppressed during voluntary movements

- associated with rigidity and bradykinesia (Box 8.D).

Box 8.D   Movement disorders associated with dopamine-receptor antagonists[48]

Parkinsonism
Coarse resting tremor of limbs, head, mouth and/or tongue
Muscular rigidity (cogwheel or leadpipe)
Bradykinesia, notably of face
Sialorrhoea (drooling)
Shuffling gait

Acute dystonias
one or more of
Abnormal positioning of head and neck (retrocollis, torticollis)
Spasms of jaw muscles (trismus, gaping, grimacing)
Tongue dysfunction (dysarthria, protrusion)
Dysphagia
Laryngo-pharyngeal spasm
Dysphonia
Eyes deviated up, down, or sideways ('oculogyric crisis')
Abnormal positioning of limbs or trunk

Acute akathisia
one or more of
Fidgety movements or swinging of legs
Rocking from foot to foot when standing
Pacing to relieve restlessness
Inability to sit or stand still for several minutes

Tardive dyskinesia
Exposure to neuroleptic medication for ≥3 months (>1 month if >60 years old)
Involuntary movement of tongue, jaw, trunk or limbs:
    choreiform (rapid, jerky, non-repetitive)
    athetoid (slow, sinuous, continual)
    rhythmic (stereotypic)

Neuroleptic malignant syndrome
Severe muscle rigidity *and*
Pyrexia
with two or more of
Tremor
Sweating
Mutism
Dysphagia
Incontinence
Drowsiness
Tachycardia
Elevated/labile blood pressure
Leucocytosis
Evidence of muscle injury, e.g. myoglobinuria, raised plasma creatine kinase

This is different from drug-induced tremors of the hands, head, mouth or tongue with a frequency of 8–12 cycles per second, and best observed with hands held outstretched and/or mouth held open (Box 8.F).

Box 8.E   Drugs which may cause extrapyramidal effects[45,49]

Palliative care	**General**
Neuroleptics	Diltiazem
butyrophenones	Fenfluramine
phenothiazines	5-hydroxytryptophan
Metoclopramide	Lithium
Ondansetron	Methyldopa
Antidepressants	Methysergide
tricyclics	Reserpine
SSRIs	
Carbamazepine	

Box 8.F   Drug-induced (non-parkinsonian) postural tremor[50]

Anti-epileptics	Methylxanthines
sodium valproate	caffeine
	aminophylline
Antidepressants	theophylline
SSRIs	
tricyclics	Neuroleptics
	butyrophenones
β-adrenoceptors	phenothiazines
salbutamol	
salmeterol	Psychostimulants
	dexamfetamine
Lithium	methylphenidate

Treatment

Use an antimuscarinic antiparkinsonian drug:

- benzatropine 1–2mg IV/IM → 2mg PO o.d.–b.d. *or*

- procyclidine 5–10mg IV/IM → 5mg PO t.d.s.

- orphenadrine 50–100mg PO b.d. is a useful alternative.

Acute dystonia

Acute dystonias occur in up to 10% of patients treated with neuroleptics. They develop abruptly within days of starting treatment, and are accompanied by anxiety (Box 8.D). They are most common in young adults.

Treatment

- benzatropine 1–2mg or procyclidine 5–10mg IV/IM for immediate relief. Benefit is seen within 10min; peak effect within 30min. If necessary, repeat after 30min

- continue treatment with a standard oral antimuscarinic antiparkinsonian drug (see above)

- some centres use IV/IM diphenhydramine 20–50mg, followed by 25–50mg b.d.–q.d.s.

- consider discontinuing or reducing dose of causal drug

- if caused by metoclopramide, substitute domperidone.

Acute akathisia

Akathisia is a form of motor restlessness in which the subject is compelled to pace up and down or to change the body position frequently (Box 8.D). It is most common in the 16–50 age range. It occurs in up to 20% of patients receiving neuroleptics. It can develop within days of starting treatment. If the drug is continued, it may progress to parkinsonism. Haloperidol and prochlorperazine carry the highest risk.[51] It is uncommon for metoclopramide to cause akathisia. Concurrent administration of morphine or sodium valproate may be additional risk factors.[50]

Treatment

- if possible, discontinue or reduce the dose of the causal drug

- switch to a neuroleptic with more antimuscarinic activity

- prescribe an antimuscarinic antiparkinsonian drug (as for acute dystonia)

- if only partial response, add diazepam 5mg o.n.

- alternatively, prescribe a lipophilic β-adrenoceptor antagonist; i.e. propranolol 10–40mg b.d. or metoprolol 50–100mg b.d.

Akathisia responds less well to antiparkinsonian drugs than drug-induced parkinsonism and dystonias. Propranolol, a highly lipophilic non-selective β-adrenoceptor antagonist, and metoprolol, a lipophilic $β_1$-adrenoceptor antagonist, are equally effective. In contrast, atenolol, a *hydrophilic* $β_1$-adrenoceptor antagonist, has no effect.

Tardive dyskinesia

Tardive (late) dyskinesia is caused by the long-term administration of drugs that block dopamine receptors, particularly D_2-receptors. It occurs in 20% of patients receiving a neuroleptic for more than 3 months. Women, the elderly and those on high doses, e.g. chlorpromazine 300mg/24h, are most commonly affected.

Tardive dyskinesia typically manifests as involuntary stereotyped chewing movements of the tongue and orofacial muscles. The involuntary movements are made worse by anxiety and reduced by drowsiness and during sleep. Tardive dyskinesia is associated with akathisia in 25% of cases.

In younger patients, tardive dyskinesia may present as abnormal positioning of the limbs and tonic contractions of the neck and trunk muscles causing torticollis, lordosis or scoliosis. In younger patients, tardive dyskinesia may occur if neuroleptic treatment is stopped abruptly.

Early diagnosis

'Open your mouth and stick out your tongue.'

The following indicate a developing tardive dyskinesia:

* worm-like movements of the tongue
* inability to protrude tongue for more than a few seconds.

Treatment

* withdrawal of the causal agent leads to resolution in 30% in 3 months and a further 40% in 5 years; sometimes irreversible particularly in the elderly
* often responds poorly to drug therapy; antimuscarinic antiparkinsonian drugs may exacerbate
* tetrabenazine, depletes presynaptic dopamine stores and blocks post-synaptic dopamine receptors; best not used in depressed patients; start with 12.5mg t.d.s. → 25mg t.d.s., increasing the dose slowly to avoid troublesome hypotension

- reserpine, depletes presynaptic dopamine stores; may be used in place of tetrabenazine but causes similar adverse effects
- levodopa, may produce long-term benefit after causing initial deterioration
- baclofen, clonazepam, diazepam and sodium valproate have all been tried with inconsistent results (all drugs which act by potentiating GABA-ergic inhibition)
- increase the dose of the causal drug; paradoxically, this may help but should be considered only in desperation.

Neuroleptic malignant syndrome

Neuroleptic malignant syndrome occurs in 1–2% of patients receiving a neuroleptic, particularly in young adults; 2/3 of cases occur <1 week after starting treatment.[52] It is more likely to occur in patients also receiving lithium.

The essential features of neuroleptic malignant syndrome are fever and muscle rigidity associated with some of the following:

- tremor
- sweating
- mutism
- dysphagia
- incontinence
- drowsiness
- tachycardia
- elevated or labile blood pressure.

Leucocytosis and evidence of muscle injury, i.e. myoglobinuria and raised plasma creatine kinase concentration, are laboratory features.

Treatment

Treatment generally comprises:

- discontinuation of the causal drug
- prescription of a muscle relaxant.

In severe cases, bromocriptine (a dopamine agonist) has been used. Death occurs in up to 20% of cases, most commonly as a result of respiratory failure.

References

1 Bruera E *et al.* (1985) Action of oral methylprednisolone in terminal cancer patients: a prospective randomized double-blind study. *Cancer Treatment Reports.* **69:**751–4.
2 Bozzetti F (1996) Guidelines on artificial nutrition versus hydration in terminal cancer patients. *Nutrition.* **12**:163–7.
3 Dropcho EJ and Soong S-J (1991) Steroid induced weakness in patients with primary brain tumours. *Neurology.* **41**:1235–9.
4 Eidelberg D (1991) Steroid myopathy. In: DA Rottenberg (ed) *Neurological Complications of Cancer Treatment.* Butterworth-Heinemann, Boston, pp 185–91.
5 Newsom-Davis J (1999) Paraneoplastic neurological disorders. *Journal of the Royal College of Physicians of London.* **33**:225–7.
6 Posner J (1997) Paraneoplastic syndromes. *Current Opinion in Neurology.* **10**: 471–6.
7 Posner J and Dalmau J (1997) Paraneoplastic syndromes affecting the central nervous system. *Annual Review of Medicine.* **48**:157–66.
8 Rees J (1998) Paraneoplastic syndromes. *Current Opinion in Neurology.* **11**: 633–7.
9 Elrington G (1992) The Lambert-Eaton myasthenic syndrome. *Palliative Medicine.* **6**:9–17.
10 Newsom-Davis J and Murray N (1984) Plasma exchange and immunosuppressant drug treatment in the Lambert-Eaton Myasthenic Syndrome. *Neurology.* **34**:480–5.
11 Motomura M *et al.* (1995) An improved diagnostic assay for Lambert-Eaton myasthenic syndrome. *Journal of Neurology, Neurosurgery and Psychiatry.* **58**: 85–7.
12 Newsom-Davis J (1998) A treatment algorithm for Lambert-Eaton myasthenic syndrome. *Annals of the New York Academy of Sciences.* **841**:817–22.
13 Bain P *et al.* (1996) Effects of intravenous immunoglobulin on muscle weakness and calcium-channel autoantibodies in the Lambert-Eaton myasthenic syndrome. *Neurology.* **47**:678–83.
14 Kramer J (1992) Spinal cord compression in malignancy. *Palliative Medicine.* **6**:202–11.
15 Loblaw D and Laperriere N (1998) Emergency treatment of malignant extradural spinal cord compression: an evidence-based guideline. *Journal of Clinical Oncology.* **16**:1613–24.
16 Bucholtz J (1999) Metastatic epidural spinal cord compression. *Seminars in Oncology Nursing.* **15**:150–9.
17 Cowap J *et al.* (2000) Outcome of malignant spinal cord compression at a cancer center: implications for palliative care services. *Journal of Pain and Symptom Management.* **19**:257–64.

18 Greenberg H *et al.* (1979) Epidural spinal cord compression from metastatic tumour: results with a new treatment protocol. *Annals of Neurology.* **8**:361–6.

19 Vecht C *et al.* (1989) Initial bolus of conventional versus high-dose dexamethasone in metastatic spinal cord compression. *Neurology.* **39**:1255–7.

20 Siegal T and Siegal T (1985) Surgical decompression of anterior and posterior malignant epidural tumours compressing the spinal cord: a prospective study. *Neurosurgery.* **17**:424–32.

21 Jansen P *et al.* (1991) Clinical diagnosis of muscle cramp and muscle cramp syndromes. *European Archives of Psychiatry and Clinical Neuroscience.* **241**: 98–101.

22 Layzer R (1994) The origin of muscle fasciculations and cramps. *Muscle and Nerve.* **17**:1243–9.

23 Steiner I and Siegal T (1989) Muscle cramps in cancer patients. *Cancer.* **63**:574–7.

24 Siegal T (1991) Muscle cramps in the cancer patient: causes and treatment. *Journal of Pain and Symptom Management.* **6**:84–91.

25 Lear J and Daniels R (1993) Muscle cramps related to corticosteroids. *British Medical Journal.* **306**:1169.

26 Warburton A *et al.* (1987) A quinine a day keeps the leg cramps away? *British Journal of Clinical Pharmacology.* **23**:459–65.

27 Man-Son-Hing M and Wells G (1995) Meta-analysis of efficacy of quinine for treatment of nocturnal leg cramps in elderly people. *British Medical Journal.* **310**:13–17.

28 Jansen P *et al.* (1997) Randomised controlled trial of hydroquinine in muscle cramps. *Lancet.* **349**:528–32.

29 Connolly PS *et al.* (1992) The treatment of nocturnal leg cramps: a crossover trial of quinine versus vitamin E. *Archives of Internal Medicine.* **152**:1877–80.

30 Kasdon D (1986) Controversies in the surgical management of spasticity. *Clinical Neurosurgery.* **35**:523–9.

31 Doraisamy P (1992) The management of spasticity – a review of options available in rehabilitation. *Annals of the Academy of Medicine of Singapore.* **21**:807–12.

32 Kita M and Goodkin D (2000) Drugs used to treat spasticity. *Drugs.* **59**:487–95.

33 Lataste X *et al.* (1994) Comparative profile of tizanidine in the management of spasticity. *Neurology.* **44**:S53–S59.

34 Wallace J (1994) Summary of combined clinical analysis of controlled clinical trials with tizanidine. *Neurology.* **44**:S60–S69.

35 Nance P *et al.* (1997) Relationship of the antispasticity effect of tizanidine to plasma concentration in patients with multiple sclerosis. *Archives of Neurology.* **54**:731–6.

36 Smith H and Barton A (2000) Tizanidine in the management of spasticity and musculoskeletal complaints in the palliative care population. *American Journal of Hospice and Palliative Care.* **17**:50–8.

37 Brin M (1997) Dosing, administration and a treatment algorithm for use of botulinum toxin A for adult-onset of spasticity. *Muscle and Nerve.* **Supplement 6**.

38 Lauterbach E (1999) Hiccup and apparent myoclonus after hydrocodone: Review of the opiate-related hiccup and myoclonus literature. *Clinical Neuropharmacology.* **22**:87–92.

39 Heafield M (2000) Managing status epilepticus. *British Medical Journal.* **320**: 953–4.

40 Lowenstein D and Alldredge B (1998) Status epilepticus. *New England Journal of Medicine.* **338**:970–6.

41 Treiman D *et al.* (1998) A comparison of four treatments for generalized convulsive status epilepticus. *New England Journal of Medicine.* **339**:792–8.

42 DiBartolomeo J (1993) Correspondence. *American Journal of Otology.* **14**:313.

43 Tonda M and Guthrie S (1994) Treatment of acute neuroleptic-induced movement disorders. *Pharmacotherapy.* **14**:543–60.

44 Zubenko G *et al.* (1987) Antidepressant-related akathisia. *Journal of Clinical Psychopharmacology.* **7**:254–7.

45 Arya D (1994) Extrapyramidal symptoms with selective serotonin reuptake inhibitors. *British Journal of Psychiatry.* **165**:728–33.

46 Mathews H and Tancil C (1996) Extrapyramidal reaction caused by ondansetron. *The Annals of Pharmacotherapy.* **30**:196.

47 Hamilton M and Opler L (1992) Akathisia, suicidality, and fluoxetine. *Journal of Clinical Psychiatry.* **53**:401–6.

48 American Psychiatric Association (1994) Neuroleptic-induced movement disorders. In: *Diagnostic and Statistical Manual of Mental Disorders, 4th edition (DSM-IV).* APA, New York, pp 736–51.

49 Anonymous (1994) Drug-induced extrapyramidal reactions. *Current Problems in Pharmacovigilance.* **20**:15–16.

50 American Psychiatric Association (1994) Medication-induced postural tremor. In: *Diagnostic and Statistical Manual of Mental Disorders, 4th edition (DSM-IV).* APA, New York, pp 749–51.

51 Gattera J *et al.* (1994) A retrospective study of risk factors of akathisia in terminally ill patients. *Journal of Pain and Symptom Management.* **9**:454–61.

52 Launer M (1996) Selected side-effects: 17. Dopamine-receptor antagonists and movement disorders. *Prescribers' Journal.* **36**:37–41.

9 Urinary symptoms

Definitions · Bladder innervation · Unstable bladder
Bladder spasms · Hesitancy · Discoloured urine

Definitions

Frequency
Passage of urine seven or more times during the day and twice or more at
night.

Urgency
A strong and sudden desire to void.

Urge incontinence
The involuntary loss of urine associated with a strong desire to void.

Detrusor instability
Detrusor contracts uninhibitedly and causes:

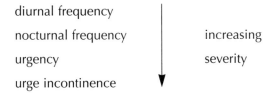

diurnal frequency

nocturnal frequency   increasing

urgency   severity

urge incontinence

Detrusor instability is the second most common cause of urinary incontinence in women.

Stress incontinence
The involuntary loss of urine associated with coughing, sneezing, laughing
and lifting.

Genuine stress incontinence (urethral sphincter incompetence)
The involuntary loss of urine when the intravesical pressure exceeds maximum urethral pressure in the *absence of detrusor activity*. The fault always
lies in the sphincter mechanisms of the bladder, and is associated with multi-
parity, after the menopause and after hysterectomy.

One or more of the following features will be present:

- descent of urethrovesical junction outside intra-abdominal zone of pressure
- decrease in urethral pressure due to loss of urethral wall elasticity and contractility
- short functional length of the urethra.

Urethral sphincter incompetence is the most common cause of urinary incontinence in women.

Dysuria
Pain during and/or after micturition. Often urethral in origin (a burning sensation) but may be caused by bladder spasm (intense suprapubic and urethral pain), or both.

Hesitancy
A prolonged delay between attempting and achieving micturition.

Bladder innervation

*'You **p**ee with your **p**arasympathetics. You **s**top with your **s**ympathetics.'*

The sphincter relaxes when the detrusor (bladder muscle) contracts, and vice versa (Table 9.1). Thus, antimuscarinic drugs not only cause contraction of the bladder neck sphincter but also relax the detrusor. Detrusor sensitivity is also:

- increased by PGs
- decreased by COX inhibitors, i.e. NSAIDs.

The urethral sphincter, under voluntary control, is innervated by the pudendal nerve (S2–4).

Table 9.1   Autonomic innervation of the bladder

Innervation	Neurotransmitter	Effect on	
		Sphincter	Detrusor
Sympathetic (T10–12, L1)	Noradrenaline (norepinephrine)	Contracts (α)	Relaxes (β)
Parasympathetic (S2–4)	Acetylcholine	Relaxes	Contracts

The urethra is derived embryologically from the urogenital sinus and is sensitive in the female to oestrogen and progesterone. Postmenopausal urge incontinence and frequency is sometimes helped by the prescription of an oestrogen, either topically or orally. Oestrogens do not improve stress incontinence.

Morphine and other opioids have several effects on bladder function:

- bladder sensation *decreased*
- sphincter tone *increased*
- detrusor tone *increased*
- ureteric tone and amplitude of contractions *increased*.

These are generally asymptomatic. Occasionally hesitancy or retention occurs.

Unstable bladder

Unstable bladder is a term encompassing three closely associated symptoms, namely, frequency, urgency and urge incontinence. The incidence in cancer patients is not known.

Causes

The causes of frequency and urgency overlap with those of urge incontinence (Box 9.A). Tiaprofenic acid (a NSAID) can cause severe cystitis with haematuria as a direct toxic effect of the drug and/or its metabolites on the bladder. Presentation is generally several months, or even years, after starting treatment with tiaprofenic acid.[1-3]

The precipitating factor in urge incontinence is delayed micturition relative to need. Delay is associated with:

- weakness and difficulty in getting to commode
- disinterest
    depression
    dejection
- lack of awareness
    confusion
    drowsiness.

Box 9.A   Causes of urgency and incontinence

Cancer
Pain
Hypercalcaemia
   (causes polyuria)
Intravesical ⎫
Extravesical ⎭ mechanical irritation
Bladder spasms
Sacral plexopathy

Treatment
Radiation cystitis
Drugs
   cyclophosphamide
   diuretics
   tiaprofenic acid

Debility
Infective cystitis

Concurrent
Idiopathic detrusor instability
Central neurological disease
   poststroke
   multiple sclerosis
   dementia
Uraemia ⎫
Diabetes mellitus ⎬ cause polyuria
Diabetes insipidus ⎭

The differential diagnosis includes:

- genuine stress incontinence

- retention with overflow

- urinary fistula

- flaccid sphincter (presacral plexopathy).

Management

Prevent the preventable

Tiaprofenic acid should not be given to patients with urinary tract disorders.[4]
Patients prescribed tiaprofenic acid should be advised to stop taking it and to
report to their doctor promptly if they develop urinary tract symptoms such
as frequency, nocturia, urgency, dysuria, haematuria.

Correct the correctable

- reduce or change diuretic

- stop tiaprofenic acid

- treat infective cystitis with the appropriate antibiotic

- for prophylaxis against cystitis, recommend cranberry juice 180ml b.d.[5]

- alternatively, prescribe a urinary antiseptic long-term, i.e.
    methenamine (hexamine) hippurate 1g b.d.[6]
    nitrofurantoin 50–100mg o.n.[7]

Cranberry juice

Cranberry (and blueberry) juice contains a large polymer of unknown structure which inhibits bacterial adherence to the bladder mucosa. It reduces the frequency of symptomatic urinary tract infections with *E. coli.*[5] Although sometimes recommended, the addition of ascorbic acid (vitamin C) is not necessary. However, two recent reviews, cast doubt on the efficacy of cranberry juice.[8,9]

Urinary antiseptics

In an acid environment (pH $<$5), methenamine is converted to formaldehyde which is responsible for the bactericidal effect.[10] Urea-splitting bacteria tend to raise the pH of urine and thereby inhibit the formation of formaldehyde; however, hippuric acid maintains an acidic environment. Nearly all bacteria are sensitive to formaldehyde at concentrations of $\geq 20\mu g/ml$. In catheterized patients, methenamine hippurate reduces sediment and catheter blockage, and doubles the interval between catheter changes.[11]

Nitrofurantoin is an alternative urinary antiseptic. Because of its rapid excretion from the blood (elimination halflife is $\leq$30min) nitrofurantoin reaches significant concentrations only in the bladder.[12] Nitrofurantoin is reduced by flavoproteins to reactive intermediates which inactivate or alter bacterial ribosomal proteins and other macromolecules. As a result, protein synthesis, aerobic metabolism, DNA synthesis, RNA synthesis and cell wall synthesis are inhibited. This broad mode of action is probably the reason why acquired bacterial resistance to nitrofurantoin is rare. Neither methenamine hippurate nor nitrofurantoin should be used to treat acute infection of the upper urinary tract. Both may cause gastro-intestinal symptoms, e.g. dyspepsia, nausea, vomiting.

Non-drug treatment

Patients with mild symptoms may respond to regular time-contingent voiding, e.g. every 1–3h. They will also be helped by:

- proximity to the toilet

- ready availability of a bottle or commode

- a rapid response by nurses to requests for help

- abstaining from caffeine and alcohol.[13]

Drug treatment

Antimuscarinic drugs are the drugs of choice but their use may be limited by adverse effects:

- oxybutynin 2.5–5mg b.d.–q.d.s., also has a topical anaesthetic effect on the bladder mucosa[14]

- tolterodine 2mg b.d., is as effective as oxybutynin 5mg t.d.s. but causes fewer adverse effects.[13]

Both drugs reduce urinary frequency by about 2/24h and incontinence episodes by 1–2/24h. If even tolterodine causes intolerable adverse effects, or if there is concurrent hepatic impairment, reduce the dose to 1mg b.d. The community cost of the two drugs is similar; contract prices generally make oxybutynin much cheaper in hospital. Other antimuscarinic drugs may sometimes be preferable:

- imipramine 25–50mg o.n.[15]

- amitriptyline 25–50mg o.n., a useful alternative in patients with concurrent insomnia

- propantheline 15mg b.d.–t.d.s.

If all antimuscarinic drugs cannot be tolerated, consider:

- a musculotropic drug, e.g. flavoxate 200–400mg t.d.s.

- a sympathomimetic, e.g. terbutaline 5mg t.d.s.

- a NSAID, e.g. flurbiprofen 50–100mg b.d. or naproxen 250–500mg b.d.

- a topical analgesic, e.g. phenazopyridine 100–200mg t.d.s. (not UK).

An antidiuretic hormone analogue, desmopressin 200–400μg PO or spray 20–40μg intranasally o.n. is often of value in refractory troublesome nocturia.[16] Because hyponatraemia is a possible complication, the plasma sodium concentration should be monitored.

Bladder spasms

Bladder (detrusor) spasms are transient, often excruciating, sensations felt in the suprapubic region and urethra. They are generally secondary to irritation or hyperexcitability of the trigone.

Causes

Bladder spasms may relate to local cancer or other factors (Box 9.B)

Box 9.B   Causes of bladder spasms

Cancer
Intravesical ⎫
Extravesical ⎭ irritation

Treatment
Radiation fibrosis

Debility
Anxiety
Infective cystitis
Indwelling catheter
    mechanical irritation by catheter balloon
    catheter sludging with partial retention

Management

Correct the correctable

Treatment options for reversible causes are listed in Table 9.2.

Table 9.2   Management of reversible causes of bladder spasms

Cause	Treatment option
Catheter irritation	Changer catheter Reduce volume of balloon

Catheter sludging	Bladder washouts (100ml)
	  0.9% saline
	  solution G[a]
	Continuous bladder irrigation

Blood clots (haematuria)	see p.243
Infection (cystitis)	Bladder washouts (if catheterized), see above Change indwelling catheter Switch to intermittent catheterization q4h–q6h Encourage oral fluids Antibiotics, systemic or by instillation Urinary antiseptics, e.g. methenamine hippurate Cranberry juice

a   costs over £2 per sachet and contains citric acid, sodium bicarbonate etc.; use if
    troublesome urinary sediment causes repeated catheter blockage despite 0.9% saline
    washouts ± methenamine hippurate or cranberry juice.

Drug treatment

Systemic analgesics should be used to control any constant background pain and, as with unstable bladder, an antimuscarinic given to reduce or prevent the spasms. Alternative antimuscarinics include:

- hyoscine (Quick Kwells) 0.3mg SL b.d.–q.d.s.

- hyoscyamine 0.15mg b.d.–q.d.s. or m/r 0.375mg b.d. (not UK); twice as potent as hyoscine

- belladonna and opium suppositories (B & O Supprettes) up to hourly (not UK); each B & O Supprette contains either 30mg (No. 15A) or 60mg (No. 16A) of powdered opium and approximately 0.2mg of belladonna alkaloids.

If the above measures are ineffective, consider:

- hyoscine butylbromide 60–160mg/24h CSCI

- intravesical morphine and bupivacaine t.d.s. (morphine 10–20mg and 0.5% bupivacaine 10ml diluted in 0.9% saline to 20ml); instil through an indwelling catheter and clamp for 30min

- spinal analgesia, e.g. epidural morphine and 0.5% bupivacaine.

Hesitancy

Hesitancy is a prolonged delay between attempting and achieving micturition.

Causes

There are many causes of hesitancy and retention (Box 9.C).

Management

Correct the correctable

Treatment options for reversible causes of hesitancy are listed in Table 9.3.

Non-drug treatment

In most patients, drug treatment should take precedence over non-drug treatment, i.e. catheterization. However, in debilitated bedbound patients, a trial

Box 9.C   Causes of hesitancy and retention

Cancer
Malignant enlargement of prostate
Infiltration of bladder neck
Presacral plexopathy
Spinal cord compression

Debility
Loaded rectum
Inability to stand to void
Generalized weakness

Treatment
Antimuscarinic drugs
Morphine (occasionally)
Spinal analgesia (particularly with bupivacaine)
Intrathecal nerve block

Concurrent
Benign enlargement of prostate

Table 9.3   Management of reversible causes of hesitancy

Cause	Treatment	
Antimuscarinic drugs	Modify drug regimen if possible	
Loaded rectum	Suppositories Enema Manual removal	→ oral laxative regimen
Inability to micturate lying down	Nursing assistance to enable more upright posture	
Benign enlargement of prostate	Transurethral resection	

of catheterization may be preferable. In such patients, perurethral catheterization will be the norm. For patients who have several months to live, suprapubic catheterization should be considered.

Drug treatment

Several options are available:

- an α-adrenoceptor antagonist
    indoramin 20mg o.n.–b.d., up to a maximum 24h dose of 100mg
    prazosin 0.5–1mg b.d.–t.d.s.
    tamsulosin 400µg o.d.
    terazosin 1–10mg o.n.

- a parasympathomimetic, e.g. bethanechol 10–30mg b.d.–q.d.s
- an anticholinesterase
  distigmine 5mg o.d.–b.d.
  pyridostigmine 60–120mg up to q4h.

Indoramin is the safest in debilitated patients; the most common adverse effect is dose-related sedation. Prazosin, tamsulosin and terazosin may all cause severe hypotension initially, particularly in patients receiving diuretics. The first dose is taken after going to bed at night. Pre-existing antihypertensive medication will need to be reduced. The only advantage in using prazosin is its cost; this has to be set against ease of compliance with tamsulosin and terazosin.

It is possible to combine either a parasympathomimetic or an anticholin-esterase with an α-adrenoceptor antagonist.

Discoloured urine

There are many causes of discoloured urine (Box 9.D). If the urine is red, it is often assumed to be haematuria and therefore is disturbing, even frightening.

Box 9.D Common causes of discoloured urine

Red/pink
Beetroot
Dantron (in co-danthramer and co-danthrusate)
Doxorubicin
Nefopam
Phenolphthalein (in alkaline urine) present in several proprietary laxatives (e.g. Agarol)
Rhubarb

Blue
Methylene blue; present in some proprietary urinary antiseptic mixtures,
    e.g. Urised (USA)
Pseudomonas aeruginosa (pyocyanin) in alkaline urine

Dark
Metronidazole

References

1 McCaffery M (1981) *Nursing Management of the Patient with Pain*. Lippincott, Philadelphia.
2 Bateman D (1994) Tiaprofenic acid and cystitis. *British Medical Journal*. **309**: 552–3.
3 Mayall F *et al*. (1994) Cystitis and ureteric obstruction in patients taking tiaprofenic acid. *British Medical Journal*. **309**:599.
4 CSM (2000) Tiaprofenic acid. In: BNF Editor *British National Formulary*. No. 39 (March). BNF, London, p.455.
5 Avorn J *et al*. (1994) Reduction of bacteriuria and pyuria after ingestion of cranberry juice. *Journal of the American Medical Association*. **271**:751–4.
6 Cronberg S *et al*. (1987) Prevention of recurrent acute cystitis by methenamine hippurate: double blind controlled crossover longterm study. *British Medical Journal*. **294**:1507–8.
7 Brumfitt W *et al*. (1981) Prevention of recurrent urinary infections in women: a comparative trial between nitrofurantoin and methenamine hippurate. *Journal of Urology*. **126**:71–4.
8 Harkins K (2000) What's the use of cranberry juice? *Age and Ageing*. **29**:9–12.
9 Jepson R *et al*. (2000) Cranberries for preventing urinary tract infections. *Cochrane Library*. **2**.
10 Strom JJ and Jun H (1993) Effect of urine pH and ascorbic acid on the rate of conversion of methenamine to formaldehyde. *Biopharmaceutics Drug Disposition*. **14**:61–9.
11 Norberg A *et al*. (1980) Randomized double-blind study of prophylactic methenamine hippurate treatment of patients with indwelling catheters. *European Journal of Clinical Pharmacology*. **18**:497–500.
12 Hooper D (1995) Urinary tract agents: nitrofurantoin and methenamine. In: G Mandell, J Bennett and R Dolin (eds) *Mandell, Douglas and Bennett's Principles and Practice of Infectious Diseases*. Churchill Livingstone, New York, pp 376–81.
13 Hills C *et al*. (1998) Tolterodine. *Drugs*. **55**:813–20.
14 Robinson T and Castledon C (1994) Drugs in focus: 11. Oxybutynin hydrochloride. *Prescribers' Journal*. **34**:27–30.
15 Castledon C (1988) Imipramine: possible alternative to current therapy for urinary incontinence in the elderly. *Journal of Urology*. **22**:525–33.
16 Matthiesen T *et al*. (1994) A dose titration and an open 6-week efficacy and safety study of desmopressin tablets in the management of nocturnal enuresis. *Journal of Urology*. **151**:460–3.

10   Skin care

Pruritus · Dry skin · Wet skin · Skin care during
radiotherapy · Sweating · Stomas · Fistulas
Fungating cancer · Decubitus ulcers

Pruritus

Pruritus is an unpleasant sensation which provokes the desire to scratch
(synonym: itch).

Neurophysiology

Pruritus is a distinct sensation which can affect the skin, conjunctivae and
mucous membranes, including the upper respiratory tract. The neuro-anatomy
of pruritus is similar to that of pain. The afferent nerve fibres mediating
pruritus are a subset of C-fibres.[1] Their terminals are more superficial than
the nociceptive C-fibres, close to the junction between the epidermis and the
dermis, and they are stimulated by histamine and other pruritogens (Box 10.A).
They project to a distinct subset of secondary neurones in the dorsal horn
of the spinal cord. The nerve endings mediating pruritus tend to be clustered
around discrete 'itch points'.

Box 10.A   Chemical mediators of pruritus

Amines, e.g.	Neuropeptides, e.g.
histamine	substance P
serotonin	calcitonin-gene-related peptide (CGRP)
Opioids	bradykinin
Eicosanoids[a]	somatostatin
Cytokines	vaso-active intestinal peptide (VIP)
Proteases	cholecystokinin
Growth factors	

---

a   collective term for metabolites of arachidonic acid, including prostanoids and leukotrienes.

Heat-induced vasodilation exacerbates pruritus, whereas cold-induced vaso-
constriction reduces it. It is also increased by attention, anxiety and boredom,

and decreased by relaxation and distraction. Pruritus can also be neuropathic, i.e. initiated centrally by brain damage, tumours and multiple sclerosis.[2]

Histamine

Histamine is the most important chemical mediator of pruritus. It reproducibly causes itching when applied to damaged skin or injected intradermally. Endogenous histamine released in the skin is mostly from mast cells. In addition to the direct stimulation of neuronal H_1-receptors, histamine probably stimulates the formation of other mediators.[3] However, the response to histamine decreases when it is injected repeatedly at the same site, casting doubt over the role of histamine in chronic itch.[4]

Serotonin

Serotonin (5HT) can also cause pruritus,[5] but is a weaker pruritogen than histamine. It is involved in pruritus associated with cholestasis and renal failure, two situations in which $5HT_3$-receptor antagonists are of benefit.[6,7]

Opioids

Endogenous opioids have a regulatory effect on pruritus and, depending on the circumstances, naloxone can either increase or decrease pruritus.[8] Morphine and other opioids can cause pruritus particularly if given spinally.[9–11] Naltrexone, an oral opioid antagonist, relieves cholestatic pruritus.[12]

In opioid-naive patients, pruritus is more common with epidural morphine (about 40%) than hydromorphone (about 10%).[11] Pruritus may be experienced in the lower half of the body or only the face, or be generalized. The pruritus is not relieved by antihistamines but $5HT_3$-receptor antagonists often help.[6] Fortunately, the incidence of pruritus with opioids by non-spinal routes is only about 1%.

Pathogenesis

About 10% of the population have dermographia, i.e. an exaggerated 'weal and flare' response to a firm linear stroke across the skin. Such people are more likely to develop a vicious circle of pruritus → scratching → more pruritus → more scratching.

Dry skin is a common cause of pruritus and may be associated with the increased expression of cytokines seen when the skin's integrity is damaged by cutaneous dehydration.[13,14] Wet macerated skin is also pruritogenic.

Primary skin disease

Pruritus is a common feature of skin disease, for example:

- atopic dermatitis
- contact dermatitis (Box 10.B)
- urticaria
- psoriasis
- scabies
- lice (pediculosis).

Box 10.B Common skin allergens

Creams and soaps containing perfume
Neomycin preparations, e.g. Cicatrin, Graneodin, Tribiotic
Antihistamine creams
Local anaesthetic creams (but not lidocaine)
Alcohol (in topical antipruritics and alcohol wipes)
Wool fat (lanolin)
Rubber, e.g. undersheets, pillow coverings

Systemic disease

Pruritus may occur in many systemic conditions (Box 10.C).

Box 10.C Systemic disease associated with pruritus[15]

Renal	**Endocrine**
Chronic renal failure	Hyperthyroidism
	Hypothyroidism
Hepatic	Carcinoid syndrome
Primary biliary cirrhosis	Diabetes mellitus (associated with
Cholestasis	genital candidiasis)
Hepatitis	
Hematological	**Other**
Lymphomas	Cancer (paraneoplastic)
Leukaemias	AIDS
Multiple myeloma	Multiple sclerosis
Polycythaemia rubra vera	
Iron deficiency	**Psychiatric**
Mastocytosis	Psychosis

Drugs

Most drugs have been implicated as the cause of a pruritic rash (Box 10.D).

Box 10.D   Common cutaneous drug reactions

Morbilliform drug rashes
Cephalosporins
Penicillins
Phenytoin
Sulphonamides

Toxic epidermal necrolysis
Allopurinol
Penicillins
Phenylbutazone
Sulphonamides

Urticaria
Cephalosporins
Penicillins
Radio-opaque dyes
Sulphonamides

Pseudolymphoma
Phenytoin

Multiple causes

In many situations, pruritus is multifactorial (Box 10.E). In patients with renal failure complicated by secondary hyperparathyroidism, correction of hypercalcaemia leads to the rapid relief of pruritus. In other circumstances hypercalcaemia is not associated with pruritus.

Box 10.E   Causal factors in pruritus

Old age
Dry skin
Increased mast cell degranulation[16]
Increased skin sensitivity to histamine[16]

Cholestasis[a]
Increased endogenous opioids
Increased release of serotonin

Renal failure[a]
Increased endogenous opioids
Mast cell proliferation $\rightarrow$ LTB_4
Increased skin vitamin A
Increased release of serotonin
   (from platelets?)

Paraneoplastic[a]
Histamine-release from basophils
Eosinophilia
Immune reaction

Increased release of substance P
Increased skin divalent ions (Ca^{2+}, Mg^{2+})

---

a   dry skin is frequently an important concurrent factor.

Evaluation

Visual appearance, pattern recognition and probability generally indicate the cause. Contact dermatitis can be caused by many different topical applications. Lanolin (wool fat) is the most common offender but preservatives and perfumes in an emollient may be the cause.

Management

Correct the correctable

Review the patient's medication:

- is the pruritus caused by a drug-induced rash (Box 10.D)?
- has an opioid been recently prescribed?

If a drug is the likely cause, it should be stopped if possible.

Virtually all patients with advanced cancer and pruritus have a dry skin. Even when there is a definite endogenous cause, rehydration of the skin may obviate the need for specific measures (see p.309). Cholestatic pruritus resolves if the jaundice is relieved by inserting a stent into the common bile duct.

Non-drug treatment

Non-drug treatment includes the following measures:

- discourage scratching but allow gentle rubbing; keep finger nails cut short
- avoid prolonged hot baths
- dry the skin gently by 'patting' with a soft towel and/or by using a hair dryer on cool setting
- avoid overheating and sweating; this can be a particular problem at night if a winter duvet is used in the summer or with nocturnal central heating.

Drug treatment

Topical

Generally, these should be applied after washing in the morning and again in the evening:

- aqueous cream + 1% menthol

- oily calamine lotion (contains 0.5% phenol) ± 0.5% phenol

- barrier cream, e.g. Comfeel

- if inflamed, clioquinol-hydrocortisone cream (or plain 1% hydrocortisone cream).

Crotamiton 10% (Eurax) cream has mild antiscabetic properties but, despite claims, it is no better than placebo as an antipruritic.[17]

The topical use of antihistamine creams should be discouraged because prolonged use may lead to contact dermatitis. If one is being used and the skin becomes inflamed, discontinue the antihistamine and apply 1% hydrocortisone cream until the inflammation has settled.

Systemic

- a corticosteroid if the skin is inflamed but not infected as a result of scratching, e.g. dexamethasone 2–4mg o.m. or prednisolone 10–20mg o.m.

- a NSAID in *en cuirass* breast cancer associated with local pruritus; this reduces the production of tumour-related PGs which sensitize nerve endings to pruritogenic substances

- an antihistamine (H_1-receptor antagonist)
    chlorphenamine 4mg t.d.s.–12mg q.d.s.; useful for rapid dose escalation to determine if an antihistamine is of benefit
    cetirizine 5mg b.d. or 10mg o.d.; a non-sedative antihistamine useful for maintenance treatment
    promethazine 25–50mg b.d.
    hydroxyzine 10–25mg b.d.–t.d.s.; 25–100mg o.n.
    alimemazine (trimeprazine) 5–10mg b.d.–t.d.s.; 10–30mg o.n.
    levomepromazine 12.5mg SC; if beneficial convert to 6–25mg PO o.n.[18]

- paroxetine and mirtazapine.[19]

Most patients with advanced cancer and pruritus never need an antihistamine or other systemic drug if appropriate skin care is undertaken; without skin care drugs are of little benefit.

In cholestatic pruritus, if relieving the obstruction is unsuccessful, alternative drug measures may be necessary. Thus, if skin care does not relieve the pruritus consider:

- ondansetron 4mg b.d., generally relieves cholestatic pruritus in 5–6h[20] and in 30min if 8mg is given IV; it is expensive

- an androgen, e.g. stanozolol 5mg PO o.d. or methyltestosterone 25mg SL b.d.

  takes 5–7 days to achieve maximum effect

  mode of action unknown

  may increase jaundice but this is not a problem in advanced cancer

  masculinization generally not a problem

- rifampicin 150mg b.d., acts by enzyme induction[21]

- naltrexone, an oral opioid antagonist, is used at some centres; it reduces the intensity of pruritus but generally does not completely relieve it and is expensive.[12] *Should not be used by patients taking opioids for pain relief.*

Colestyramine (an anion exchange resin which binds bile acids) is *not* recommended; it is often ineffective, is unpalatable and can cause diarrhoea.

Dry skin

Rough scaly skin, either fine or coarse (synonym: xerosis).

Pathogenesis

The most superficial layer of the skin (stratum corneum or keratin layer) needs to be hydrated in order to function as a protective layer. Water is held in the layer of oil secreted by sebaceous glands. Dried out keratin contracts and splits, exposing the dermis and forming fine scales which flake off. The exposed dermis becomes inflamed and itchy, possibly as a result of increased cytokine expression.[13,14] Scratching increases inflammation and a vicious circle is created. This is broken by adding moisture and retaining it in a lubricant (emollient), thereby enabling the keratin layer to reconstitute.

Management

Apply an emollient cream to the skin (Table 10.1); the greater the concentration of oil the more wetting power a preparation has.[22] Aqueous cream o.d.–b.d. is generally adequate and much cheaper than most proprietary preparations. For mobile patients, if the emollient is applied at bedtime it is fully absorbed before the next morning. With dry flaky skin, an ointment may be needed for a few days. Other measures include:

- stop using soap

- use a non-detergent soap substitute, e.g. aqueous cream BP (emulsifying ointment 30%, phenoxyethanol 1% in water)

- add an emollient to bath water, e.g. Balneum bath oil

- wet wrapping of localized pruritic area
    apply emollient cream
    cover with a wet dressing
    cover wet dressing with a dry dressing.

Table 10.1   Composition of emollients: least oily to most oily

	Preservative	Perfume	Lanolin
Lotion (suspension of oil-in-water)			
Keri lotion	+	+	+
Light creams (suspension of water-in-oil)			
Aveeno cream	–	–	–
Aqueous cream BP	+	–	–
Diprobase cream	+	–	–
Hydromol cream	+	–	–
E45 cream	+	–	+
Ultrabase cream	+	+	–
Oilatum cream	+	+	+
Rich creams (more oily)			
Aquadrate cream	–	–	–
Unguentum Merck cream	+	–	–
Lipobase cream	+	–	–
Oily cream BP (hydrous ointment)	+	–	+
Ointments (most oily)			
White soft paraffin BP	–	–	–
Liquid paraffin in white soft paraffin	–	–	–
Coconut oil BP	–	–	–
Diprobase ointment	–	–	–
Neutrogena dermatological cream	+	–	–

Wet skin

Wet skin means maceration, often compounded by blisters, exudate or pus from secondary infection.

Pathogenesis

Because the skin is wet, the epidermal keratin absorbs water, swells and becomes macerated. Once the protective barrier is broken, infection follows, commonly with yeasts and less commonly with Staphylococcus and/or Streptococcus. The result is inflammation and pruritus.

Maceration occurs particularly where two layers of skin are apposed. For example:

- perineum
- between buttocks   } particularly in incontinent bedbound patients
- groins
- under pendulous breasts
- between fingers, particularly if arthritic
- around ulcers
- around stomas.

Management

The first step is to dry excess moisture:

- pat with a soft towel
- use a hair dryer on a cool setting
- dust carmellose (Orahesive) powder over the affected area
- apply an aqueous solution topically t.d.s., either alone or as a compress, and allow it to dry out completely
- if infected, use an antifungal solution, e.g. clotrimazole 1%
- if very inflamed, use 1% hydrocortisone solution for 3–4 days.

Be careful with adsorbent powders, e.g. starch, talc, zinc oxide; in excess they can form a hard abrasive coating on the skin. However, the use of a proprietary preparation such as Ster-Zac dusting powder is often satisfactory.

Particularly where two areas of skin are apposed, protect with an appropriate barrier:

- a wipe-on protective skin barrier, e.g. CliniShield, Peri-Prep; these contain an alcohol and sting if the skin is excoriated
- Cavilon No Sting Barrier Film; this is sprayed on and does not sting on broken skin
- a barrier cream, e.g. Comfeel, Drapolene, or ointment, e.g. Morhulin (zinc oxide 38%).

Although a barrier cream or ointment is of little value if the excess moisture is caused by sweating, a wipe-on protective skin barrier may help. Barrier creams and ointments should not be used under the breasts or in the groins unless it is to protect the skin from exudate from a local ulcer or from urine.

Monitor for allergic contact dermatitis secondary to topical agents; this may look like the initial problem. Morhulin, Comfeel and Drapolene all contain lanolin.

Skin care during radiotherapy

Guidelines 10.1: Skin care for radiotherapy patients (p.391).

In the past, overstrict advice about skin care was given to patients receiving radiotherapy. It is important not to burden patients with unnecessary restrictions while, at the same time, providing them with clear instructions.

Sweating

Sweat is skin moisture which has been secreted by sweat glands. Sweating (synonyms: diaphoresis, hyperhydrosis) is a normal part of thermoregulation and aids cooling by evaporation from the skin surface. Sweating also occurs in response to noxious stimuli, fear and embarrassment. In cancer patients, sweating ranges from mild to severe. Severe sweating necessitates a change of clothing or bedlinen, or both.[23]

Physiology

Two types of gland secrete moisture onto the surface of the body:

- apocrine
- eccrine.

Apocrine glands develop at puberty and their ducts empty into hair follicles. They occur in the scalp, axillae, around the nipples and in the anogenital area. Secretions contain proteins and complex carbohydrates, and are under adrenergic control.[24]

The eccrine glands secrete sweat, a watery fluid containing chloride, lactic acid, fatty acids, glycoproteins, mucopolysaccharides and urea, directly onto the skin surface. There are two functionally separate sets of eccrine glands. One set populates the entire skin except the palms and soles and is responsible for thermal regulation; secretion is controlled by cholinergic postganglionic sympathetic fibres. The other set is confined to the palms, soles and axillae and is controlled by adrenergic fibres. Those on the palms and soles respond mostly to emotion whereas those in the axillae respond to both heat and emotion.

Evaporation of secretions occurs constantly from the skin and the mucous membranes of the mouth and respiratory tract. The basal level of 'insensible' water loss is about 50ml/h, i.e. about 1200ml/24h.[25] The maximal secretion from the 3–4 million eccrine glands in the skin is 2–3L/h.[26]

Causes

A high ambient temperature, exercise, emotion and fever are the common causes of sweating. In some patients, sweating is a paraneoplastic phenomenon. It ranges in severity from a mild nuisance to a major symptom with repeated drenching sweats, particularly during the night. Paraneoplastic sweating may or may not be associated with a remittent temperature. Several hypotheses have been adopted to explain the phenomenon:

- the release of pyrogens as a result of leucocyte infiltration or necrosis of the tumour
- a substance released by the tumour which acts either directly on the hypothalamus or indirectly via endogenous pyrogen.

The pyrogens then induce a PG cascade which results in sweating ± fever.[26–28] Drugs are sometimes responsible for sweating, either *ab initio* or by exacerbating a concurrent cause:

- ethanol (vasodilation)
- tricyclic antidepressants (paradoxical effect)
- morphine.

Metastatic hepatomegaly and morphine seem to be a potent combined risk factor for sweating.

Sweating also occurs at the menopause as a hormone deficiency phenomenon distinct from hot flushes.[29] Sweating occurs in men after chemical or surgical castration.

Management

Correct the correctable

* lower the ambient temperature
    reduce heating
    increase ventilation
    use fan
    use cotton clothing (aids surface evaporation)

* treat infection with the appropriate antibiotic

* hormone deficiency after castration, prescribe
    medroxyprogesterone 5–20mg b.d.–q.d.s.
    megestrol acetate 20–40mg o.m.[30]   ⎫
    diethylstilbestrol 1mg o.m.   ⎬ effect manifests
    cyproterone (has weak progestogen activity)[31] after 2–4 weeks
    clonidine 100µg o.n.[32]   ⎭

* if a tricyclic antidepressant or an SSRI is the cause, switch to venlafaxine or mirtazapine

* if morphine is the cause, consider switching to an alternative strong opioid (see p.42).

Non-drug treatment

Although local treatment with aluminium chloride hexahydrate (axillae) and formalin or gluteraldehyde (feet) are of value in emotional sweating,[33] they are generally irrelevant in advanced cancer. Such treatments work by blocking or destroying sweat glands. Iontophoresis,[34] botulinum toxin and surgical approaches such as undercutting the axillary skin, excision and sympathectomy, are also irrelevant.[35,36]

Drug treatment

This is summarized in Box 10.F.

Box 10.F   Drugs to relieve cancer-related sweating

If the sweating is associated with fever, prescribe an antipyretic (and an antibiotic if appropriate):
    paracetamol 500–1000mg q.d.s. or p.r.n.
    NSAID, e.g. ibuprofen 200–400mg t.d.s. or p.r.n., or the locally preferred alternative.

Naproxen 250–500mg b.d. may be the NSAID of choice for persistent paraneoplastic sweating associated with a remittent temperature;[28] however, this view has been challenged.[37] NSAIDs are probably more effective than paracetamol and corticosteroids in this situation.

Paradoxically, some people transiently sweat more after taking an antipyretic, possibly as part of the body's way of cooling down.

If sweating is not associated with fever or fails to respond to a NSAID, consider an antimuscarinic drug:
    amitriptyline 25–50mg o.n.
    propantheline 15–30mg b.d.–t.d.s.

Stomas

A stoma is an artificial opening on the surface of the body. About 5% of patients with advanced cancer have one:

- colostomy after resection of the rectum or to palliate incontinence associated with a rectovaginal or rectovesical fistula

- ileostomy after total colectomy or panproctocolectomy

- gastrostomy for venting or feeding

- urostomy (ileal conduit) after cystectomy

- tracheostomy.

Long-term metabolic complications of an ileostomy, such as urolithiasis and cholelithiasis, are not seen in advanced cancer because of the short prognosis. Vitamin B_{12} absorption will cease if an ileostomy excludes the distal 90–120cm of ileum but body stores are adequate for about 5 years.

Management

In the UK, a patient with a stoma will receive advice and support from a trained stoma care nurse.[38] In some oncology departments and palliative care units other nurses may develop a special interest in stoma care. In the community, district nurses provide much ongoing support. Stoma care includes:

- psychological support
- rehabilitation
- skin care
- faecal consistency
- flatus control.

Psychological support

Psychological preparation before the stoma operation is important and is the key to postoperative rehabilitation. Explanation about the use of stomas in various conditions helps the patient to feel less strange and less isolated from 'normal' people. Contact with other stoma patients before and after the stoma operation helps. Several support organizations have been established in the UK, generally run by patients (or former patients) for patients, including:

- British Colostomy Association
- Ileostomy Association
- National Association of Laryngectomee Clubs
- Urostomy Association.

In addition to these national organizations there are self-financing local groups or fellowships for ostomy patients in most counties and the large metropolitan areas.

Rehabilitation

Rehabilitation includes addressing issues such as clothing, physical activity, sexual relationships and travel. Close relatives also need an opportunity to talk with nursing and/or medical staff about the stoma. This reduces misunderstandings and increases the likelihood of positive support for the patient from the family.

Skin care

Care of the peristomal skin includes the careful replacement of a new ap-pliance. Mild solvents, e.g. Clear Peel, Lift, can be used to reduce discomfort in patients with sensitive skin. Warm water is used to clean the surrounding skin. The skin is dried by placing paper tissues or kitchen roll over the stoma and pressing lightly with an open hand over the stoma and surrounding area. Any residual mucus from the stoma should be dabbed away; if it gets under the flange it reduces the bonding of the adhesive to the skin.

A skin barrier, e.g. Comfeel barrier cream, may be applied sparingly if the effluent is liquid or if the appliance/flange is being changed more than once daily. It is gently rubbed in and any excess wiped off. A barrier preparation is also useful around the anus in patients with a rectal discharge despite having a defunctioning colostomy.

A template/cutting guide should be used to help prepare the opening for the stoma in the flange of the appliance. This reduces the chance of a poorly fitting appliance and is particularly helpful when several different people are involved in the care of the stoma. All modern appliances have hydrocolloid in the flange which helps to protect the skin. In the UK, patients can receive their own personalized supply precut by the manufacturers.

Serious skin problems are uncommon with modern standards of care and are mainly the result of liquid faeces coming into contact with the skin (Box 10.G). Poorly fitting appliances can lead to 'pancaking', i.e. faeces ooze into a gap between the flange of the appliance and the skin and become trapped there.

Box 10.G Risk factors for peristomal skin problems

Poor skin hygiene	Poorly fitting appliance
Sweating	Retraction
Diarrhoea	Prolapse
Skin reactions	Herniation
Abdominal radiotherapy	Stenosis

If the skin becomes red and sore, there is a reason for it. Steps must be taken immediately to stop faecal leakage. The use of a wipe-on skin barrier, e.g. CliniShield, Peri-Prep is often sufficient to allow resolution of early skin changes. Skin wipes may also be used prophylactically. The wipes dry quickly and do not leave a greasy surface. Because they contain alcohol, wipes should not be applied to excoriated skin; Cavilon No Sting Barrier Film should be used instead.

Cavilon No Sting Barrier Film is a polymeric solution containing two siloxanes and acrylate copolymer which dries about 30 seconds after application. The film is colourless, transparent and is permeable to oxygen and moisture vapour. It acts as a barrier against irritation from body fluids, protecting intact or damaged skin from urine and/or faecal incontinence, digestive juices and wound drainage. It also reduces skin damage by adhesives, friction and shear. Cavilon No Sting Barrier Film can be applied to apposing skin surfaces provided the surfaces are held apart and the coating allowed to dry thoroughly before the surfaces are in contact again.

When used as a protection against body fluids or incontinence, Cavilon No Sting Barrier Film is generally applied every 2–3 days. Daily application may be necessary if there is need for frequent cleaning of the area, e.g. with frequent incontinent diarrhoea. If covered by an adhesive, re-application is necessary every time the adhesive dressing is changed.

If necessary, a two-piece appliance can be used until the skin has healed; the flange is left in place for 4–5 days before removal, thereby facilitating healing. To help appliances adhere to moist areas, Orahesive powder (carmellose, gelatin and pectin) can be dusted onto raw skin. The powder adheres to the raw surface; excess powder is removed by blowing.

If peristomal skin infection is confirmed, it is best treated with a combination antibiotic-corticosteroid cream:

- miconazole 2% + hydrocortisone 1% (Daktacort)
- fusidic acid 2% + betamethasone 0.1% (Fucibet).

Faecal consistency

Most patients with a distal colostomy achieve normal faecal consistency spontaneously or with the help of a hydrophilic bulking agent. Consistency and quantity also depend on diet. With an ileostomy normal faeces are never possible; the aim is an effluent with the consistency of soft porridge.

The average effluent from an ileostomy is about 700ml/24h and sodium and water loss is only about three times that in the faeces of normal subjects. Normal dietary intake can compensate for such losses. However, a high output (>1L/24h) from an ileostomy leads to sodium and water depletion. These can be corrected by prescribing oral rehydration salts, e.g. Diorylate, Rehidrat (contain potassium as well as sodium salts). Another option is Boot's Isotonic powder which contains no potassium. For patients paying their own prescription charges, a home-made rehydration solution is cheaper (Box 10.H).

Output can be reduced with an opioid antidiarrhoeal such as loperamide (see p.128). Although hydrophilic bulking agents PO do not reduce ileostomy

---

Box 10.H   Home-made rehydration solution: instructions for patients

---

Make a fresh solution every day:

glucose	6 × flat 5ml spoonfuls	
sodium chloride	1 × flat 5ml spoonful	in 1L of tap water.
sodium bicarbonate	1 × heaped 2.5ml spoonful	

You can buy the powders from any community pharmacy and some supermarkets.

Sodium chloride is table salt which you have already.

Sodium bicarbonate is also known as bicarbonate of soda.

---

output, adding a sachet of a bulking agent, e.g. Fybogel, Regulan, to the ostomy bag makes the effluent firmer and more manageable. Vernagel sachets, marketed to solidify urine standing in a urine bottle, are even more effective.

If an ostomy patient complains of troublesome diarrhoea:

- review the patient's medication (*see* p.126)
- identify foods which increase stoma output and remove them from the diet (Table 10.2)
- encourage foods which decrease output (Table 10.2)
- recommend marshmallows 5–6 b.d., these make faeces more solid
- if the diarrhoea persists, culture the faeces for possible infection.

Constipation with a colostomy generally relates to:

- the use of analgesics and other constipating drugs
- an inadequate fluid intake
- a failure to eat a moderately high residue diet and/or eating too many constipating foods
- immobility
- depression
- obstruction caused by cancer.

If receiving an opioid or other constipating drug, in the first instance recommend oral laxatives (*see* p.117). However, digital examination of the colostomy, is necessary before proceeding to suppositories or an enema. If indicated,

Table 10.2 Foods which affect stoma function

Increase output	Decrease output	Cause skin/ anal irritation	Increase flatus	May block stomas[a]
Fruit juices	Apple sauce	Citrus fruits and juices	Milk and milk products	Onion	Mushroom
Beer and alcohol	Bananas	Coconut	Instant coffee	Cucumber	Sweetcorn
Caffeinated beverages	Boiled rice	Nuts	Carbonated drinks	Lentils	Potato skins
Chocolate	Tapioca	Oriental vegetables	Dark beer	Carrots	Nuts
Raw fruits	Suet pudding	Some raw fruits and	Red wine	Peppers	Tomato
Beans	Cheese	vegetables, e.g.	Apricots	Aubergines	Raw fruit skin
Greens	Peanut butter	apples, oranges	Prunes	Dahl	Celery
Spicy foods	White bread	celery, coleslaw	Greens	Ghee	
Wholemeal food	Potatoes	sweetcorn	Beans	Molasses	
Wholegrain cereals	Pasta		Chick peas	Tempeli	
	Noodles				

a these foods in particular need to be chewed well.

a phosphate enema is almost always effective. With faecal impaction, an oil enema may be necessary first.

Flatus control

Flatus is normal but is influenced by various factors, including diet. If problematic, discussion about foods, fluids and eating habits which increase the volume of flatus may help to reduce the unwanted embarrassment. Habits which contribute to flatulence include:

* rushed eating

* chewing gum

* smoking

* breathlessness

* missing meals

* eating and drinking at the same time

* certain types of foods (Table 10.2)

* carbonated drinks.

Most 1-piece and 2-piece closed systems have an inbuilt vent with a charcoal filter which adsorbs flatus and odour. Many drainable systems are also now designed with an integral filter. Some bags contain deodorant pellets.

If malodour remains a problem, adding a de-odorizer to the appliance bag is preferable to oral medication, e.g. Atmocol, Citrus Fresh, Limone (Table 10.3). If two puffs of a de-odorizer into the bag are not sufficient, they can also be used as room sprays. However, with such agents there should be no malodour except when the bag is changed.

Most so-called de-odorizers are in fact counter-odours. In contrast, NaturCare is an odourless deodorant. It works in a confined space by chemically denaturing malodourous organic molecules. Because it does not harm normal or damaged skin, NaturCare can be sprayed around an ostomy appliance or a malodourous wound dressing when it is being changed, and onto the stoma or wound itself, although the benefit of this is questionable.

Mechanical complications

Mechanical complications can occur with a stoma (Box 10.I). Apart from impaction, management will generally require consultation with the stoma

Table 10.3   Selected agents for odour control in colostomy patients

Formulation	Name
Tablets	Amplex-C
	Chlorophyll
	Charcoal
	Lactobacillus acidophilus[a]
Capsules	Peppermint oil (Colpermin, Mintec)
Spray[b]	Atmocol
	Citrus Fresh
	Limone
	NaturCare
Liquid[b]	Chironair liquid
	Forest Breeze oil drops
	Nilodor
	Noroma
Powder[b]	Ostobon

a   alters the intestinal flora and reduces the number of colonic bacteria
b   put in the appliance bag or, if liquid, it can be put on a tissue inserted into the bag.

Box 10.1   Complications of a stoma

Retraction	Bleeding	Granulation
Prolapse	Necrosis	Recurrent cancer
Herniation	Perforation	obstruction
Stenosis	Fistula	fungation

care nurse and possibly the surgeon who fashioned the stoma. However, in patients with a very poor prognosis simple supportive measures are all that is appropriate.

Fistulas

A fistula is an abnormal communication between two hollow organs or between a hollow organ and the skin. Most fistulas in advanced cancer develop as a result of postoperative infection and/or radiotherapy. A few are caused solely by tumour progression and necrosis.

Rectovaginal and rectovesical fistulas

Management is either conservative or surgical. A colostomy or ileostomy provides complete relief. On the other hand, stomas are not always trouble-free. Because of this or for psychological reasons, some patients prefer not to have surgery.

Enterocutaneous fistulas

Enterocutaneous fistulas can be divided into four broad categories:

1   A single orifice in an otherwise intact abdominal wall or healed scar around which the skin is flat and in reasonably good condition.

2   Single or multiple orifices in the abdominal wall near to bony prominences, surgical scars, other stomas or the umbilicus.

3   Fistulas into a small dehiscence of a surgical wound or scar.

4   Fistulas into a large gaping wound dehiscence.[39]

Management comprises:

• effluent collection

• monitoring plasma electrolytes

• skin protection

• odour control.

IV hyperalimentation may need to be considered in patients with a prognosis of >3 months. This prevents malnutrition through loss of nutrients in the effluent and promotes healing. About 50% of enterocutaneous fistulas will close spontaneously, particularly with a defunctioning ileostomy.[40]

Effluent collection

Categories 1 and 3 are managed like a stoma. With Category 2, a 2-piece appliance with a hard flange is unsuitable because it will not lie flat; a 1-piece appliance is used instead. Sometimes, if a fistula has two surface exits, it may be necessary to use two appliances.

Categories 2 and 4 both present a major nursing challenge. Management is time-consuming and frequent leakage demoralizes both nurses and patient.

A stoma care or tissue viability nurse should be consulted. Acknowledgement by the doctors of the difficulties faced by the patient and the nurses is supportive.

High output fistulas are generally ileocutaneous. The effluent is caustic because of the presence of proteolytic and other enzymes; contact with the skin leads to erythema in <1h and excoriation in 3–4h. Effluent can be reduced by:

- loperamide ≤30mg/24h (i.e. more than the manufacturer's recom-mendation) is useful in low ileal fistulas because it allows more ileal absorption as a result of a prolonged transit time and a pro-absorptive effect
- hyoscine butylbromide 60–120mg/24h by CSCI, reduces gastro-intestinal secretions[41]
- octreotide 100μg SC t.d.s. or 250–500μg/24h by CSCI; reduces gastro-intestinal secretions.[42]

Skin protection

Skin protection is essential. When the appliance is changed, it helps if the fistula can be plugged temporarily[43] or the flow of effluent removed by suctioning. The shape of the orifice is cut out of a sheet of hydrocolloid but before application any crevices are filled in with Stomahesive paste (carmellose, gelatin, pectin, alcohol) (Figure 10.1). The alcohol in Stomahesive paste stings the raw areas transiently. After applying the paste, the appliance is attached. Alternatively, a Cohesive seal can be used; this moulds to the contours of the body surface.

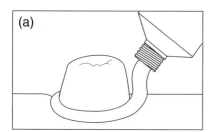
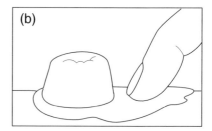

Figure 10.1   (a) Stomahesive paste is used to fill depressions and irregular skin contours. (b) If the paste needs to be spread more evenly, use a moistened finger or spatula. If more paste is required to form an even surface, wait 30 seconds before it is added.

Special high output bags are available with an extension bag for use overnight. This enables a patient to sleep through the night without having to
worry about overfilling and leakage.

Odour control

If the effluent is faecal there is the added problem of odour. This is embar-
rassing for the patient, the family and visitors, other patients and staff, and
appropriate measures should be introduced (see p.321).

Buccal fistulas

Fistulas can occur between the mouth and the face or neck. In addition to the
inevitable psychological distress associated with a visible deformity, buccal
fistulas cause problems with leakage of saliva and of ingested fluids. If the
fistula is of small diameter, a wad of gauze changed regularly may suffice.
Neonatal stoma appliances can sometimes be used and are often acceptable
to the patient. It may be helpful to reduce the volume of saliva with an antisecretory drug, e.g. hyoscine butylbromide, octreotide.

With a larger fistula, the use of a silicone foam casting should be considered.
Silicone foam is available as Cavicare. The use of plastic film results in a
smoother surface to the casting. If a second casting is made, this can be
inserted when the dressing is changed and the first one washed and dried.
Silicone foam castings have also been used in the management of enterocutaneous fistulas.[44]

Fungating cancer

A fungating cancer is a primary or secondary malignant tumour which
has ulcerated the skin. The tumour may be proliferative or cavitating and is
associated with:

*   stinging, soreness, pain
*   pruritus, particularly in breast cancer
*   exudate
*   malodour ($\rightarrow$ nausea)
*   bleeding
*   infection.

A fungating cancer is distressing to the patient and is repulsive to the carers, family and friends. Malodour can lead to social isolation and despair.

Management

Guidelines 10.2: Fungating cancer (India) (p.392).

The treatment of pain and bleeding are discussed elsewhere (*see* p.25 and p.237). Topical morphine is a theoretical option but not always feasible because of the extent of the ulceration (*see* p.60). Pruritus is probably caused by inflammatory substances, e.g. PGs and may respond to a NSAID. Measures for dealing with exudate and infection are the same as those used with decubitus ulcers (*see* p.331).

Malodour

Controlling malodour is often the biggest challenge. Malodour is caused partly by tumour necrosis and partly by deep anaerobic infection. Treatment options include:

- metronidazole, topical or systemic
- live yoghurt b.d. topically
- manuka honey b.d. topically (available in UK from the New Zealand Natural Food Company, London)
- an occlusive dressing
    film, e.g. Opsite (totally occlusive)
    hydrocolloid, e.g. Granuflex (almost totally occlusive).

The benefit of charcoal activated dressings, e.g. Actisorb, is questionable.

Domestic air fresheners are generally unsatisfactory. Even if these mask the malodour, it is generally a case of replacing one disgusting odour by another one. Weather permitting, fresh air through a wide-open window is the best option. Air filter systems are generally impractical and/or too costly for routine use. Most patients need to be nursed in a single room.

Oxidizing agents are no longer widely used because of concern for the surrounding healthy tissue. However, occasionally, such agents may have a part to play, for example:

- irrigation with 3% hydrogen peroxide
- packing a deep malignant ulcer with 10–20% benzoyl peroxide (Box 10.J).

Box 10.J   Use of benzoyl peroxide to reduce malodour in deep malignant ulcers

Benzoyl peroxide is a powerful organic oxidizing agent; it often causes an irritant dermatitis and may cause a contact allergic dermatitis.

Normal skin surrounding the ulcer must be protected with petroleum jelly or zinc oxide ointment, e.g. Morhulin.

A large cavity or an undercut margin is firmly packed with surgical gauze soaked with 10–20% benzoyl peroxide.

A dressing is cut from sterile terry towelling to fit the ulcer exactly and saturated with benzoyl peroxide; the terry towelling must not overlap normal skin.

A plastic film is placed over the dressing, e.g. Clingfilm, and allowed to adhere to the ointment or paste protecting the surrounding normal skin.

An abdominal pad dressing is taped over the plastic film with hypo-allergenic tape, e.g. Hypafix, Micropore.

Unless there is excessive exudate, the dressing need be changed only o.d.

The wound surface is cleaned with 0.9% saline at each change of dressing.

Occasionally a patient complains of burning in the ulcer when the new dressing is applied; this subsides within 30min.

Decubitus ulcers

A decubitus ulcer is an ulcer of the skin $\pm$ subcutaneous tissue caused by ischaemia secondary to extrinsic pressure and/or shear.

Pathogenesis

Tissue ischaemia is caused by extrinsic pressure if it is greater than capillary pressure, i.e. >25mmHg. Pressure for periods as short 1–2h may produce irreversible cellular changes leading to cell death. This occurs particularly over bony prominences (Box 10.K). Many other factors make tissue ischaemia more likely, for example:

- emaciation
- anaemia
- skin fragility
- incontinence

Box 10.K   Sites of decubitus ulcers in terminally ill patients

Major	Minor
Ear	Occipital
Spine	Mastoid
Sacrum	Acromion
Greater trochanter	Spine of scapula
Head of fibula	Lateral condyle of humerus
Malleolus	Ischial tuberosity
	Knees

- immobility
- old age.

Pressure on the skin over the ischial tuberosities when sitting is about 300mmHg. The pressure on the skin when lying on a hospital foam mattress is about 160mm.[45]

Prevention

A scoring system, such as the Waterlow card, should be used to determine the patient's risk status (Figure 10.2).[46] It prompts the carers to be vigilant and facilitates the introduction of specific preventive measures. However, some decubitus ulcers are inevitable in terminally ill patients. Further, patient comfort is paramount and there must be flexibility rather than automatic adherence to a rigid nursing protocol.

Pressure redistribution

Mattresses vary in their pressure reducing properties (Table 10.4).

Feather pillows can reduce pressure considerably. In countries where airbeds are not readily available, consider using a camping mattress filled with water (Box 10.L); this reduces pressure more than a standard foam mattress. Carefully laundered natural sheepskin also helps but is now rarely used in the UK.

Sheets should not be tucked in tightly. For some patients, a bed cradle to raise the bedding off the body helps. Rolled towels or pillows can be used to 'fine-tune' the patient's position.

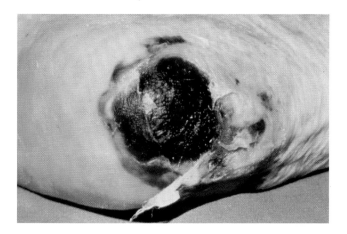

Plate 1   Black necrotic decubitus ulcer.

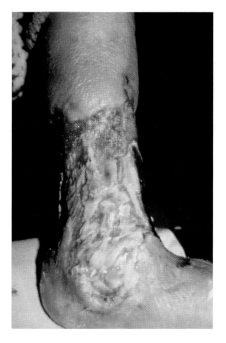

Plate 2   Yellow sloughy decubitus ulcer.

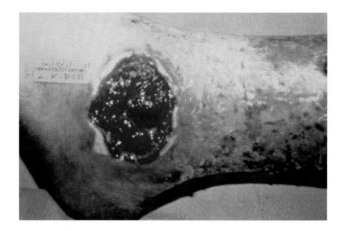

Plate 3   Deep red granulating decubitus ulcer.

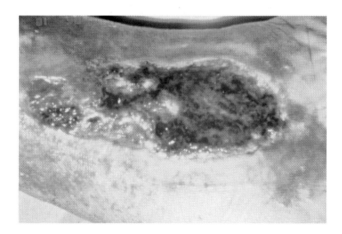

Plate 4   Superficial red epithelializing decubitus ulcer.

Build/weight for height		Skin type/visual risk areas		Sex and age		SPECIAL RISKS	
Average	0	Healthy	0	Male	1	**Tissue malnutrition**	
Above average	1	Tissue paper dry	1	Female	2	Terminal cachexia	8
Obese	2	Oedematous	1	14–49	1	Cardiac failure	5
Below average	3	Clammy (increased temperature)	1	50–64	2	Peripheral vascular disease	5
		Discoloured	2	65–74	3	Anaemia	2
Continence		Broken/spot	3	75–80	4	Smoking	1
Complete/catheterized	0			81+	5		
Occasional incontinence	1					**Neurological deficit**	
Catheterized/incontinent of faeces	2	**Mobility**		**Appetite**		Diabetes, multiple sclerosis, cerebrovascular accident, motor/sensory paraplegia	4–6
Doubly incontinent	3	Fully mobile	0	Average	0		
		Restless/fidgety	1	Poor	1		
		Apathetic	2	Nasogastric tube/fluids only	2	**Major surgery/trauma**	
		Restricted	3	Nil by mouth/anorexia	3	Orthopaedic, below waist or spinal	2
		Inert/traction	4			On table>2h	3
		Chairbound	5				5
						Medication	
						Cytotoxics	
						High-dose corticosteroids	
						NSAIDs	4

Ring the appropriate scores in the table and add them up.
More than one score can be ringed per section if more than one score is provided.

| Total score | 10+ at risk | 15+ high risk | 20+ very high risk |

Figure 10.2 Waterlow pressure sore risk assessment card. Modified with permission from Waterlow, 1998.[46]

Table 10.4   Hospital mattresses in descending order of skin surface pressures

Type	Examples
Foam	Standard hospital mattress (UK)
Profiled foam	Cyclone
Foam + fibre overlay	Spenco
Static pressure airbed	First Step, Roho, Vicair
Alternating pressure airbed	Pegasus, Ripple
Low loss airbed	Kinair, Mediscus[a]
Air fluidized bed	Clinitron[a]

a   pressure less than capillary pressure; patient need not be turned.

Box 10.L   Using a camping mattress as a makeshift water bed

Fill with warm water instead of air and cover with a sheet.

When the patient lies on the mattress, the top and bottom surfaces should not meet at any point, nor should the mattress present a hard surface because of overfilling.

The patient will maintain the water at body temperature. When the patient is out of bed in a temperate climate, heat is retained by an electric blanket or heating pad; this is not used when the patient is in bed.

A camping mattress weighs about 120kg when filled; it can be used at home where floors may not be able to stand the weight of a commercial water bed.

Mattresses are washed with soap and water before re-use.

Holes are mended with a bicycle puncture repair kit.

When sitting in a chair or wheelchair, a pressure-relieving cushion should be used for patients at risk of developing a decubitus ulcer, or with one, for example:

- profiled foam (Eggcrate)
- inflatable cushion (Roho).

If strong enough, patients should be encouraged to raise themselves off the seat and shift their weight every 15–20min. Short walks should be encouraged if the patient is capable.

The tradition of repositioning very ill and unconscious patients q2h probably stems from the fact that this was the time it took the nurses to work their way round a Nightingale ward of 24–30 bedbound patients. Nowadays, the frequency of repositioning depends on various factors, including:

- distress when moved, e.g. pain or breathlessness

- discomfort when lying for long periods unmoved

- presence of risk factors (*see* Box 10.K)

- level of consciousness.

Skin care

- inspect the skin every time the patient's position is changed

- maintain optimal hygiene and hydration
    dry skin (*see* p.309)
    wet skin (*see* p.311).

- avoid trauma
    place pillows between the patient and bedrails
    patients lifted when repositioned, not dragged
    loose clothing and smooth bedding
    avoid overheating and sweating
    use loose bandaging instead of firmly adherent tape.

Nutrition

Nutritional goals can be modified in dying patients. It is not always possible to achieve the ideal of a plasma albumin concentration of $>30g/L$ and a haemoglobin concentration of $>10g/dL$.

Management

An ulcer will not heal without an adequate blood supply. Local pressure must be avoided as much as possible. However, healing may be impossible and preventing further deterioration is often a more appropriate aim.

For the purposes of management, decubitus ulcers may be classified as follows:

- black and necrotic, i.e. covered with a hard, dry black necrotic layer (Plate 1)

- yellow and sloughy, i.e. covered or filled with a soft yellow slough (Plate 2)
- red and clean with significant tissue loss, i.e. granulating (Plate 3)
- red and clean and superficial, i.e. epithelializing (Plate 4).

In addition, ulcers may be malodourous and infected. This classification represents both the different *types* of wound and the various *stages* through which an ulcer passes as it heals.

Non-drug treatment

Growth of clean red granulation tissue will occur only after the elimination of local infection and necrotic tissue (eschar). Because it is normal for skin to be colonized with some bacteria, bacterial growth from a swab is not an indication for antibiotics unless there are clinical signs of infection. Systemic antibiotics should be used if there is surrounding cellulitis. Antiseptics are used less than in the past because they too may have adverse effects (Table 10.5). Cleanse with 0.9% saline or even tap water if it is safe to drink.

Granulation tissue must be protected from prolonged cooling, drying out and trauma when the dressing is changed (Box 10.M). *Desloughing agents can cause maceration of normal skin and must be used with great care.* The value of proprietary preparations, e.g. dextranomer polysaccharide beads or paste and cadexomer iodine polysaccharide, is questionable.[47] Further, in none of five trials of enzymatic agents was there a significant outcome in favour of the desloughing agent.[47]

As the condition of the wound changes, the type of dressing also changes (Table 10.6).

Drug treatment

Vitamin C 500–1000mg o.d. aids healing in malnourished patients.[48] Zinc supplements help in zinc deficient patients and may be worth checking in a patient with a prognosis of several months.

Table 10.5 Properties of antiseptics[45]

	Bactericidal (++) Bacteriostatic (+)	Fungicidal (++) Fungistatic (+)	Virucidal (++) Virustatic (+)	Other characteristics
Alcohols	++	++	+	Rapid onset of action at high concentrations; painful if skin broken
Phenol derivatives, e.g. hexachlorophene (Ster-Zac) chloroxylenol (Dettol)	++	++		Some absorption may occur
Iodine	++	++	++	Some iodine is absorbed; less effective in the presence of organic material; may cause contact dermatitis
Povidone-iodine	++	++	+	Some iodine is absorbed; has an inhibitory effect on wound healing
Chlorhexidene	++	+	+	Some iodine is absorbed; has an inhibitory effect on wound healing
Cationic compounds, e.g. benzalkonium chloride cetrimide cetylpyridinium (Merocet)	++	++		Adsorption at the surface; weak antibacterial action against Gram-negative bacteria
Quinoline derivatives, e.g. dequalinium	+	+		
Heavy metals	+	+		Enzyme blocking; coagulatory action
Light metals	+			Astringent
Gentian (crystal) violet	+	+		Strong inhibition of wound healing *and risk of carcinogenesis*
Brillant green	?	?		Strong inhibition of wound healing
Eosin	?	?		No inhibition of wound healing

Box 10.M   Commonly used wound dressings[49]

Films, e.g. Bioclusive, Opsite, Tegaderm
Totally occlusive; maintain wound hydration and temperature, contain malodour but permeable to water vapour and oxygen.

Cannot absorb exudate but allow observation of the wound surface without removal.

Stretching the film eases removal but even so may be difficult to remove without causing trauma. Often used as an 'extra layer of skin' to help prevent ulceration, particularly on the elbows and spine.

Hydrocolloids, e.g. Aquacel, Comfeel, Granuflex
Hydrocolloid dressings generally comprise an absorbent layer on a semipermeable film or foam; also available as a paste for filling cavities. Maintain wound hydration and temperature. May be left in place for up to 1 week.

Suitable for softening eschars or for promoting granulation and as a preventive measure, particularly over the sacrum. The occlusive nature of their backing means that they are not suitable for heavily exuding wounds. Despite contrary advice in the BNF, hydrocolloid dressings can be used on infected wounds (see manufacturer's literature).

When applied to non-flat surfaces, a warm hand placed on the dressing for 1–2min helps to mould them to the body shape and improves adherence.

Hydrogels, e.g. Granugel, Intrasite gel
Hydrogel dressings are generally supplied as an amorphous cohesive material which takes up the shape of a wound. They are easily inserted into and removed from cavities. However, because they can damage healing tissue if allowed to dry out, they must be covered with an occlusive film dressing to maintain wound hydration.

They absorb large amounts of exudate and facilitate autolysis of slough and eschar.

Alginates, e.g. Kaltostat, Sorbsan
These are highly absorbent and are suitable for moderately exuding wounds. They are also haemostatic.

Form a gel in contact with fluid but even so may require copious amounts of warm saline to remove them without trauma. Not suitable for eschars or dry wounds.

Foams, e.g. Alleyn, Lyofoam
These are highly absorbent and are useful for desloughing. Formulations available for deep cavities.

Low adherent, e.g. Release, Mepore
These protect the wound surface and absorb some exudate. If allowed to dry out, removal causes skin damage; if wet, they are easily removed.

Table 10.6 Choice of dressing for decubitus ulcers

Wound type	Aim	Dressing
Necrotic	Debride/remove eschar	Hydrogel *or* Hydrocolloid ± hydrocolloid paste
Sloughy	Remove slough; provide clean base for epithelialization	Hydrogel *or* Hydrocolloic ± hydrocolloid paste
Granulating	Promote granulation	Hydrogel *or* Hydrocolloic ± hydrocolloid paste *or* Foam *or* Alginate sheet ± rope
Epithelializing	Wound maturation	Hydrocolloic *or* Low-adherent dressing *or* Film

Infected	Treat infection and thereby reduce odour	*Infection*
		 Antibiotics
		   metronidazole PO or topical
		   (for anaerobes)
		   silver sulfadiazine
		   (for pseudomonas)
		
		 Dressing
		 Low adherent dressing *or*
		 Alginate sheet ± rope *or*
		 Polyurethane foam *or*
		 Actisorb (for odour)

References

1 Teofoli P et al. (1996) Itch and pain. International Journal of Dermatology. 35: 159–66.
2 Kimyai-Asadi A et al. (1999) Poststroke pruritus. Stroke. 30:692–3.
3 Yao G et al. (1992) Histamine-caused itch induces Fos-like immunoreactivity in dorsal horn neurons: effect of morphine pretreatment. Brain Research. 599:333–7.
4 Hagermark O and Wahlgren C (1992) Some methods for evaluating clinical itch and their application for studying pathophysiological mechanisms. Journal of Dermatology and Science. 4:55–62.
5 Lowitt M and Bernhard J (1992) Pruritus. Seminars in Neurology. 12:374–84.
6 Sanger GJ and Twycross R (1996) Making sense of emesis, pruritus, 5HT and 5HT₃ receptor antagonists. Progress in Palliative Care. 4:7–8.
7 Weisshaar E et al. (1997) Can a serotonin type 3 (5-HT₃) receptor antagonist reduce experimentally-induced itch? Inflammation Research. 46:412–16.
8 Summerfield J (1980) Naloxone modulates the perception of itch in man. British Journal of Clinical Pharmacology. 10:180–3.
9 McQuay HJ et al. (1980) Demand analgesia to assess pain relief from epidural opiates. Lancet. 1:768–9.
10 Moulin D et al. (1984) The analgesic efficacy of intrathecal D-Ala2-D-Leu5 Enkephalin (DADL) in cancer patients with chronic pain. Pain Supplement 2. 2:343.
11 Chaplan SR et al. (1992) Morphine and hydromorphone epidural analgesia. Anesthesiology. 77:1090–4.
12 Jones E and Bergasa N (1996) Why do cholestatic patients itch? Gut. 38:644–5.
13 Wood L et al. (1997) Barrier disruption increases gene expression of cytokines and the 55kD TNF receptor in murine skin. Experimental Dermatology. 6:98–104.
14 Man M-Q et al. (1999) Cutaneous barrier repair and pathophysiology following barrier disruption in IL-1 and TNF type I receptor deficient mice. Experimental Dermatology. 8:261–6.
15 Greaves M (1992) Itching-research has barely scratched the surface. New England Journal of Medicine. 326:1016–17.
16 Guillet G et al. (2000) Increased histamine release and skin hypersensitivity to histamine in senile pruritus: study of 60 patients. Journal of the European Academy of Dermatology and Venereology. 14:65–8.
17 Smith E et al. (1984) Crotamition lotion in pruritus. International Journal of Dermatology. 23:684–5.
18 Closs S (1997) Pruritus and methotrimeprazine. Personal communication.
19 Zylicz Z et al. (1998) Paroxetine for pruritus in advanced cancer. Journal of Pain and Symptom Management. 16:121–4.
20 Raderer M et al. (1994) Ondansetron for cholestatic jaundice due to cholestasis. New England Journal of Medicine. 300:1540.
21 Ghent C and Carruthers S (1988) Treatment of pruritus in primary biliary cirrhosis with rifampin. Results of a double-blind crossover randomized trial. Gastroenterology. 94:488–93.

22   Cork M (1998) Complete emollient therapy. In: *The National Association of Fundholding Practices Official Yearbook.* BPC Waterlow, Dunstable, pp 159–68.

23   Quigley C and Baines M (1997) Descriptive epidemiology of sweating in a hospice population. *Journal of Palliative Care.* **13**:22–6.

24   Kirby K (1990) Dermatology. In: P Kumar and M Clarke (eds) *Clinical Medicine.* Baillière Tindall, London, pp 1000–1.

25   Ganong WF (1979) *Review of Medical Physiology.* Lange Medical Publications, pp 177–81.

26   Ryan T (1996) Diseases of the skin. In: DJ Weatherall (ed) *Oxford Textbook of Medicine.* Oxford University Press, Oxford, pp 3765–7.

27   Tabibzadeh S *et al.* (1989) Interleukin-6 immunoreactivity in human tumours. *American Journal of Pathology.* **135**:427–33.

28   Tsavaris N *et al.* (1990) A randomized trial of the effect of three nonsteroidal anti-inflammatory agents in ameliorating cancer-induced fever. *Journal of Internal Medicine.* **228**:451–5.

29   Hargrove J and Eisenberg E (1995) Menopause. *Medical Clinics of North America.* **79**:1337–56.

30   Quella SK *et al.* (1998) Long term use of megestrol acetate by cancer survivors for the treatment of hot flashes. *Cancer.* **82**:1784–8.

31   Miller J and Ahmann F (1992) Treatment of castration-induced menopausal symptoms with low dose diethylstilbestrol in men with advanced cancer. *Urology.* **40**:499–502.

32   Pandya K *et al.* (2000) Oral clonidine in postmenopausal patients with breast cancer experiencing tamoxifen-induced hot flashes: a University of Rochester Cancer Center community clinical oncology program study. *Annals of Internal Medicine.* **132**:788–93.

33   Simpson N (1988) Treating hyperhidrosis. *British Medical Journal.* **296**:1345.

34   Murphy R and Harrington C (2000) Iontophoresis should be tried before other treatments. *British Medical Journal.* **321**:702–3.

35   Collin J and Whatling P (2000) Treating hyperhidrosis: surgery and botulinum toxin are treatments of choice in severe cases. *British Medical Journal.* **320**: 1221–2.

36   Atkins J and Butler P (2000) Treating hyperhidrosis: excision of axillary tissue may be more effective. *British Medical Journal.* **321**:702.

37   Johnson M (1996) Neoplastic fever. *Palliative Medicine.* **10**:217–24.

38   Meadows C (1997) Stoma and fistula care. In: L Bruce and T Finlay (eds) *Nursing in Gastroenterology.* Churchill Livingstone, London, pp 85–118.

39   Irving M and Beadle C (1982) External intestinal fistulas: nursing care and surgical procedures. *Clinics in Gastroenterology.* **11**:327–36.

40   Lange M *et al.* (1989) Management of multiple enterocutaneous fistulas. *Heart and Lung.* **18**:386–91.

41   De-Conno F *et al.* (1991) Continuous subcutaneous infusion of hyoscine butyl-bromide reduces secretion in patients with gastrointestinal obstruction. *Journal of Pain and Symptom Management.* **6**:484–6.

42   Fallon M (1994) The physiology of somatostatin and its synthetic analogue, octreotide. *European Journal of Palliative Care.* **1**:20–2.

43   Walls A *et al.* (1994) The closure of an abdominal fistula using self-polymerizing silicone rubbers – case study. *Palliative Medicine.* **8**:59–62.

44   Streza G *et al.* (1977) Management of enterocutaneous fistulas and problem stomas with silicone casting of the abdominal wall defect. *American Journal of Surgery.* **134**:772–6.

45   Hatz R *et al.* (1994) *Wound Healing and Wound Management.* Springer-Verlag, London.

46   Waterlow J (1998) The history and use of the Waterlow card. *Nursing Times.* **94**:63–7.

47   Bradley M *et al.* (1999) The debridement of chronic wounds: systematic review. *Health Technology Assessment.* **3**: Part 1.

48   Breslow R (1991) Nutritional status and dietary intake of patients with pressure ulcers: review of the research literature 1943–1989. *Decubitus.* **4**:16–21.

49   VFM-Unit (1996) *A prescriber's guide to dressings and wound management materials.* Welsh Office Health Department, Cardiff.

11   Lymphoedema

Clinical features · Evaluation · Management
Complications

This chapter deals with lymphoedema in advanced cancer. A more comprehensive account of lymphoedema and its management is available elsewhere.[1]

Lymphoedema is tissue swelling caused by a failure of lymph drainage. It is the result of an imbalance between influx and efflux in the lymphatic system. It can occur in any part of the body but generally it affects one or more limbs ± the adjacent trunk.

In the UK, cancer and cancer treatment account for most cases of lymphoedema. A combination of two or more of the following factors greatly increases the likelihood of lymphoedema:

- axillary or groin surgery
- postoperative infection
- radiotherapy
- lymph node metastases, e.g. axillary, groin, intrapelvic or retroperitoneal.[2]

After radical hysterectomy for cancer of the cervix (which includes excision of the pelvic lymph nodes) and postoperative radiotherapy, about 40% of women develop lymphoedema.[3]

Although described as 'protein-rich', the protein content of chronic lymphoedema is about 5g/L lower than that of interstitial fluid in the contralateral normal limb.[4] Further, the protein content is relatively low in early lymphoedema (10–20g/L) compared with long-established lymphoedema (>30g/L).[5] However, the protein content of lymphoedema is much higher than the protein content of cardiac and venous oedemas (<5g/L and 5–10g/L respectively).[5] The protein in lymphoedema stimulates fibrosis.

Clinical features

Symptoms include:

- tightness

- heaviness

- a bursting feeling if there is an acute exacerbation

- pain caused by
    shoulder strain (because of the weight of the arm)
    inflammation
    brachial or lumbosacral plexopathy

- impaired function/mobility

- psychosocial distress
    altered body image
    problems in obtaining well-fitting clothes or shoes.

The impact on the patient psychosocially is not always obvious. Specific enquiry is needed to elicit the extent of the patient's distress.

Unlike other types of oedema, chronic lymphoedema results in changes in the skin and subcutis. Clinical signs include:

- persistent swelling of part or all of the limb which in time becomes non-pitting as a result of interstitial fibrosis and which does not decrease with elevation overnight

- increased tissue turgor

- Stemmer's sign (the inability to pick up a fold of skin at the base of the second toe); *the absence of this sign does not necessarily exclude more proximal lymphoedema*

- distorted limb shape

- lymphangiomas (dilated skin lymphatics which look like blisters)

- deep skin creases associated with cutaneous fibrosis

- hyperkeratosis (a build-up of surface keratin resulting in a warty scaly skin)

- papillomatosis (a cobblestone effect caused by dilated skin lymphatics surrounded by fibrosis)

- acute inflammatory episodes (AIE, *see* p.396)

- lymphorrhoea (leakage of lymph).

Hyperkeratosis and papillomatosis are seen mainly in lymphoedema of the leg. Lymphorrhoea is more common in lymphovenous stasis, IVC obstruction and chronic congestive cardiac failure. Ulceration is uncommon unless there is associated venous or arterial disease.

When the trunk is involved:

- the subcutis feels thickened on palpation
- when a fold of skin is pinched up simultaneously on both sides on the trunk, the skin is more difficult to grip on the affected side
- underwear leaves deeper markings on the affected side
- in unilateral leg lymphoedema, the ipsilateral buttock is bigger when examined with the patient standing
- in females, there may be genital wetness from leaking lymphangiomas.

Radiotherapy also causes subcutaneous thickening but it is qualitatively different from that in lymphoedema, i.e. it is firmer and completely non-pitting.

Evaluation

Oedema is a common symptom of advanced malignant disease (Box 11.A). Because muscle activity is essential to maintain both venous and lymph return from dependent limbs, lymphatic failure is also inevitable in immobile patients who sit for many hours day after day and have little or no exercise ('armchair legs').

Box 11.A   Causes of oedema in advanced malignant disease

General	**Local**
Cardiac failure ± anaemia	Venous obstruction
Hypoproteinaemia	Lymphovenous oedema
End-stage renal failure	immobility and dependency
Drugs	paralysis, e.g. hemiplegia,
salt and water retention,	paraplegia
e.g. NSAIDs, corticosteroids	Lymphatic obliteration/obstruction
vasodilation, e.g. nifedipine	surgery
Malignant ascites, associated with	radiotherapy
secondary hyperaldosteronism	repeated infections
(see p.131)	metastatic tumour in lymph nodes

The extra load placed on the lymphatics as a result of venous incompetence also leads to lymphatic failure. Thus, patients with chronic venous leg ulcers and swelling have a combination of venous oedema and lymphatic failure, often called lymphovenous stasis.

If the clinical features do not suggest a likely cause, investigations should be considered:

- full blood count

- plasma albumin concentration

- plasma electrolytes and creatinine concentrations

- ultrasound, CT or MRI to determine disease status and to identify lymphadenopathy.

In patients who have months or years ahead of them, it may be helpful to check venous function with ultrasound and possibly a venogram.

Management

In advanced cancer it is generally not possible to reduce the size of a lymph-oedematous limb.

Emphasis should be placed on preventing deterioration and relieving discomfort (Box 11.B).

Box 11.B   Palliative lymphoedema management

Correct the correctable
Skin care
Treatment of infection

Non-drug treatment
Positioning
Containment
Exercise
Massage
Pneumatic compression

Drug treatment
Analgesics
Corticosteroids
Diuretics ?
Oxerutins ?

Correct the correctable

Skin care

Guidelines 11.1: Dry skin in lymphoedema (p.394).

The aim of skin care is to prevent debilitating infections which exacerbate the oedema. In chronic lymphoedema the skin becomes dry, warty and discoloured. A break in the skin, often invisible, enables bacteria to gain access to an ideal growth medium, protein-rich lymph. Infection accelerates fibrosis and causes more damage to the lymphatics. Careful hygiene reduces the risk of infection by reducing the bacteria resident on the skin. After washing, preferably every day, the swollen limb should be dried carefully, paying particular attention to between the digits and any skin folds (Box 11.C).

Box 11.C   Written information for patients about skin care[6]

General information
If an arm is swollen, protect hands when washing up or gardening.

If a leg is swollen, wear protective footwear at all times. Do not walk in bare feet.

Wear a thimble when sewing.

Dry well between digits after bathing to protect from fungal infections.

Keep the skin supple by applying oil or bland cream.

Take care when cutting toe or finger nails; use clippers rather than scissors.

Treat any cuts or grazes promptly by washing and applying antiseptic, e.g Savlon, TCP.

Notify your general practitioner immediately if the limb becomes hot or more swollen.

Use an electric razor to reduce the risk of cutting the skin.

Other important points about the swollen limb:
   do not have blood taken from it
   do not have injections into it
   do not allow your blood pressure to be taken on it.

Summer advice
Avoid insect bites; use repellent sprays.

Treat bites with antiseptics and/or antihistamines.

Protect the swollen limb from the sun:
   sit in the shade when possible
   use a high-factor sun block, e.g. 15–30.

Equipment to take on holiday:
   emollient
   high-factor sun block
   insect repellents/sprays
   antihistamine tablets
   antiseptic solutions.

If you have had recurrent infections, take antibiotics with you when you go on holidays in case of need.

An emollient (moisturizing) cream should be applied daily to prevent drying and cracking. If applied at bedtime it is fully absorbed before the next morning. It is best not to use one containing lanolin because of the possibility of contact dermatitis.[7] Perfumed creams or lotions should not be used for the same reason. Aqueous cream, made from emulsifying ointment, does not contain lanolin and is cheap. However, any bland hand cream or body lotion will probably be satisfactory. If the skin is flaky or scaly, additional topical measures may be necessary (*see* p.395).

Treatment of infection

Guidelines 11.2: Acute inflammatory episodes (p.396).

Recurrent infections, called acute inflammatory episodes (AIE), are a feature of chronic lymphoedema. A hot red tender area and a rapid increase in swelling suggests infection which requires prompt treatment with antibiotics. AIE may develop rapidly without warning and can be frightening. Severe attacks cause malaise, fever, rigors, headache, vomiting and even delirium.

Presentation varies considerably and the diagnosis may be missed. Some patients recall an accidental skin puncture, e.g. a gardening injury or an insect bite, which preceded the attack but most do not. The redness varies from multifocal inflamed spots to confluent erythema. Pain may occur without any obvious inflammation and any constitutional upset may be minimal. Sometimes the condition 'grumbles' in a chronic manner for weeks and a firm diagnosis is made only with recovery after prolonged antibiotic treatment.

AIE tend to recur. The interval between episodes may be several months or just a few weeks. With each attack, a stepwise deterioration in the lymphoedema occurs as a result of fibrosis and further damage to lymphatics. Unlike cellulitis in a non-lymphoedematous arm, the causal agent in AIE is generally a Streptococcus. Empirical antibiotic therapy is based on this supposition (*see* p.396). Because lymphoedema is stagnant, treatment is for a minimum of 2 weeks. If there is significant constitutional upset, bed rest, limb elevation and IV antibiotics are all necessary. With patients who have repeated episodes of infection, long-term prophylaxis is the best way of preventing recurrent attacks and minimizing fibrosis secondary to infection (*see* p.397).

Fungal infections are also common, e.g. tinea pedis (Athlete's foot), and should be treated with an appropriate antifungal agent.

Non-drug treatment

Positioning

In very ill patients, swollen limbs should be supported with pillows to provide comfort. If possible, avoid the use of a sling in ambulant patients with arm oedema because it tends to cause pooling of fluid at the elbow and stiffness of the elbow and shoulder joints.[8] However, in ambulant patients with gross arm oedema and weakness from brachial plexopathy, a broad arm sling (e.g. Poly sling) to take the weight off the shoulder and neck and distribute it across the back provides comfort and may also improve mobility by improving balance. The sling should be removed when the patient is not ambulant, and the arm provided with full-length support of the limb, preferably with some elevation. *Do not use a collar and cuff sling*; it does not provide enough support and tends to act as a tourniquet.

At rest, patients benefit by placing the arm in specially made foam supports so that the limb, including the hand, is fully supported in a horizontal position.[9] Similarly, elevation of the legs with support is comforting to patients with lymphoedema of the legs. The patient's back also needs to be well-supported to prevent back pain, possibly by using a reclining chair.

Keeping the affected limb elevated as much as possible reduces venous hyper-tension and enhances drainage of the venous and lymphatic systems, thereby reducing swelling. Maximum benefit is achieved by elevation to the level of the heart. Arms should not be raised above 90% because further elevation reduces the space between the clavicle and the first rib, and may obstruct venous return.

Containment

Apply a wrapping to help contain the swollen limb:

- if the limb shape is still fairly normal and the patient is ambulant, apply elastic compression garments of International Class 1 or 2 (Figure 11.1)

- if the limb is misshapen and the patient is ambulant, use Shaped Tubigrip

- if the limb is misshapen and the patient is immobile, apply a light support bandage o.d. (e.g. crepe) which is neither short-stretch nor elasticated.

It is important to ensure that Shaped Tubigrip does not form ridges or roll down the limb and act as a tourniquet, thereby exacerbating the swelling and increasing discomfort. Shaped Tubigrip is often uncomfortable if the foot or hand is very swollen; *it should not be used if the digits are swollen.*

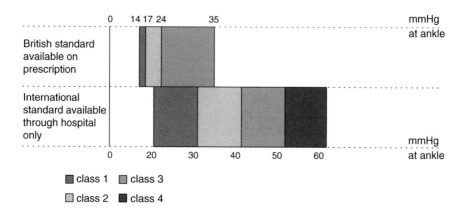

Figure 11.1 Compression garments: British and International compression classes.

In patients with fungating breast cancer affecting the axilla or chest wall, the application of pressure to the adjacent swollen arm may improve lymph drainage from the arm and increase the load on the neighbouring superficial lymphatics around the shoulder and chest wall. With damaged lymphatics exposed to the surface in fungating tumours, increased flow will result in increased leakage. In these circumstances, it may still be appropriate to use containment to relieve symptoms but the patient should be warned that the discharge from the chest wall or axilla may increase. In addition, the district nurse should be advised that the dressings may need to be changed more than once a day, at least in the short-term.

Further, in advanced pelvic malignancy with bilateral leg swelling, genital and truncal oedema, compression of the legs may lead to increased truncal and genital swelling. Compression garments can be used to provide support to the genitalia, e.g. support tights, maternity garments (panty girdles), cycling shorts.

Compression garments should fit snugly around the limb to prevent:

- a tourniquet effect if too tight, particularly if there are deep skin folds or crevasses
- the collection of fluid if too loose.

In patients with swelling of the fingers, a compression glove should be worn. Garments are worn all day and removed at night. It is worth spending time finding a suitable garment because a patient will not wear it unless it is comfortable. Compression garments do not fit comfortably on awkwardly shaped limbs; padding and bandaging may need to be used instead.[10]

Modern garments are lightweight, extremely strong and machine washable. Most sleeves last 3 months; stockings 4–6 months. Garments can have their life extended if allowed to 'rest' for a week every month; in this way they regain some elasticity.

Exercise

The skin is so designed that the health of the outer 0.3mm of its surface (mainly the epidermis) is maintained by low amplitude body movements.[11] These are the kind of movements which occur during normal activity, e.g. blinking, yawning, stretching, walking. Yawning, stretching and abdominal breathing all alter the intra-thoracic pressure and help to empty the thoracic and abdominal lymphatics. Walking and other limb movements help to empty the peripheral lymphatics. Static activity, e.g. carrying a heavy object for more than a few metres, should be discouraged because it reduces both venous and lymphatic return.

Movement of the skin also helps the superficial non-contractile initial lymphatics to empty into the deeper muscular contractile collecting lymphatics. Normal use of the affected limb and gentle active movements should be encouraged. On the other hand, vigorous exercise damages the superficial fine vasculature with consequential overload of the lymphatics and should be avoided.

Specific exercises should be carefully tailored to the patient's abilities and general condition:

- joints are put through a full range of movements to maintain, and possibly improve, function
- limb muscles are used to improve lymph drainage
- fibrosis may be disrupted.

If active exercises are impossible, passive exercises should be carried out at least b.d. Passive movements of a swollen limb (including hand and fingers or feet and toes) in a severely ill, bedbound patient can reduce stiffness and discomfort. In more active patients, exercise may maintain rather than improve function. A complex exercise regimen is inappropriate in advanced cancer.[12]

To enable patients to continue to function as normally as possible with severely swollen limbs, various appliances may be helpful, for example:

- aids for walking and dressing for those with swollen legs
- special cutlery, tin openers, scissors etc. for those with swollen hands and arms.

Massage

Massage of the skin with associated deep breathing is an important component of lymphoedema management. It is the only way of reducing truncal lymphoedema but is not possible in areas of cutaneous metastasis, e.g. *en cuirass* spread in breast cancer.

Specialized forms of massage are used in lymphoedema clinics.[13,14] These are generally inappropriate in patients with a short prognosis; instead a more straightforward form of self-massage should be encouraged. In this circumstance, 'self-massage' includes massage by a relative, close friend or carer.

When contained by a bandage or compression garment, limb movements automatically massage the limb. Self-massage is therefore confined to the trunk. It is appropriate even if there is no detectable truncal oedema because it clears the abdominal and thoracic lymphatics, and thereby facilitates the movement of lymph from the limbs into the empty truncal lymphatics. Truncal massage takes about 20min. The following points should be noted:

- the patient should lie in a comfortable position with the head supported with a pillow or cushion but leaving the neck free

- hands should be clean and dry if they are to move the skin effectively (use non-scented talcum powder if sweaty); always keep your hands in contact with the skin

- movements should be light, slow and rhythmic; the hands, fingers and wrists are kept straight with the movement coming from the arms and body

- use only enough pressure to move the skin over the underlying tissue; massage should not cause any reddening of the skin or discomfort to the patient

- the neck should always be massaged first, i.e. empty the neck lymphatics into the venous system via the thoracic duct

- in unilateral limb oedema, the contralateral upper half of the trunk is massaged next, followed by the ipsilateral side before proceeding to the lower half

- the area adjacent to a lymphoedematous limb is massaged last

- as well as a practical demonstration, the patient should be given written instructions (Boxes 11.D and 11.E).

Box 11.D   Self-massage for arm lymphoedema: advice to patients

---

Recline comfortably but, before starting the session, make sure that the hands and the area to be massaged are free of oils and creams so as to allow good contact between the hand and the skin.

The hand moves the skin over the underlying tissues:
  if you just glide over the surface of the skin, you are not being firm enough
  if the skin reddens, you are being too firm.

The massage is slow and gentle with the hand moving the skin in semicircles away from the affected arm, and then allowing the elasticity of the skin to return the hand to the starting position.

Both sides of the neck below the ears are massaged for 2min using a slow circular motion (Figure 11.2a).

Place the hand of your unaffected arm behind your head and massage the unaffected axilla for 1min (Figure 11.2b).

Starting close to the unaffected arm (Figure 11.2c), massage across the chest towards the swollen arm, changing hands when you cross the midline (Figure 11.2d); this takes 5–10min. Finish by massaging over the affected shoulder.

If someone can help you, ask them to do the same across the upper back starting close to the unaffected arm, moving across towards the swollen arm; this takes 5–10min.

Finish with abdominal breathing to clear the deep lymphatic channels. Place both hands in the gap between your ribs (Figure 11.2e). Without arching the back, breathe in slowly and deeply. You should feel your fingers rise as your abdomen expands. Count 1 and 2, then breathe out slowly. Repeat 4 times, then relax for a few minutes before getting up.

Deep abdominal breathing is an important part of the massage. To help the patient do this effectively, ask the patient to bend their knees and then:

- place your flat hand in the centre of their abdomen to offer a little resistance

- ask the patient to inhale so that their abdomen balloons out, and pushes against your hand

- ask them to exhale and let your hand sink

- ask them to inhale again and repeat several times.

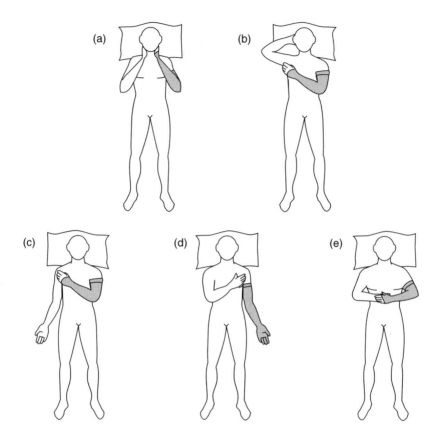

Figure 11.2 Self-massage for arm lymphoedema.

Pneumatic compression

Guidelines 11.3: Pneumatic compression therapy (p.398).

Pneumatic compression therapy is used less in lymphoedema than in the past.[15] It is particularly helpful in venous oedema, but should be avoided in cardiac failure. In advanced cancer, it may soften a hard oedema and ease discomfort. There is a risk of increasing truncal or genital oedema if pneumatic compression therapy is used alone. Care should also be taken if the patient has impaired sensation. The use of pneumatic compression therapy without the use of support bandaging or a compression garment between applications is generally not helpful.

Pneumatic compression consists of an inflatable sleeve connected to a motor driven air pump. The limb is inserted into the sleeve which inflates and deflates cyclically. A multichamber sequential intermittent pneumatic compression

---

Box 11.E   Self-massage for leg lymphoedema: advice to patients

---

Recline comfortably but, before starting the session, make sure that the hands and the area to be massaged are free of oils and creams so as to allow good contact between the hand and the skin.

The hand moves the skin over the underlying tissues:
  if you just glide over the surface of the skin, you are not being firm enough
  if the skin reddens, you are being too firm.

The massage is slow and gentle with the hand moving the skin in semicircles away from the affected leg, and then allowing the elasticity of the skin to return the hand to the starting position.

Both sides of the neck below the ears are massaged for 2min using a slow circular motion (Figure 11.3a).

Place the hand of one arm, behind your head and massage the lymph glands under the arm in the same way for 1min; repeat with the other arm (Figure 11.3b).

Massage your chest on the side of the unaffected leg, starting from below the collar bone and progressing down to the groin (Figure 11.3c); this takes 5–10min. The lymph glands in the groin of the unaffected leg are then massaged for 1min. Repeat on the affected side.

If someone can help you, ask them to do the same on the upper back, progressing downwards; this takes 10–15min.

Finish with abdominal breathing to clear the deep lymphatic channels. Place both hands in the gap between your ribs (Figure 11.3d). Without arching the back, breathe in slowly and deeply. You should feel your fingers rise as your abdomen expands. Count 1 and 2, then breathe out slowly. Repeat 4 times, then relax for a few minutes before getting up.

---

pump is preferable. A compression pump used on low pressure, i.e. 20–30mmHg, can help by massaging the legs. However, if containment is not applied between treatments, fluid will seep back into the overstretched tissues.

Various makes and models are available, e.g. Centromed, Flowtron, Lymphapress, Jobst, Talley, ranging from small portable pumps with a single chamber sleeve to larger models with multichamber sleeves which inflate and deflate sequentially. The smaller models generally operate on a predetermined inflation/deflation cycle whereas the larger models offer a selection of cycle times. The machines have a pressure dial which may range from 20mmHg to as high as 300mmHg.

The ripple effect of a multichamber sequential pump is more effective at shifting fluid than the simple squeezing effect of single chamber pumps. Single

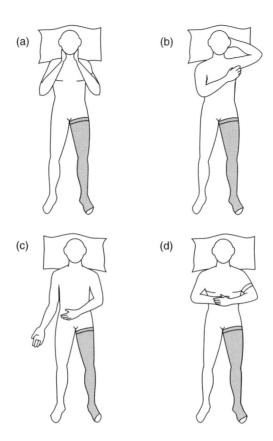

Figure 11.3   Self-massage for leg lymphoedema.

chamber pneumatic compression has no direct effect on lymph flow; it simply forces fluid out of the limb via tissue planes and veins. The sequential action of multichamber pneumatic compression may also help to disrupt tissue fibrosis.

Compression pumps can be used for as many hours as is practical but most patients will not cope with more than about 4h/day.[15] Allow the patient to find the highest comfortable pressure; this may be only 20–30mmHg but could be 40–60mmHg. Pressures higher than this may result in the obstruction of blood flow, increased venous leakage and increased lymph production. High pressure also leads to oxygen deprivation and, if sustained, will cause nerve damage,[16,17] particularly with single chamber pumps.

Indications

A compression pump is particularly useful in non-obstructive leg oedemas:

*   lymphovenous stasis
      immobility
      venous incompetence

*   hypoproteinaemia.

Sometimes in non-obstructive oedema, treatment overnight may be the best way of achieving a good result rapidly.[18]

There is a theoretical danger of a systemic overload and heart failure. In practice this is not a problem provided treatment is limited to 30min initially. As in lymphoedema, containment should be used between treatments to prevent the overstretched tissues rapidly refilling. A low pressure garment is adequate, e.g. Shaped Tubigrip.

Contra-indications

Absolute contra-indications comprise:

*   extensive cutaneous metastases around upper arm and shoulder or upper thigh and groin

*   infection (it is too painful)

*   venous thrombosis (may dislodge recent thrombus).

Trunk oedema is a relative contra-indication; fluid is pushed from the limb into an already congested area. Remember:

*   normally, do not use pressures higher than 30–40mmHg

*   fit compression garments, Shaped Tubigrip or support bandages to the limb between treatments

*   do not start pneumatic compression for 6 weeks after a venous thrombosis.

Initially, the use of pneumatic compression therapy should be closely monitored.

Drug treatment

Analgesics

Analgesics should be prescribed for pain associated with lymphoedema in advanced cancer. A NSAID, paracetamol and/or an opioid should be tried and are often helpful.[19] If analgesics are of little benefit, resting the arm in a well-supported position gives relief. For those having difficulty sleeping at night, ensure that adequate nocturnal sedative-cum-analgesic drugs are prescribed, e.g. morphine.

Corticosteroids

A trial of dexamethasone 4–8mg o.d. for one week should be considered in advanced cancer if tumour recurrence is the main cause of the lymphoedema. By reducing peritumour inflammation, lymphatic obstruction may be reduced. If improvement is noted, dexamethasone 2–4mg o.d. can be continued indefinitely. Occasionally, in breast and prostate cancer or lymphoma, corticosteroids have a direct antitumour effect.

Diuretics

Diuretics are not of value in lymphoedema unless:

- the swelling has developed or increased since the prescription of a NSAID or a corticosteroid
- there is a cardiac or venous component.

In these circumstances, prescribe furosemide 20–40mg o.d. for 1 week initially; the dose is then adjusted according to response.

Oxerutins

Oxerutins, licensed in the UK for use in venous disease, are probably beneficial in lymphoedema, e.g. oxerutins 1.5mg b.d. or 1g t.d.s.[19] Capillary permeability to protein is reduced, macrophage activity is increased and interstitial proteolysis enhanced.[20–22] Protein reduction results in less swelling and less fibrosis. However, because it takes several months to detect benefit,[23] oxerutins have little place in lymphoedema associated with advanced cancer.

Complications

Ulceration

Ulceration is more a feature of venous and arterial disease.[24] When it occurs in lymphoedema in advanced cancer, it is generally associated with:

- fragile skin and/or skin damage as a result of a poorly fitting compression garment or poorly applied support bandaging
- severe infection with blistering and desquamation
- fungating cutaneous secondaries.

If the skin is thin and fragile, the shearing forces created when putting on an elastic compression garment and taking it off can tear the skin and make matters worse. In this situation, light support is more appropriate, e.g. Shaped Tubigrip. With very fragile skin, any dressings should be non-adherent but, even so, will need to be soaked off with sterile saline to avoid further damage to the skin. Haemostatic dressings may be needed to control bleeding (e.g. calcium alginate) or topical adrenaline (epinephrine) solution 1 in 1000 (1mg in 1ml) applied when dressings are changed (*see* p.237).

Lymphorrhoea

Lymphorrhoea refers to leakage of lymph through the skin surface. If severe, lymphorrhoea can soak through dressings and pool in shoes. It occurs mainly when the skin is thin and fragile. It may also occur in an acute exacerbation when the skin is rapidly stretched. Apart from the discomfort and inconvenience, lymphorrhoea places the patient at risk of infection. Treatment comprises:

- normal skin care, including emollients
- elevation of the limb to reduce venous hypertension and to increase venous return
- bandaging to prevent or minimize further leakage until the skin heals.

Lymphorrhoea generally responds to these measures in a few days. The bandages should be applied around the clock but replaced when they become soaked.

References

1   Twycross R *et al.* (2000) *Lymphoedema.* Radcliffe Medical Press, Oxford.
2   Kissin M *et al.* (1986) The risk of lymphoedema following treatment of breast cancer. *British Journal of Surgery.* **73**:580–4.
3   Werngren-Elgstrom M and Lidman D (1994) Lymphoedema of the lower extremities after surgery and radiotherapy for cancer of the cervix. *Scandinavian Journal of Plastic Reconstruction and Hand Surgery.* **28**:289–93.
4   Bates D *et al.* (1993) Change in macromolecular composition of interstitial fluid from swollen arms after breast cancer treatment, and its implications. *Clinical Science.* **86**:737–46.
5   Crockett D (1956) The protein levels of oedema fluids. *Lancet.* **ii**:1179–82.
6   Linnitt N (2000) Skin management in lymphoedema. In: R Twycross, K Jenns and J Todd (eds) *Lymphoedema.* Radcliffe Medical Press, Oxford, pp 118–29.
7   Ryan T and Mallon E (1995) Lymphatics and the processing of antigen. *Clinical Dermatology.* **13**:485–92.
8   Badger CMA (1987) Lymphoedema management of patients with advanced cancer. *Professional Nurse.* **2**:100–2.
9   O'Brien A and Hickey J (1995) *Poster.* British Lymphology Interest Group Annual Conference. Oxford.
10   Todd J (2000) Containment in the management of lymphoedema. In: R Twycross, K Jenns and J Todd (eds) *Lymphoedema.* Radcliffe Medical Press, Oxford, pp 165–202.
11   Ryan T (1998) The skin and its response to movement. *Lymphology.* **31**: 128–9.
12   Hughes K (2000) Exercise and lymphoedema. In: R Twycross, K Jenns and J Todd (eds) *Lymphoedema.* Radcliffe Medical Press, Oxford, pp 140–64.
13   Bellhouse S (2000) Self-massage appendix. In: R Twycross, K Jenns and J Todd (eds) *Lymphoedema.* Radcliffe Medical Press, Oxford, pp 223–35.
14   Leduc A and Leduc O (2000) Manual lymphatic drainage. In: R Twycross, K Jenns and J Todd (eds) *Lymphoedema.* Radcliffe Medical Press, Oxford, pp 203–16.
15   Gray R (1987) Management of limb oedema in advanced cancer. *Nursing Times.* **83**:39–41.
16   Rydevik B *et al.* (1981) Effects of graded compression on intraneural blood flow. *The Journal of Hand Surgery.* **6**:3–12.
17   Ogata K and Naito M (1986) Blood flow of peripheral nerve effects of dissection, stretching and compression. *The Journal of Hand Surgery.* **11**:10–14.
18   Holt P and Bennett R (1972) Pneumatic stockings to treat 'rheumatic oedema'. *Lancet.* **ii**:688–9.
19   Twycross R (2000) Drug treatment for lymphoedema. In: R Twycross, K Jenns and J Todd (eds) *Lymphoedema.* Radcliffe Medical Press, Oxford, pp 244–70.
20   Piller N (1980) Lymphoedema, macrophages and benzopyrones. *Lymphology.* **13**:109–19.
21   Casley-Smith J and Casley-Smith J (1990) The effects of O-(beta-hydroxy-ethyl)-rutosides (HR) on acute lymphoedema in rats' thighs, with and without macrophages. *Microcirculation Endothelium Lymphatics.* **6**:457–63.

22   Wadworth A and Faulds D (1992) Hydroxyethylrutosides. A review of its pharmacology, and therapeutic efficacy in venous insufficiency and related disorders. *Drugs.* **44**:1013–32.

23   Casley-Smith J and Casley-Smith J (1997) *Venous disease, ulcers, palliative and geriatric care and acute injuries in modern treatment of lymphoedema.* The Lymphoedema Association of Australia, Australia, pp 280–1.

24   Chant A (1992) Hypothesis: Why venous oedema causes ulcers and lymph-oedema does not. *European Journal of Plastic Surgery.* **6**:427–9.

12 Therapeutic emergencies

Anaphylaxis · Respiratory · Infection · Pain · Psychiatric

A sense of urgency is important in symptom management. This is helped by setting goals and by regular reviews at appropriate intervals. However, there are several circumstances when one is faced with a *therapeutic emergency* which demands an even greater sense of urgency and speed of action (Box 12.A).

Box 12.A Therapeutic emergencies in palliative care

Haemorrhage (see p.244)

Anaphylaxis

Respiratory
  choking
  superior vena caval obstruction
  acute tracheal compression

Pain
  biliary and ureteric colic
  intrahepatic haemorrhage
  bladder spasm (see p.296)
  acute vertebral collapse
  spinal instability
  fracture of long bone

Neurological
  spinal cord compression (see p.267)
  grand mal seizures (see p.277)
  multifocal myoclonus in the moribund
    (see p.276)

Psychiatric
  suicidal ideas
  panic (see p.188)
  delirium (see p.206)
  delirium in the last days of life

Anaphylaxis

Anaphylaxis is a potentially life-threatening systemic allergic reaction. It manifests as a constellation of features but there is disagreement over which are essential. The confusion about definition arises partly because systemic allergic reactions can be mild, moderate or severe. In practice, the term 'anaphylaxis' should be reserved for cases where there is:

- respiratory difficulty (related to laryngeal oedema or bronchoconstriction) *or*

- hypotension (presenting as fainting, collapse or loss of consciousness) *or*

- both.[1]

Urticaria, angioedema or rhinitis alone are best not described as anaphylaxis because neither respiratory difficulty nor hypotension is present.[1]

Causes

In anaphylaxis, an allergic reaction results from the interaction of an allergen with specific IgE antibodies bound to mast cells and basophils. This leads to activation of the mast cell with release of chemical mediators stored in granules (including histamine) as well as rapidly synthesized additional mediators. A rapid major systemic release of these mediators causes capillary leakage and mucosal oedema, resulting in shock and respiratory difficulty.[1]

In contrast, anaphylactoid reactions are caused by activation of mast cells and release of the same mediators, but without the involvement of IgE antibodies. For example, certain drugs act directly on mast cells. In terms of management it is not necessary to distinguish anaphylaxis from an anaphylactoid reaction. This difference is relevant only when investigations are being considered.

Anaphylaxis is rare in palliative care and is generally associated with antibiotics, aspirin or another NSAIDs. A possible case has been recorded in a woman with known peanut allergy who received an arachis (peanut) oil enema (Pharmax 1998). Anaphylaxis is:

- specific to a given drug or chemically-related class of drugs
- more likely after parenteral administration
- more frequent in patients with aspirin-induced asthma or systemic lupus erythematosus.

Clinical features

Clinical manifestations of anaphylaxis typically develop *within minutes* of taking the causal drug (Box 12.B). Bronchospasm occurs in only 10% of patients.

Box 12.B   Clinical features of anaphylaxis

Essential
Hypotension *and/or* bronchospasm

Possible

Flushing	Tingling of the extremities
Urticaria	Weakness
Angioedema	Agitation

Management

Anaphylaxis requires urgent treatment with adrenaline (epinephrine) followed up with an antihistamine and hydrocortisone (Box 12.C). *However, because their impact is not immediate, corticosteroids are only of secondary value.*

Box 12.C   Management of anaphylaxis[2,3]

Adrenaline (epinephrine) 1 in 1000, 0.5–1ml (0.5–1mg) IM:
   if the patient is unconscious, double the dose
   repeat every 10min until pulse and blood pressure satisfactory.

Oxygen.

Chlorphenamine (chlorpheniramine):
   10–20mg IV over 1min
   4–8mg PO q.d.s. for 24–48h to prevent relapse.

Hydrocortisone 200mg IV to prevent further deterioration.

Respiratory

Choking

Choking is the sudden inability to breathe because of an acute obstruction of the pharynx, larynx or trachea.

Many specialist palliative care services care for patients with motor neurone disease (MND)/amyotrophic lateral sclerosis. Pseudobulbar palsy (dysfunction of the lower cranial nerves) is common in advanced disease and manifests as increasingly severe dysphagia and dysarthria; sometimes there are bouts of choking when eating.

Neuropathic dysphagia is also a problem for patients with dysfunction of the lower cranial nerves associated with metastases in the base of the skull and with head and neck cancers, or as a result of a brain primary or secondary cancer and after hemiplegia. Dementia and a reduced level of consciousness are other common causes of aspiration; this can occur silently, i.e. without causing cough.

Apart from episodes of choking, aspiration of oral bacteria and gastric contents increases the risk of pneumonia, abscess formation, airway obstruction, pulmonary fibrosis and adult respiratory distress syndrome (non-cardiogenic pulmonary oedema).[4,5] Aspiration of water alone is well-tolerated if it does not cause bouts of coughing, and patients should not be denied sips of water or ice chips to relieve a dry mouth or momentary thirst.[5]

Choking because of aspiration of food at mealtimes or of saliva at night is distressing. Patients are extremely fearful of a recurrence. A strategy is necessary to give the patient confidence that he will not choke to death.

Management

Explanation

Validate the patient's fear by telling them that you can imagine how terrifying a choking attack must be. Emphasize that there are measures which will reduce the probability and intensity of any choking attacks. In MND, these measures mean that they will *not* die from choking.[6] As always, prevention is better than cure.

Prophylaxis

Oral morphine should be introduced as an antitussive. Many patients need only morphine 5–6mg t.d.s. a.c. and o.n., a few take it q4h. The use of oral morphine is one reason why choking need not be a problem for patients with MND.[6]

Patients can also be supplied with hyoscine hydrobromide 0.3mg SL to use if they start to cough when drinking or eating and have difficulty in clearing matter from the trachea.[6] Hyoscine hydrobromide acts quickly, probably as a sedative. 'Sublingual' does not need to be literally under the tongue; placing it in a cheek or by the gums is equally satisfactory. Only about 1/3 of patients ever need to use SL hyoscine.

In an emergency

Generally the above measures are sufficient to make coughing during eating or drinking and at night much less disturbing. However, it is recommended that ampoules of the following drugs are kept in the patient's home for emergency use and used if the patient becomes distressed as a result of a prolonged episode of coughing:

- diamorphine 5mg or morphine 10mg
- midazolam 10mg
- hyoscine hydrobromide 400–600µg *or*
- glycopyrrolate 200µg.

Superior vena caval obstruction

Superior vena caval (SVC) obstruction is generally caused by extrinsic compression by metastases in the upper mediastinal lymph nodes (Box 12.D). Lung cancer is responsible for 80% of cases. It occurs in about 15% of patients with lung cancer, particularly small cell. It is also associated with other malignancies such as lymphoma, breast cancer and testicular seminoma.[7,8] Venous thrombosis can cause an acute onset.

Box 12.D   Clinical features of superior vena caval obstruction

Common symptoms
Dyspnoea (50%)
Neck and facial swelling (40%)
Trunk and arm swelling (40%)
A sensation of choking
A feeling of fullness in the head
Headache

Other potential symptoms
Chest pain
Cough
Dysphagia
Cognitive dysfunction
Hallucinations
Seizures

Common physical signs
Thoracic vein distension (65%)
Neck vein distension (55%)
Facial oedema (55%)
Tachypnoea (40%)
Plethora of face (15%)
Cyanosis (15%)
Arm oedema (10%
Vocal cord paresis (3%)
Horner's syndrome (3%)

If severe
Laryngeal stridor
Coma
Death

Management

SVC obstruction with severe symptoms is an emergency. The usual treatment consists of high-dose corticosteroids (e.g. dexamethasone 16mg o.d./8mg b.d. PO) and radiotherapy to the mediastinum. Corticosteroids reduce peritumour oedema and thereby reduce extrinsic compression. Chemotherapy may be used for patients with lymphoma and small cell lung cancer.

In patients who fail to improve with the above, or in whom SVC obstruction recurs, a self-expanding metal stent can be introduced into the SVC via a brachiocephalic or femoral vein.[9,10] All patients are anticoagulated with heparin before stent insertion. If there is associated thrombosis, thrombolytic treatment, e.g. streptokinase, may also be necessary.[11] Long-term anticoagulation is advisable.[12] Over 90% of patients die without recurrence of the obstruction.

Acute tracheal compression

This is a rare palliative care emergency. It should be responded to in the same way as severe haemorrhage (*see* p.244):

- IV diazepam/midazolam until the patient is unconscious (5–20mg)
- PR diazepam or SC/buccal midazolam 10–20mg if IV administration is not possible
- continuous company.

Infection

Many cancer patients eventually develop pneumonia as a complication of extreme debility. Antibiotics are inappropriate in this situation (*see* p.4). However, there are situations where antibiotics should be prescribed urgently:

- acute inflammatory episode in lymphoedema (*see* p.396)
- ascending cholangitis in patients with a biliary stent.

Ascending cholangitis

Ascending cholangitis should be treated with a combination of an appropriate cephalosporin and metronidazole:

- cefuroxime 1500mg IV t.d.s. for 48h *followed by*
- cefradine 1g PO b.d. for 5 days
- metronidazole 400mg PO t.d.s. (tablets are taken with or after food but the suspension is taken on an empty stomach 1h a.c.).

If oral administration is unreliable because of nausea and vomiting, metronidazole should be given 1g PR t.d.s. or 500mg IV t.d.s. Prolonged rectal use causes proctitis; use by this route should be limited to 2–3 days. If IV administration is not possible, cefuroxime can be given IM but 1500mg means an injection of 6ml.

Pain

Biliary and ureteric colic

The treatment of choice for biliary colic is an IM or IV injection of a NSAID, e.g. diclofenac 75mg.[13] If this fails to provide relief in 20–30min, it should be supplemented by diamorphine 5mg SC/IV or morphine 10mg SC/IV.

Alternatively, if already receiving PO morphine for cancer pain give:

- a double dose of morphine PO *or*
- an injection of diamorphine/morphine equal in mg to the previous regular PO dose; this will have treble/double the effect of the oral dose.

Intrahepatic haemorrhage

Occasionally with malignant hepatomegaly, the patient experiences increasingly severe right upper quadrant pain. Unless associated features suggest an alternative diagnosis, e.g. perforated peptic ulcer or cholecystitis, the most likely diagnosis is an intrahepatic haemorrhage causing acute distension of the hepatic capsule. When this is the case:

- explain the cause to patient
- give *double* the previous oral analgesic morphine requirement *or*
- if the patient has already taken an extra rescue dose of morphine with inadequate relief, *treble* the previous oral morphine dose; the presence of severe pain despite an additional dose of morphine indicates that the dose can be safely increased to this level.[14]

This is an acute phenomenon which resolves as the hepatic capsule adapts and the haematoma is resorbed. Therefore advise the patient that, in about a week, analgesic requirements are likely to be similar to that needed before the haemorrhage. Tentative dose reductions can be made after 3 days or sooner if the patient is comfortable but complaining of drowsiness. Failure to reduce the dose may result in increased adverse opioid effects:

- drowsiness
- nausea and vomiting
- constipation.

Acute vertebral collapse

Typically the patient is already taking regular analgesics for bone pain and, before being seen by a doctor, will already have taken one or more rescue doses of oral morphine. If these have failed to give adequate relief, it may be necessary to *treble* the previous satisfactory dose of morphine for up to several weeks.

Palliative radiotherapy is generally beneficial but it may take 4–6 weeks to achieve maximal relief. In patients with secondary muscle spasm, diazepam 5mg stat and 5–10mg o.n. may help.

For those with associated nerve compression pain, dexamethasone 4–8mg o.d. may also help. Alternatively, some patients benefit by epidural depot methylprednisolone 80mg in 2ml. This can be repeated once or twice at daily or weekly intervals.

Spinal instability

In terms of distress, spinal instability related to metastatic cancer is comparable to a pathological fracture of a long bone. Instability of an affected spinal segment is suggested by one or more of the following signs:

*   collapse or fracture of the vertebral body

*   kyphotic angulation

*   destruction of intervertebral joints with luxation and listhesis.[15]

Spinal instability can cause excruciating back pain on even slight movement; this overwhelms the patient. *Spinal cord compression must be excluded*; this is suggested by radicular pain, motor weakness, sensory symptoms and bladder dysfunction (*see* p.267).

Management options for spinal instability include:

*   nitrous oxide (50% with oxygen) before and during movement

*   epidural analgesia with morphine and bupivacaine

*   orthopaedic surgery, particularly when instability is accompanied by neurological symptoms or signs.[16]

Patients with breast, kidney, thyroid and prostate cancer are more likely to benefit from surgery than patients with cancers of the lung, bowel, melanoma and unknown primary. Surgery is generally considered only when there is localized spinal involvement, i.e. when there are robust vertebrae above and below the affected area. Surgery may involve:

- spinal cord decompression

- tumour resection

- replacement of destroyed bone with synthetic material

- stabilization with metal implants via an anterior approach (cervical spine in particular) or posterior approach (thoracic and lumbar spine in particular), and sometimes both.[15,17]

Surgery will generally be followed by radiotherapy, chemotherapy or hormone therapy. These should also be considered for patients unable to undergo surgery.

Pathological fracture of a long bone

Conservative management of pathological fractures of a long bone may well be unsatisfactory, with pain and reduced mobility continuing for many weeks if the fracture does not heal. Surgery should be considered for impending or established fractures in all patients because it offers the most reliable and rapid means of relieving pain and restoring function. Surgery requires the patient to be willing and generally fit enough to undergo an operation and the presence of enough bone for stable fixation. Radiotherapy should be considered after surgical stabilization.[18] Even in cases of non-union of the fracture, the inserted device (e.g. an intramedullary nail) can give sufficient stability for pain relief and satisfactory function.

While awaiting surgery, it is important to ensure that sufficient analgesia is provided together with night sedation. If surgery is planned, ensure that pre-fracture analgesics are continued and that additional p.r.n. postoperative medication is prescribed at an appropriate level. This includes giving advice on the dose of SC diamorphine or morphine to replace PO morphine in the immediate postoperative period.

Humerus

Immediate care (or if surgery inappropriate):

- use a standard triangular sling *or*

- splint arm to trunk with Netelast and/or Velcro *or*

- fracture braces (humeral shaft)
- give adequate analgesics (*see above*).

Consider a nerve block or epidural analgesia if pain remains a major problem. Arrange for radiotherapy.

Femur

Immediate care (or if surgery inappropriate):

- immobilize leg with pillows or skin traction
- use appropriate nursing techniques for turning the patient in bed, e.g. 'logrolling'
- administer a local anaesthetic femoral nerve block with 10ml of 0.5% bupivacaine before obtaining a radiograph
- use a Thomas splint or bandage the legs together if transferring to orthopaedic/accident service (plus local anesthetic block)
- if treating conservatively, consider epidural diamorphine and bupivacaine by CSCI
- consider radiotherapy.

Psychiatric

Nearly 1/2 of patients with cancer have a psychiatric disorder as judged by criteria in the *Diagnostic and Statistical Manual*.[19] However, in 2/3 of these it is a transient adjustment disorder with depressed, anxious or mixed mood rather than a florid psychiatric illness. The other 1/3 comprise, in order of occurrence, depression, delirium, anxiety disorders, personality disorders or psychoses. Unrelieved pain is particularly associated with depression and delirium.

Suicidal ideas

Suicidal statements range from comments which merely reflect the 'heat of the moment' to ones which are an expression of despair. Suicidal ideas are relatively common in patients with cancer, and the risk of suicide is increased compared to the general population.[20] Suicidal cancer patients are likely to be suffering from:

- an adjustment disorder with anxious and depressed features (50%)

- major depression (30%)

- delirium (20%).

Depression, a sense of hopelessness and exhaustion (physical, psychological, social, spiritual or financial) greatly increase the risk of suicide. There are also many other risk factors (Box 12.E).

Box 12.E   Risk factors for suicide[2]

Historical
Family history of suicide
Previous attempt
Pre-existing psychiatric disorder

Diagnostic
Cancer (particularly head and neck)
AIDS
Spinal cord injury
Multiple sclerosis
Huntington's chorea
Systemic lupus erythematosus

Psychological
Depression
Other psychiatric disorder
Recent bereavement
Social isolation
Fear of serious physical deformity or
   suffering
A sense of helplessness associated with
   physical dependency and loss
   of control

Physical
Severe pain
Multiple physical symptoms

Exploring suicidal thoughts is imperative; find out if definite plans to commit suicide have been made and take note of any risk factors (Box 12.E). Obtain help from a psychiatrist in evaluation and in formulating a management plan (Box 12.F).

Although more common than in the general population, suicide among cancer patients is still uncommon. In patients supported by a specialist palliative care service suicide is rare, less than 1 in 3000.[22,23]

Delirium in the last days of life

Delirium in the last days of life is often associated with progressive multiple organ failure and is generally not reversible. Medication is generally necessary. An antipsychotic is the drug of choice:

- haloperidol 5mg PO/SC

- repeat after 30min, if the patient has not settled

Box 12.F   Dealing with suicidal cancer patients[20]

Preliminaries
Establish rapport.

Explore the patient's understanding of their illness and present symptoms.

Evaluation
Mental status, e.g. cognitive function, mood, fears.

Uncontrolled pain or other distressing symptoms?

Any past major psychiatric disorders (patient or family), suicide threats, suicide attempts?

Seriousness of suicidal thoughts/intent/plans.

Presence of other risk factors?

Level of supervision required.

Management
If the patient is actively suicidal, constant supervision is required.

Indicate what can be done to improve the quality of life by relieving pain, other physical symptoms, delirium, anxiety, depression etc.

As far as possible, give the patient some degree of control.

Make use of the patient's social network.

- give a double dose after a further 30min if necessary
- sometimes 10–20mg PO/SC/IV is necessary
- add midazolam 10mg SC if the patient does not settle.

Occasionally, heavy sedation is necessary to control agitation, keeping the patient asleep for much or all of the time until death comes.[24] In one study the incidence of heavy sedation for agitated delirium was 3%.[25] In this situation, it is generally best to prescribe both a benzodiazepine and an antipsychotic drug, for example:

- midazolam 10–20mg SC and haloperidol 10–20mg SC stat *and*
- midazolam 30–60mg/24h and haloperidol 20–30mg/24h by CSCI *and*
- midazolam 10mg SC with haloperidol 5mg SC p.r.n.

Occasionally larger doses are necessary, particularly in a patient previously extremely anxious or who has been using denial as a main coping mechanism. As the patient becomes less able to control his thoughts, unresolved fears break through into the now confused mind with devastating impact.

Some centres use levomepromazine up to 200–300mg/24h or chlorpromazine 50–100mg q4h IM. In situations where seizures are a definite risk, i.e. patients with multifocal myoclonus or a cerebral tumour, midazolam should be prescribed as well, e.g. 30–60mg/24h by CSCI (Figure 12.1).

Phenobarbital can be used for sedation in terminal delirium not responding to midazolam 60mg and *either* haloperidol 30mg/24h *or* levomepromazine 200mg/24h:

- give a stat dose of 100–200mg IV
- then 600–1200mg/24h by CSCI.

It has no effect upon delusions or hallucinations and can lead to paradoxical agitation.

Propofol, an ultrafast-acting anaesthetic agent, provides yet another option.[26,27] Propofol is given IV as a 1% solution (10mg/ml) in doses ranging from 5–70mg/h (0.5–7ml) using a computer-controlled volumetric infusion pump. 10mg/h (1ml) is a typical starting dose with 10mg/h increments every 15min until a satisfactory level of sedation is achieved. Any change in rate has an effect in 5–10min. If it is necessary to increase the level of sedation quickly, boluses of 20–50mg can be given by increasing the rate to 1ml/min for 2–5min. If the patient is too sedated, the infusion should be turned off for 2–3min and then restarted at a lower rate. It is important to replenish the infusion quickly when a container empties, otherwise the sedation will wear off after a few minutes.

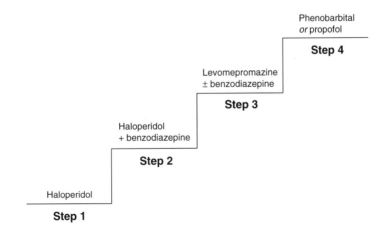

Figure 12.1   Drug treatment for irreversible agitated delirium in the last days of life.

References

1 Ewan P (1998) ABC of allergies: anaphylaxis. *British Medical Journal.* **316**: 1442–5.

2 Szczeklik A (1986) Analgesics, allergy and asthma. *Drugs.* **32**:148–63.

3 Anonymous (1999) *British National Formulary.* No. 37 (March) British Medical Association and the Royal Pharmaceutical Society of Great Britain, London, pp 150–2.

4 Terry P and Fuller S (1989) Pulmonary consequences of aspiration. *Dysphagia.* **3**:179–83.

5 Garon (1997) A randomized control study to determine the effects of unlimited oral intake of water in patients with identified aspiration. *Journal of Neurological Rehabilitation.* **11**:139–48.

6 O'Brien T *et al.* (1992) Motor neurone disease: a hospice perspective. *British Medical Journal.* **304**:471–3.

7 Tabbarah H (1988) Intrathoracic complications. In: D Casciato and B Lowitz (eds) *Manual of Clinical Oncology.* Little Brown, Boston, pp 435–52.

8 Kee S *et al.* (1998) Superior vena cava syndrome: treatment with catheter-directed thrombolysis and endovascular stent placement. *Radiology.* **206**:187–93.

9 Nicholson A *et al.* (1997) Treatment of malignant superior vena cava obstruction: metal stents or radiation therapy. *Journal of Vascular and Interventional Radiology.* **8**:781–8.

10 Renwick I (1999) Metallic stents in palliative care. *CME Bulletin of Palliative Medicine.* **1**:41–4.

11 Jackson J and Brooks D (1995) Stenting of superior vena caval obstruction. *Thorax.* **50**:531–6.

12 Stock K *et al.* (1995) Treatment of malignant obstruction of the superior vena cava with the self-expanding wallstent. *Thorax.* **50**:1151–6.

13 Anonymous (1987) NSAIDs for renal and biliary colic: intramuscular diclofenac. *Drug and Therapeutics Bulletin.* **25**:85–6.

14 Hagen N *et al.* (1997) Cancer pain emergencies: a protocol for management. *Journal of Pain and Symptom Management.* **14**:45–50.

15 Klekamp J and Samii H (1998) Surgical results for spinal metastases. *Acta Neurochirurgica (Wein).* **140**:957–67.

16 Fallon M and O'Neill W (1993) Spinal surgery in the treatment of metastatic back pain: three case reports. *Palliative Medicine.* **7**:235–8.

17 Magerl F and Jeanneret B (1988) Surgical management of tumour-related spinal instability. *Recent Results in Cancer Research.* **108**:163–71.

18 Townsend P *et al.* (1995) Role of postoperative radiation therapy after stabilization of fractures caused by metastatic disease. *International Journal of Radiation Oncology, Biology and Physics.* **31**:43–9.

19 American Psychiatric Association (1994) *Diagnostic and Statistical Manual of Mental Disorders.* APA, Washington DC.

20 Roth A and Breitbart W (1996) Psychiatric emergencies in terminally ill cancer patients. *Haematology and Oncology Clinics of North America.* **10**:235–59.

21 Harris E and Barraclough B (1994) Suicide as an outcome for medical disorders. *Medicine (Baltimore).* **73**:281–96.

22   Grzybowska P and Finlay I (1997) The incidence of suicide in palliative care patients. *Palliative Medicine.* **11**:313–16.
23   Ripamonti C *et al.* (1999) Suicide among patients with cancer cared for at home by palliative-care teams. *Lancet.* **354**:1877–8.
24   Chater S *et al.* (1998) Sedation for intractable distress in the dying – a survey of experts. *Palliative Medicine.* **12**:255–69.
25   Morita T *et al.* (2000) Terminal sedation for existential distress. *American Journal of Hospice and Palliative Care.* **17**:189–95.
26   Mercadante S *et al.* (1995) Propofol in terminal care. *Journal of Pain and Symptom Management.* **10**:639–42.
27   Moyle J (1995) The use of propofol in palliative medicine. *Journal of Pain and Symptom Management* **10**:643–6.

13   Clinical guidelines

Except where indicated, the clinical guidelines in this chapter have been produced to guide practice at Sir Michael Sobell House. They are *not* in the same league as well-referenced guidelines produced by a national or international consensus panel, nor are they set in 'tablets of stone'. Indeed, their fluidity is partly their strength; their content is reviewed at least annually.

In preparing the guidelines, we have the self-imposed discipline of not exceeding two pages; if guidelines are to be implemented they must be short enough to be read rapidly. The use of these guidelines remains the responsibility of the practitioner.

The topics included are listed below. The numbering of the guidelines relates them to the relevant chapters in this book.

2.1   Starting patients on oral morphine
2.2   Switching opioids
2.3   Transdermal fentanyl
2.4   Use of methadone
2.5   Use of syringe drivers at Sobell House
3.1   Nausea and vomiting in palliative care
3.2   Opioid-induced constipation
5.1   Depression
10.1   Skin care for radiotherapy patients
10.2   Fungating cancer (India)
11.1   Dry skin in lymphoedema
11.2   Acute inflammatory episodes
11.3   Pneumatic compression therapy

2.1: Starting patients on oral morphine

1   Morphine is indicated in patients with pain which does not respond to the combined optimized use of a non-opioid and a weak opioid.

2   The starting dose should provide greater analgesia than the previous medication:
- if the patient was previously receiving a weak opioid, give 10mg q4h or m/r 30mg q12h PO
- if changing from an alternative strong opioid, a much higher dose of morphine may be needed (see Guidelines 2.2: Switching opioids).

3   If the patient is frail and elderly, a lower starting dose, e.g. 5mg q4h, titrated upwards every 2–3 days helps to reduce initial drowsiness, confusion and unsteadiness.

4   If ≥2 p.r.n. doses are taken in 24h, the regular dose should be increased 30–50%.

5   Upward titration of the dose of morphine stops when the pain is relieved or intolerable adverse effects supervene. In the latter case, it is generally necessary to consider alternative measures.

6   The aim is to have the patient free of pain and mentally alert.

7   Supply an anti-emetic for regular use if the patient becomes nauseated, e.g. haloperidol 1.5mg stat & o.n.

8   Prescribe laxatives, e.g. co-danthrusate or senna ± docusate. Adjust the dose as necessary. Suppositories and enemas continue to be necessary in about 1/3 of patients. Constipation may be more difficult to manage than the pain.

9   Warn patients about the possibility of initial drowsiness.

10   For outpatients, write out the drug regimen in detail with times, names of drugs and amount to be taken; arrange for follow-up.

11   M/r morphine may not be satisfactory in patients with frequent vomiting or those with diarrhoea or an ileostomy.

12   If swallowing is difficult or vomiting persists, morphine may be given PR by suppository (same dose as PO). Alternatively give:
- 1/2 of the oral dose of morphine by SC injection or
- 1/3 of the oral dose as SC diamorphine.

Scheme 1: ordinary (normal-release) morphine tablets or solution
- morphine given q4h 'by the clock' with p.r.n. doses of equal amount
- after 1–2 days, recalculate q4h dose based on total used in previous 24h (regular + p.r.n. use)
- continue q4h and p.r.n. doses
- increase the regular dose until there is adequate relief throughout each 4h period, taking p.r.n. use into account
- *a double dose at bedtime obviates the need to wake the patient for a q4h dose during the night.*

Scheme 2: ordinary (normal-release) morphine and modified-release (m/r) morphine
- begin as for Scheme 1
- when the q4h dose is stable, replace with m/r morphine q12h, or o.d. if a 24h preparation is prescribed
- the q12h dose will be *three times* the previous q4h dose; an o.d. dose will be *six times* the previous q4h dose, rounded to a convenient number of tablets
- continue to provide ordinary morphine solution or tablets for p.r.n. use.

Scheme 3: m/r morphine and ordinary (normal-release) morphine
- starting dose generally m/r morphine 20–30mg b.d.
- use ordinary morphine tablets or solution for p.r.n. medication; give about 1/6 of the total daily dose
- increase the dose of m/r morphine every 2–3 days until there is adequate relief throughout each 12h period, taking p.r.n. use into account.

2.2: Switching opioids

1   It is occasionally necessary to switch strong opioids because of:
    • poor response to morphine (→ methadone)
    • intractable constipation (→ transdermal fentanyl)
    • intolerable adverse effects
    • poor compliance (→ transdermal fentanyl).

Oral and other non-injectable routes

2   Multiply the dose of opioid by its potency ratio to determine the dose of morphine sulphate.

Approximate analgesic equivalence to oral morphine		
Analgesic	Potency ratio with morphine	Duration of action (h)[a]
Codeine		
Dihydrocodeine	1/10	3–6
Dextropropoxyphene		
Pethidine	1/8	2–4
Tramadol	1/5[b]	4–6
Oxycodone	1.5–2[b]	4–5
Methadone	5–10[c]	8–12
Hydromorphone	7.5	4–5
Buprenorphine (*sublingual*)	60	6–8
Fentanyl (*transdermal*)	100–150[d]	72

a   dependent in part on the severity of pain and on the dose; often longer-lasting in the very elderly and those with renal impairment
b   tramadol and oxycodone are both relatively more potent by mouth because of high bio-availability; parenteral potency ratios with morphine are 1/10 and 3/4 respectively
c   methadone: a single 5mg dose is equivalent to morphine 7.5mg (approximately 1:1). However, its long plasma halflife and its broad-spectrum receptor affinity result in a much higher than expected potency ratio when given repeatedly
d   manufacturers in UK state 150; in Germany they state 100.

Injections

3   The following conversion ratios are approximate and should be regarded only as a general guide. Subsequent adjustment up or down may be necessary:
    • PO → SC/IV morphine, give 1/2–1/3 the PO dose
    • PO morphine → SC diamorphine, give 1/3 of the PO dose.

Switching at high doses

4   The recommended equivalent doses of the strong opioids are approximate, and cannot be exact for everyone. Further, they relate to typical doses, e.g. up to 600mg of PO morphine and possibly higher.

5   Inequivalence also stems from the fact that it is not possible to compare chalk with cheese. In other words, all strong opioids are not just morphine in a different guise; they often possess distinct properties.

6   If the dose of morphine has been escalated to very high levels, say >2g/24h, the recommended equivalent doses will be progressively more erroneous, partly because the main metabolite of morphine, M3G, cumulates and neutralizes the analgesic effect of morphine. Thus, when converting at high dose levels it is best to give 1/2–1/4 of the calculated equivalent dose.

7   A separate strategy is necessary for methadone (see Guideline 2.4).

2.3: Transdermal fentanyl

1   Transdermal (TD) fentanyl is an alternative strong opioid which can be used in place of both PO morphine and CSCI morphine/diamorphine in the management of cancer pain.

2   Indications for using TD fentanyl patches include:
   • intractable morphine-induced constipation
   • intolerable adverse effects with morphine e.g. nausea and vomiting (despite the appropriate use of anti-emetics) and/or hallucinations (despite the use of haloperidol)
   • 'tablet phobia' or difficulty swallowing oral preparations
   • poor compliance with oral medication.

3   TD fentanyl is *contra-indicated* in patients who need rapid titration of their medication for severe uncontrolled pain.

4   *Warning*: pain not relieved by morphine will **not** be relieved by fentanyl. If in doubt, seek specialist advice before prescribing TD fentanyl.

5   TD fentanyl is available in 4 strengths: 25, 50, 75, 100µg/h *for 3 days*:
   • patients with inadequate relief from **codeine, dextropropoxyphene** or **dihydrocodeine ≥240mg/day** should start on 25µg/h
   • patients on **oral morphine**: *divide 24h dose in mg by 3* and choose nearest patch strength in µg/h
   • patients on **SC diamorphine**: choose nearest patch strength in µg/h.
   Note: the latter two doses are slightly higher than the manufacturer's recommendations.

6   An alternative method of deciding the initial patch strength is to use a potency ratio of 100 (as in Germany) and to round down to the nearest convenient patch size. [Example: morphine daily dose 120mg ÷ 100 = fentanyl daily dose 1.2mg, i.e. patch strength 50µg/h.]

7   Apply the patch to *dry, non-inflamed, non-irradiated, hairless skin* on the upper arm or trunk; body hair may be clipped but not shaved. May need micropore to ensure adherence.

8   Systemic analgesic concentrations are generally reached within 12h; so if converting from:
   • **4-hourly oral morphine**, continue to give regular doses for 12h
   • **12-hourly m/r morphine**, apply the patch at the same time as giving the final 12-hourly dose
   • a syringe driver, continue the syringe driver for about 12h after applying the patch.

9   Steady-state plasma concentrations of fentanyl are achieved only after 36–48h; the patient should use p.r.n. doses liberally during the first 3 days, particularly during the first 24h. Rescue doses should be approximately half the fentanyl patch strength given as normal-release morphine in mg. [Example: with fentanyl 50µg/h, use morphine 20–30mg p.r.n.]

10   After 48h, if a patient continues to need 2 or more rescue doses of morphine a day, the patch strength should be increased by 25µg/h. When using the manufacturer's recommended starting doses, about 50% of patients need to increase the patch strength after the first 3 days.

11   About 10% of patients experience opioid withdrawal symptoms when changed from morphine to TD fentanyl. Patients should be warned that they may experience symptoms like flu for a few days after the change, and that rescue doses of morphine will relieve them.

12   Fentanyl is less constipating than morphine; halve the dose of laxatives when starting fentanyl and titrate according to need. Some patients develop diarrhoea; if troublesome, use rescue doses of morphine to control it, and completely stop laxatives.

13   Fentanyl probably causes less nausea and vomiting than morphine but, if necessary, prescribe haloperidol 1.5mg stat & o.n.

14   In febrile patients, the rate of absorption of fentanyl increases, and occasionally causes toxicity, principally drowsiness. Absorption may also be enhanced by an external heat source over the patch, e.g. electric blanket or hot-water bottle; patients should be warned about this. Patients may shower with a patch but should not soak in a hot bath.

15   Remove patches after 72h; change the position of the new patches so as to rest the underlying skin for 3–6 days.

16   A reservoir of fentanyl accumulates in the skin under the patch, and significant blood levels persist for 24h, sometimes more, after removing the patch. This only matters, of course, if TD fentanyl is discontinued.

17   In moribund patients, it is best to continue TD fentanyl and give rescue doses of SC diamorphine based on the 'rule of 5', i.e. divide the patch strength by 5 and give as **mg of diamorphine**. [Example: with fentanyl 100µg/h, use diamorphine 20mg p.r.n.]

18   In moribund patients, if the patch is replaced by **CSCI diamorphine**:
   • give *half the patch strength as mg/24h* rounded up to a convenient ampoule size
   • after 24h, give *the whole of the previous patch strength as mg/24h* rounded up to a convenient ampoule size.

19   TD fentanyl is unsatisfactory in some patients, generally because of failure to remain adherent or allergy to the silicone adhesive.

20   Used patches still contain fentanyl. After removal, fold the patch adhesive side inwards and discard, preferably in a sharps container; wash hands. Any unused patches should be returned to a pharmacy.

2.4: Use of methadone

In additiion to being an opioid agonist, methadone is a NMDA-receptor-channel blocker and a presynaptic blocker of serotonin re-uptake. Its plasma half-life varies from about 8–80h.

Indications for use

1   Methadone is used in the following situations:
   - severe/intolerable adverse effects with morphine at any dose, e.g. sedation, hallucinations, dysphoria, delirium, myoclonus, allodynia, hyperalgesia, as an alternative to low dose spinal morphine or if these effects complicate spinal morphine use
   - increasing pain despite increasingly high doses of morphine compounded by intolerable adverse effects
   - neuropathic cancer pain not responding to a typical regimen of a NSAID, morphine, amitriptyline and sodium valproate
   - renal failure, where it may be used as the opioid of choice because its metabolism and excretion are unchanged in this circumstance
   - only in patients with a prognosis of ⩾10 days.

Therapeutic inequivalence

2   Because methadone is very different from morphine, when switching from high-dose morphine to methadone it is necessary to be aware of opioid *inequivalence*, i.e. the two drugs do *not* have a single potency ratio. In practice the 24h dose of methadone is 5–10 times *smaller* than the previous dose of morphine, and sometimes even smaller.

Dose titration

3   For patients in renal failure who have not been on PO morphine, commence on methadone 5–10mg q12h *and* q3h p.r.n. If necessary, titrate the regular dose upwards every 4–6 days.

4   For patients already receiving morphine, use Scheme 1.

Scheme 1 (Morley and Makin, UK)
Stop morphine abruptly; i.e. do *not* reduce progressively over several days.
Prescribe a dose of methadone that is 1/10 of the 24h PO morphine dose *up to a maximum of 30mg.*
Allow the patient to take the prescribed dose *q3h p.r.n.*
On day 6, the amount of methadone taken over the previous 2 days is noted and converted into a regular q12h dose, with provision for a similar or smaller dose q3h p.r.n.
If p.r.n. medication is still needed, increase the dose of methadone by 1/2–1/3 every 4–6 days [Example: 10mg b.d. → 15mg b.d.; 30mg b.d. → 40mg b.d.]; it is uncommon to need more than 40mg b.d.

5   Because many patients (and staff) have become used to morphine by-the-clock, they are not comfortable with a total p.r.n. regimen. In this case, Scheme 2 may be preferable.

Scheme 2 (Nauck, Germany)

Stop morphine abruptly; i.e. do *not* reduce progressively over several days.
Initially prescribe methadone 5–10mg PO q4h *and* q1h p.r.n. *whatever the dose of morphine.*

After 12–24h, if frequent p.r.n. doses are still needed and the pain is not easing, increase methadone to 10–15mg q4h and q1h p.r.n.

After 72h, reduce regular methadone to q8h *and* q3h p.r.n.

Subsequently, increase the dose of methadone every 4–5 days if still needing multiple p.r.n. doses. [Maintenance doses of methadone typically range from 10–50mg q8h.]

---

6   With both schemes, morphine (or other opioid) is stopped abruptly.

7   *Particularly over the first 48h, the patient may experience significant pain but if the switch is successful, the pain steadily diminishes and p.r.n. doses of methadone similarly.* A failed conversion is obvious: pain remains unrelieved and the intervals between doses do not lengthen, or the patient experiences undue adverse effects without adequate analgesia.

8   When the b.d. dose has been determined, methadone can continue to be used as rescue medication for break-through pain.

SC methadone

9   CSCI methadone causes a skin reaction; this is reduced if:
   • a more dilute solution is used, e.g. a 20–30ml syringe
   • the syringe is changed b.d.
   • the site is changed every day.

10   An arbitrary SC methadone dose of 1/20 the previous dose of SC morphine is a safe dose. In patients on morphine ≤1g/24h, it is generally safe to give 1/10. When converting from PO methadone to SC methadone, give 1/2 the PO dose.

11   Additional rescue doses of methadone can be given for break-through pain, using 1/5–1/6 of the 24h infusion dose q3h p.r.n.

12   If necessary, p.r.n. doses of morphine (or other previously used strong opioid) can be given q1h, based on previous morphine requirements.

13   The dose of methadone should be increased if p.r.n. doses are still needed after several days.

2.5: Use of syringe drivers at Sobell House

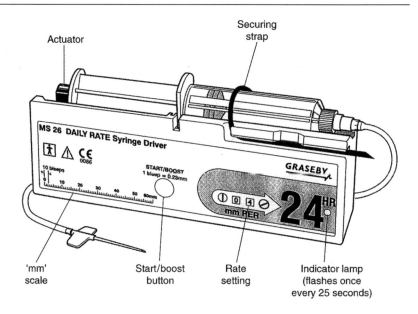

The Graseby Medical MS26 battery-driven portable syringe driver

General information

1   Battery-driven portable syringe drivers are used when oral administration is unreliable or impossible.

2   Syringe drivers are set up and monitored by nurses; a second nurse checks the rate of administration to prevent mistakes.

3   The normal route is subcutaneous; the epidural route is occasionally used for intractable pain.

4   Common indications for use are:
   • persistent nausea and vomiting
   • intestinal obstruction
   • dysphagia
   • patient moribund.

Prescribing

5   When a syringe driver is prescribed, indicate this on the regular side of the Drug Chart and enter details in the space provided.

6   The drugs most commonly given by CSCI are:
    • metoclopramide (*anti-emetic*)
    • haloperidol (*anti-emetic/antipsychotic*)
    • hyoscine butylbromide (*anti-spasmodic/antisecretory*)
    • midazolam (*sedative/anti-epileptic*)
    • diamorphine (*analgesic*).

    Cyclizine is sometimes used either as the sole anti-emetic or in conjunction with hyoscine.

> Because antimuscarinics block the prokinetic effect of metoclopramide, cyclizine and metoclopramide should not be prescribed concurrently.

7   Most drugs are diluted in Water for Injections (WFI); a few are diluted in 0.9% saline:
    • levomepromazine (*but see 8*)
    • ketorolac
    • octreotide
    • tropisetron (*but see 8*).

8   Drugs with a long duration of action do not need to be infused but can be given o.d. by separate SC injection:
    • dexamethasone
    • haloperidol (*but in practice it is often given by infusion*)
    • levomepromazine (*if given by infusion, dilute in saline*)
    • tenoxicam
    • tropisetron.

9   In epidural analgesia, the following are often given concurrently:
    • diamorphine/morphine
    • bupivacaine
    • clonidine.

Incompatibility

10 Cyclizine may precipitate at concentrations above 20mg/ml or at temperatures above 37.5°C, or in the presence of saline, or as the concentration of diamorphine relative to cyclizine increases. Mixtures of diamorphine and cyclizine are also liable to precipitate after 24h.

11 Cyclizine generally precipitates if mixed with metoclopramide, but should not be combined because antimuscarinic drugs block the intestinal action of metoclopramide.

12 Mixtures of haloperidol and diamorphine are liable to precipitate after 24h if the concentration of haloperidol is above 2mg/ml.

3.1: Nausea and vomiting in palliative care

1   After clinical evaluation, document the most likely cause(s) of the nausea and vomiting in the patient's case notes.

2   Ask the patient to record symptoms and response to treatment, preferably using a diary.

3   Correct correctable causes/exacerbating factors, e.g. drugs, severe pain, infection, cough, hypercalcaemia. (*Correction of hypercalcaemia is not always appropriate in a dying patient.*) Anxiety exacerbates nausea and vomiting from any cause and may need specific treatment.

4   Prescribe the most appropriate anti-emetic stat, regularly & p.r.n. Give by SC injection if continuous nausea or frequent vomiting, preferably by CSCI.

Commonly used anti-emetics

Prokinetic anti-emetic (about 50% of prescriptions)
For gastritis, gastric stasis, functional bowel obstruction (peristaltic failure):
metoclopramide 10mg PO stat & q.d.s. or 10mg SC stat & 40–100mg/24h CSCI, & 10mg p.r.n.

Anti-emetic acting principally in chemoreceptor trigger zone (about 25% of prescriptions)
For most chemical causes of vomiting, e.g. morphine, hypercalcaemia, renal failure:
haloperidol 1.5–3mg PO stat & o.n. or 2.5–5mg SC stat & 2.5–10mg/24h CSCI, & 2.5–5mg p.r.n.
Metoclopramide also has a central action.

Antispasmodic and antisecretory anti-emetic
If bowel colic and/or need to reduce gut secretions:
hyoscine butylbromide 20mg SC stat, 80–200mg/24h CSCI, & 20mg SC hourly p.r.n.

Anti-emetic acting principally in the vomiting centre
For raised intracranial pressure (in conjunction with dexamethasone), motion sickness and in organic bowel obstruction:
cyclizine 50mg PO stat & b.d.–t.d.s. or 50mg SC stat & 100–150mg/24h CSCI, & 50mg p.r.n.

Broad-spectrum anti-emetic
For organic bowel obstruction and when other anti-emetics are unsatisfactory:
levomepromazine 6.25–12.5mg SC or 3–25mg PO stat, o.n. & p.r.n.

---

5   Review anti-emetic dose every 24h, taking note of p.r.n. use and the patient's diary.

6   Anti-emetics for inoperable bowel obstruction are best given by CSCI: Levomepromazine is the exception ; it is generally given as a single SC dose o.n.:

No colic → metoclopramide ── **If fails** ──▶ Substitute ⎫ Levomepromazine[b] *or*
Severe colic → hyoscine butylbromide[a] ── **If fails** ──▶ Add ⎭ cyclizine ± haloperidol[c]

  a   can use glycopyrrolate 600–1200µg/24h instead
  b   if not available, consider olanzapine 1.25–5mg PO o.n.
  c   if levomepromazine too sedative.

7   If little benefit despite optimizing the dose, have you got the cause right?
   • if no, change to an alternative anti-emetic and optimize
   • if yes, provided the anti-emetic has been optimized, add or substitute a second anti-emetic.

8   In patients who fail to respond to the commonly used anti-emetics, consider:

Other drugs for nausea and vomiting

Corticosteroid
Adjuvant anti-emetic for chemotherapeutic vomiting, bowel obstruction and when all else fails:
dexamethasone 8–16mg PO/SC stat & o.d.; consider reducing the dose after 7 days.

5HT$_3$-receptor antagonist
Use when massive release of serotonin (5HT) from enterochromaffin cells or platelets, e.g. chemotherapy, abdominal radiation, bowel obstruction (distension), renal failure:
tropisetron 5mg PO/SC stat & o.d.

Somatostatin analogue
An anti-secretory agent without antispasmodic effects; use in obstruction if hyoscine inadequate:
octreotide 100µg stat, 250–500µg/24h CSCI, & 100µg p.r.n.

---

9   Some patients with nausea and vomiting need more than one anti-emetic.

10   *Antimuscarinic drugs block the cholinergic pathway through which prokinetics act; concurrent use antagonizes the prokinetic effect of metoclopramide and is best avoided.*

11   Continue anti-emetics unless the cause is self-limiting.

12   Except in organic bowel obstruction, consider changing to PO after 72h of good control with CSCI.

3.2: Opioid-induced constipation

All opioids constipate, although to a varying extent. Morphine is more constipating than methadone and fentanyl.

1   Ask about the patient's past (premorbid) and present bowel habit and use of laxatives; record the date of last bowel action.

2   Palpate for faecal masses in the line of the colon; do a rectal examination if the bowels have not been open for >3 days or if the patient reports rectal discomfort.

3   For inpatients, keep a daily record of bowel actions.

4   Encourage fluids generally, and fruit juice and fruit specifically.

5   When an opioid is prescribed, prescribe co-danthrusate 1 capsule o.n. prophylactically; although occasionally it is appropriate to optimize a patient's existing bowel regimen, rather than change automatically to co-danthrusate.

6   If already constipated, prescribe co-danthrusate 2 capsules o.n.

7   Adjust the dose every few days according to results, up to 3 capsules t.d.s.

8   If the patients prefers a liquid preparation, use co-danthrusate suspension (5ml = 1 capsule).

9   If >3 days since last bowel action, 'uncork' with suppositories, e.g. bisacodyl 10mg and glycerine 4g or a micro-enema. If these are ineffective, administer a phosphate enema and possibly repeat the next day.

10   If co-danthrusate causes intestinal colic, divide the total daily dose into smaller more frequent doses, e.g. change from co-danthrusate 2 capsules b.d. to 1 capsule q.d.s. Alternatively, change to an osmotic laxative, e.g. lactulose syrup 20–40ml o.d.–t.d.s. or magnesium hydroxide + liquid paraffin 25–50ml o.m.–b.d.

11   If the maximum dose of co-danthrusate is ineffective, halve the dose and add an osmotic laxative, e.g. lactulose 20ml b.d. or magnesium hydroxide + liquid paraffin 25ml o.m.–b.d.

12   Lactulose may be preferable to co-danthrusate in patients with a history of colic with other colonic stimulants, e.g. senna.

Notes

- co-danthrusate 50/60 capsules contain dantron 50mg + docusate sodium 60mg; dantron is a colonic stimulant and docusate sodium is a surface wetting agent/ faecal softener
- lactulose is a non-absorbable sugar which acts as an osmotic laxative in both the small and large bowel
- magnesium hydroxide is generally also considered to be an osmotic laxative but in fact may act by stimulating the release of cholecystokinin-pancreozymin (CCK-PZ)
- liquid paraffin is a lubricant and makes the evacuation of constipated faeces less painful.

5.1: Depression

Sadness and tears on their own, even if associated with transient suicidal thoughts, do not justify the diagnosis of depression or the prescription of an antidepressant; many are part of an adjustment reaction. Other patients are demoralized rather than medically depressed and respond to symptom management and psychosocial support.

Evaluation

1   *Screening*: about 5–10% of patients with advanced cancer develop a major depression. Cases will be missed unless specific enquiry is made of all patients:

    'What has your mood been like lately?' … 'Are you depressed?'
    'Have you had serious depression before? Are things like that now?'

2   *Assessment interview:* if depression is suspected, explore the patient's mood more fully by encouraging the patient to talk further with appropriate prompts. Symptoms suggesting clinical depression include:
    *   *sustained* low mood (i.e. most of every day for several weeks)
    *   *sustained* loss of pleasure/interest in life (anhedonia)
    *   diurnal variation (i.e. worse in mornings and better in evenings)
    *   waking significantly earlier than usual (e.g. 1–2 hours) and feeling 'awful'
    *   feelings of hopelessness/worthlessness
    *   excessive guilt
    *   withdrawal from family and friends
    *   persistent suicidal thoughts and/or suicidal acts
    *   requests for euthanasia.

3   *Differential diagnosis:* the symptoms of depression and cancer, and of depression and sadness overlap. If in doubt whether the patient is suffering from depression, an adjustment reaction or sadness, review after 1–2 weeks and/or seek the help of Dr Malmberg (psycho-oncologist).

4   *Medical causes of depression:* depression may be the consequence of:
    *   a medical condition, e.g. hypercalcaemia, cerebral metastases
    *   a reaction to severe uncontrolled physical symptoms
    *   drugs, e.g. cytotoxics, benzodiazepines, antipsychotics, corticosteroids, antihypertensives.

Management

5   *Correct the correctable*: prescribe specific treatment for medical causes.

6   *Non-drug treatment:*
    *   explanation and assurance that symptoms can be treated
    *   depressed patients often benefit from the ambience of the Day Centre
    *   psychological treatments available through the *Psycho-oncology Service*
    *   other psychosocial professionals, e.g. chaplain and creative therapists, have a therapeutic role but avoid overwhelming the patient with simultaneous multiple referrals.

7 *Drug treatment:*
- prescribe a first-line antidepressant if the patient is clinically depressed and is expected to live for >4 weeks (*see* Box)
- a tricyclic antidepressant (TCA) is probably more effective for severe depression; otherwise the choice depends on adverse effects and the patient's symptoms
- *the initial and continuing doses of antidepressants are generally lower in debilitated patients compared with the physically fit*
- if the patient is unable to tolerate adverse effects or there is no response after 4 weeks, change from TCA → SSRI or vice versa, or consider a second-line antidepressant (*see* Box)
- generally, a second-line antidepressant should be prescribed only after consultation with Dr Malmberg.

First-line antidepressants

Tricyclic antidepressant (TCA)
Amitriptyline (mixed noradrenaline and serotonin re-uptake inhibitor):
- universally available and minimal cost
- 10–25mg o.n. initially, increasing to 25–50mg o.n.
- if no benefit after 2 weeks, increase to 75–150mg o.n. in steps
- dose escalation often limited by adverse effects, e.g. dry mouth and sedation.

Selective serotonin re-uptake inhibitors (SSRIs)
Paroxetine:
- some antimuscarinic effects; initial increase in anxiety *less* likely; greater likelihood of a withdrawal (discontinuation) syndrome
- 10–20mg o.m. initially, preferably after food (but give o.n. if it causes daytime sedation)
- if no benefit after 2 weeks, increase to 20–30mg, occasionally 40mg.

Sertraline:
- no antimuscarinic effects; initial increase in anxiety *more* likely; less likelihood of a withdrawal (discontinuation) syndrome
- standard dose = 50mg o.m., preferably after food
- occasionally necessary to increase the dose to 100–200mg o.m.

Second-line antidepressants

Venlafaxine (mixed noradrenaline and serotonin re-uptake inhibitor):
- a good choice for patients with psychomotor retardation
- 37.5mg b.d., increasing to 75mg b.d. after 2 weeks if necessary
- can use m/r preparations, i.e. 75mg or 150mg capsules o.m.
- fewer adverse effects than amitriptyline but much more expensive.

Mirtazapine (noradrenaline and specific serotonergic antidepressant):
- a good choice for patients with marked anxiety/agitation
- is not a mono-amine re-uptake inhibitor; acts on receptors
- 15mg o.n. initially, increasing to 30mg o.n.
- concurrent H_2-receptor antagonism leads to sedation *but this may decrease with higher dose because of noradrenergic effects*
- fewer adverse effects than amitriptyline but much more expensive.

10.1: Skin care for radiotherapy patients

Your treatment may result in some soreness of the skin overlying the part of the body being treated. The risk of this happening should be discussed with your radiotherapy doctor and radiographer, but in most cases skin reactions are mild. They develop some days after starting treatment and may well worsen until the end of treatment. In most cases the reaction heals within 4 weeks.

1   Bath or shower using warm, not hot, water; don't spend more than 5 minutes in the bath or shower.

2   Don't use soap in the area being irradiated.

3   Pat your skin dry with a soft towel, do not rub it. You may blow-dry your skin with a hairdryer on a cool setting.

4   Dust lightly with baby talc if you like to use powder.

5   Do not put anything else on the skin unless recommended by the radiotherapy staff. Certain products may irritate your skin, so please ask the staff before using anything on the treatment area.

6   Use an electric shaver, not a razor for shaving in the treatment area.

7   Wear loose clothing next to the skin in the treatment area. Underwear made from natural fibres are best, e.g. cotton.

8   Protect your skin from wind, sun and direct heat. You risk making the skin in the treatment area very sore if you expose it to direct sunshine, hot water bottles, electric blankets etc.

Remember
- always ask for advice if you develop a problem
- it may be necessary to change this general advice in certain situations
- if you have any questions, please ask.

These guidelines may be relaxed when the reaction is diminishing, generally about 2 weeks after finishing treatment. Continue to avoid exposure of treated skin to intense sunlight either by keeping it covered or by using a sun-barrier cream.

10.2: Fungating cancer (India)

A fungating cancer is a primary or secondary malignant tumour which has ulcerated the skin. The tumour may be proliferative or cavitating, and is associated with pain, exudate, bleeding, infection and malodour. A fungating cancer generally has a major negative psychological impact on the patient and family. Malodour can cause or exacerbate nausea and anorexia.

Anticancer treatment

1   Discuss possibilities with oncologists (radiotherapy, chemotherapy, hormonal manipulation, debulking surgery, plastic surgery).

Correct the correctable

2   Antibiotics for deep anaerobic infection:
   • metronidazole 200mg tablet *crushed* and applied to the ulcerated area mixed in KY jelly or 2% lidocaine jelly; *benefit often noticed within 12h*
   • proprietary metronidazole jelly 0.75% (75mg/10ml) can also be used but is more expensive and benefit is generally observed only after several days.
   Metronidazole and surface cleansing generally also resolve any concurrent aerobic infection.

3   Maggots: apply one of the following to the ulcerated area after cleansing:
   • di-ethylether (an anaesthetic agent)
   • turpentine (may cause burning pain)
   • mercurochrome 2–4% solution.

Topical treatment

4   Wound care can be done by doctor, nurse or family:
   • wash hands
   • cleanse ulcerated areas using tap water with added salt
   • apply gamgee pad or several layers of cotton pads (more if much exudate) and retain in position with a light bandage and/or adhesive tape.

5   Control of bleeding:
   • apply cotton pads and gentle hand pressure
   • if still bleeding after 10–15min, pour diluted Hemolek onto pads and allow to soak in; use 1ml from 10ml ampoule diluted to 100ml; repeat after several hours if still bleeding
   • subsequently, apply sucralfate 1g tablet crushed and mixed in KY jelly; cover with a cotton pad and repeat daily; soak pad with tap water before removing it.

6   Control of malodour (caused by necrosis and anaerobic infection):
   • cleanse and debride the surface
   • topical metronidazole (*see above*)
   • use strong pleasant odours to counter malodour, e.g. lavender, herbs, incense.

Systemic treatment

7   If bleeding continues, prescribe etamsylate 500mg q.d.s. for 3 days; continue if helpful.

8   Relieve pain using WHO 3-step analgesic ladder; *if infected, the best analgesic may be the antibiotic.*

11.1: Dry skin in lymphoedema

Many elderly and/or malnourished patients have a dry skin – which can cause pruritus. In lymphoedema a healthy skin is crucial in prophylaxis against local infection (acute inflammatory episodes/AIE); moisturising the skin regularly is most important.

1   *Emollients* soothe, smooth and hydrate the skin. They are indicated for all causes of dry skin and scaling disorders. Because effects are short-lived, emollients should be applied frequently (up to q.d.s.). Less frequent use, e.g. o.d., should continue indefinitely.

2   The choice of emollient depends mainly on the state of the skin. The stepladder below is used in patients with lymphoedema. *For patients without lymphoedema, aqueous cream b.d. may be adequate as step 2.* For normally active people, o.d. application is best at bedtime.

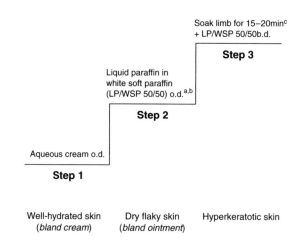

Soak limb for 15–20min[c]
+ LP/WSP 50/50b.d.

Step 3

Liquid paraffin in
white soft paraffin
(LP/WSP 50/50) o.d.[a,b]

Step 2

Aqueous cream o.d.

Step 1

Well-hydrated skin   Dry flaky skin   Hyperkeratotic skin
(*bland cream*)   (*bland ointment*)

a   ointments are generally not necessary for more than a few days
b   some people prefer coconut oil BP because it has a skin-cooling effect. Use the plain variety; added fragrance can cause allergic dermatitis
c   after soaking in a bucket of warm water (to which 15–20ml of LP/WSP 50/50 has been added) and after drying the limb, apply LP/WSP 50/50 using a circular motion; this tends to lift off hyperkeratotic skin.

3   Other options for hyperkeratotic skin:
- use jacuzzi or shower spray to penetrate into the crevasses
- to reduce bacterial and fungal colonization in the crevasses, add sufficient *potassium permanganate tablets or granules* to achieve a rose wine colour (note: it stains skin and material brown)
- if culture of a skin swab indicates superficial infection with pseudomonas, add *vinegar* 30ml/4L to the soaks
- if there is fungal infection, apply *hydrocortisone 1% and miconazole 2%* (Daktacort) to the affected areas.

4   For areas resistant to treatment, consider applying LP/WSP 50/50 and covering with a hydrocolloid dressing (Comfeel, Granuflex) for 2 days and then soak etc. (*see* 2c).

5   Topical creams and ointments can cause folliculitis if massaged into the hair follicles; the likelihood of this is reduced by massaging in the direction of hair growth.

6   Avoid the use of emollients which:
- contain lanolin/wool fat or are strongly scented (can cause allergic dermatitis)
- are expensive, e.g. E45 cream (contains hypo-allergenic lanolin; 500g = £5.61) (aqueous cream 500g = £1.10).

7   Soap should *not* be used because it dries the skin; use aqueous cream as a soap substitute.

8   *Emollient bath additives:* Balneum (soya) bath oil is the preferred choice at Sobell House. Oilatum emollient bath additive contains lanolin/wool fat.

9   *Antipruritic emollients:* if pruritus is caused by the dry skin, rehydration of the skin will correct it. Thus, all emollients are anti-pruritic in this sense. Preparations which have more specific anti-pruritic properties include:
- aqueous cream + 1% menthol (or 2%)
- colloidal oatmeal cream (Aveeno); popular with children.

Addendum Topical applications		
Ointments	**Creams**	**Lotions**
Grease-based	Water-in-oil emulsion	Oil-in-water suspension
Most hydrating	Less hydrating	Least hydrating; cools as it evaporates
Messy to apply; difficult if skin very hairy	Massage well into skin; cosmetically more acceptable	Shake well before use

11.2: Acute inflammatory episodes

In lymphoedema acute inflammatory episodes (AIE), often called cellulitis, are common. AIE are frequently associated with fever, flu-like symptoms or even greater constitutional upset (e.g. nausea and vomiting). In AIE it is often difficult to isolate the pathogen responsible. However, Streptococcus is the mostly likely infective agent.

Evaluation

1   *Clinical features:*
   - mild – pain, increased swelling, erythema (well-defined *or* blotchy)
   - severe – extensive erythema with well-defined margins, increased swelling, blistering and weeping skin; often accompanied by fever, nausea and vomiting, pain and, when the leg is affected, difficulty in walking.

2   *Diagnosis* is based on pattern recognition and clinical judgement. The following information should be solicited:
   - present history – date of onset, precipitating factor (e.g. insect bite or trauma), treatment received to date
   - past history – details of previous AIE, precipitating factors, antibiotics taken
   - examination – include the sites of lymphatic drainage to and from the inflamed area.

Antibiotics

3   All AIE should be treated promptly with antibiotics to prevent increased morbidity associated with increased swelling and accelerated fibrosis. In the UK, there is no standard regimen for AIE. The following is current practice in the Lymphoedema Service at Sobell House.

4   *No systemic upset:*

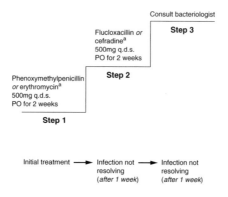

a   alternatives for patients with a history of penicillin allergy (rash); if a history of penicillin anaphylaxis, do not use cefradine but jump from step I to step 3

b   some centres use co-amoxiclav 625mg t.d.s. instead. This is active against both Streptococci and Staphylococci but causes more rashes and diarrhoea, and is more expensive.

5   *Systemic upset:* bed rest is crucial and may necessitate inpatient admission. Blood cultures, aspirates of bullae and surface swabs (if the skin is broken) should be taken to guide treatment in case the infection does not resolve. Meanwhile, prescribe IV antibiotics for 1 week followed by antibiotics PO for 1 week, i.e. 2 weeks in total.

6   *Week 1:*

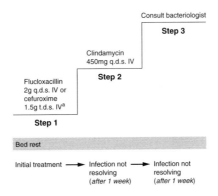

a   alternative for patients with a history of penicillin allergy (rash); if a history of penicillin anaphylaxis, proceed to step 2.

7   *Week 2:* if the infection is resolving, continue with PO medication for a second week:
    • flucloxacillin injections are replaced by capsules *500mg* q.d.s. PO
    • cefuroxime injections are replaced by *cefradine* 1g b.d. PO
    • clindamycin injections are replaced by capsules 300mg q.d.s. PO.

8   *Antibiotic prophylaxis:* if an AIE recurs within a year, prescribe phenoxymethylpenicillin *500mg o.d. for 1 year* or cefradine if a history of penicillin rash. If a history of penicillin anaphylaxis, prescribe clindamycin 150mg o.d.

General

9   Remember:
    • AIE are painful; analgesics should be prescribed regularly and p.r.n.
    • compression garments should not be worn until limb is comfortable
    • daily skin hygiene should be continued: washing and gentle drying
    • emollients should not be used in the affected area if the skin is weeping or cracked
    • the affected limb should be elevated in a comfortable position, supported on pillows.

10 Patients should be educated about:
    • why they are susceptible to AIE, i.e. skin less robust, stagnant fluid, reduced immunity
    • the consequence of AIE, i.e. increased swelling, more fibrosis, reduced response to treatment
    • the importance of daily skin care, i.e. to improve and maintain the integrity of the skin
    • reducing risk, e.g. protect hands when gardening, cleanse cuts, treat fungal infections
    • prophylaxis with antibiotics.

11.3: Pneumatic compression therapy

1   Centromed Macro pptt (10 chambers) sequential compression pump. Can operate three compression garments simultaneously, e.g. two stockings and one abdominal girdle:
   - fixed options for treatment duration: 20, 30, 60min or continuous
   - cycle time: 40, 60 or 120sec (*normally use 60*)
   - pressure: variable.

2   Intermittent pneumatic compression is used mainly *for leg swelling other than lymphoedema*; it must be medically prescribed and monitored.

3   Explain the procedure to the patient:
   - remove rings and watch from the hand and arm to be treated
   - advise patient to empty their bladder
   - ensure that the patient is in a comfortable lying position with the affected limb supported
   - during treatment the patient should wear Tubifast (cylindrical cotton bandage) or pyjama trousers or light-weight trousers.

4   External compression should be maintained between treatments during the day, using Shaped Tubigrip or compression garments; the foot of the bed should be elevated at night.

5   *First session*: pressure 20–30mmHg for 30min on the swollen leg(s); use the session to familiarize the patient with the multichamber stockings and pump, and to make sure that the treatment is comfortable.

6   *Subsequent sessions*: pressure 40mmHg for 60min b.d. on the swollen leg(s), *but not all patients can tolerate this.*

7   If the limb size does not reduce, consider increasing pressure to 60mmHg for 1–2h t.d.s.; overnight is also a possibility.

8   *Hygiene*: the inflatable garments should be cleaned with soap and water between use by different patients.

9   Stop the treatment and contact a doctor:
   - if the patient becomes breathless when using the pump
   - if the limb becomes red, hot or painful.

10   Reconsider if swelling develops around:
   - the shoulder or chest wall (with arm oedema)
   - the groin, genitalia or buttock (with leg oedema).

11   Monitor progress by making circumferential limb measurements before starting the treatment and then once or twice a week using three fixed points, for example:
   •   10cm proximal to the base of the nail of the big toe
   •   30cm above the base of the heel (inner aspect)
   •   60cm above the base of the heel (inner aspect).
   It is *not* necessary to measure limb volume.

Index